Treating Difficult Couples

*Helping Clients with Coexisting Mental
and Relationship Disorders*

Edited by

DOUGLAS K. SNYDER
MARK A. WHISMAN

THE GUILFORD PRESS
New York   London

Library of Congress Cataloging-in-Publication Data

Treating difficult couples : helping clients with coexisting mental and
relationship disorders / edited by Douglas K. Snyder, Mark A. Whisman.
      p. cm.
Includes bibliographical references and index.
  ISBN 1-57230-882-6 (alk. paper)
  1. Marital psychotherapy.   2. Mentally ill—Marriage.   I. Snyder,
Douglas K.   II. Whisman, Mark A.
RC488.5.T7184 2003
616.89′156—dc21

                                                    2003005211

In honor of my parents, Audrey and Henry Snyder,
and my parents-in-law, Marcile and Vaughn Rinard.
You showed us the meaning of commitment and grace.
— D. K. S.

To my wife, Emily, and my children, Hannah and Henry,
for their unconditional love and support.
— M. A. W.

About the Editors

Douglas K. Snyder, PhD, is Professor and Director of Clinical Psychology Training at Texas A&M University in College Station. He has been recognized internationally for his programmatic research on couple therapy and is the author of the widely used Marital Satisfaction Inventory. In 1992, the American Association for Marriage and Family Therapy honored Dr. Snyder with its Outstanding Research Award for his 4-year follow-up study (along with Robert Wills), funded by the National Institute of Mental Health, comparing behavioral and insight-oriented approaches to couple therapy. Dr. Snyder is a Fellow of the American Psychological Association and has served as Associate Editor of the *Journal of Consulting and Clinical Psychology* and *Journal of Family Psychology,* and on the editorial boards of numerous journals, including *Clinical Psychology: Science and Practice, Journal of Clinical Psychology, Journal of Marital and Family Therapy, Journal of Marriage and the Family,* and the *American Journal of Family Therapy.*

Mark A. Whisman, PhD, is Associate Professor of Psychology at the University of Colorado at Boulder. His research, which has been supported by the National Institute of Mental Health, has focused on the reciprocal association between relationship functioning and mental health. His other areas of research interest include cognitive-behavioral and interpersonal perspectives on the onset, maintenance, and treatment of depression and relationship distress. Dr. Whisman is a Founding Fellow of the Academy of Cognitive Therapy, and has served as Associate Editor of *Contemporary Psychology* and on the editorial boards of the *Journal of Consulting and Clinical Psychology, Journal of Family Psychology,* and *Clinical Psychology: Science and Practice.*

Contributors

Claudia Avina, MA, is a doctoral student in clinical psychology at the University of Nevada, Reno, and is working in the research lab of Dr. William O'Donohue. Her research interests include sexual assault prevention, the treatment of victimized women and children, and sexual dysfunctions.

Carl Bagnini, MSW, serves on the clinical faculty of the Postdoctoral Program in Couple and Family Therapy at St. John's University in Queens, New York, as well as Chair of the Child, Couple and Family Therapy Program at the International Institute of Object Relations Therapy in Washington, DC. His clinical and research interests include object relations couple therapy and affective learning in psychotherapy training. He maintains a clinical practice in Port Washington, New York.

Donald H. Baucom, PhD, is Professor of Psychology at the University of North Carolina at Chapel Hill, where he has also served as Director of Clinical Psychology Training. He has published over 120 scholarly papers on treating couple distress and on couple-based treatments for a range of individual emotional, behavioral, and health problems. Along with Norman Epstein, he is coauthor of *Enhanced Cognitive-Behavioral Therapy for Couples: A Contextual Approach.* Dr. Baucom is also an experienced clinician and recipient of the Mary G. Clarke Award for outstanding lifetime contributions to psychology in North Carolina.

Steven R. H. Beach, PhD, is Professor of Psychology at the University of Georgia, where he also serves as Associate Director of the Institute for Behavioral Research. He has published more than 100 scholarly papers on marital processes, close relationships, and depression, and is the author of *Depression in Marriage* and *Marital and Family Processes in Depression: A Scientific Foundation for Clinical Practice.* Dr. Beach is also an experienced clinician in outpatient, hospital, and independent practice settings and is a Fellow of the American Psychological Association.

Gary R. Birchler, PhD, is a clinical psychologist and a Clinical Professor of Psychiatry at the University of California, San Diego School of Medicine. He serves as the Director of the Family Mental Health Program at the VA San Diego Healthcare System. His clinical, teaching, and research interests emphasize marital, family, and sex therapy, about which he has written over 75 publications; he is a frequent presenter of clinical workshops in these areas.

Mary F. Brunette, MD, is Assistant Professor of Psychiatry at the Dartmouth Medical School. She participates in research on services for people with severe mental illness at the New Hampshire–Dartmouth Psychiatric Research Center. Dr. Brunette became interested in services for families in which parents have a mental illness through her clinical work with adults who were struggling with parenting. She writes and lectures about services for adults and families with severe mental illness.

W. Jeffrey Canar, PhD, is a staff psychologist in the Spinal Cord Injury Service at the Veterans Hospital in Hines, Illinois. He is also an Instructor for the Department of Health Systems Management at Rush University in Chicago. His research interests include psychosocial oncology, rehabilitation psychology, and adaptation to illness as it relates to individual and family systems.

Angela M. Castellani, MS, is a doctoral candidate in clinical psychology at Texas A&M University. Her current research interests include assessing couples' relationship functioning and conceptual models of matching treatment to individual differences.

Norman B. Epstein, PhD, is Professor in the Department of Family Studies at the University of Maryland, College Park. His teaching, research, and publications have focused on cognitive factors in marital dysfunction, development of assessment and treatment methods for couple relationship problems, relations between individual psychopathology and relationship functioning, family stress and coping, and cross-cultural research on families. He is a Clinical Member and an Approved Supervisor of the American Association for Marriage and Family Therapy, a Fellow of the American Psychological Association, a Diplomate of the American Board of Assessment Psychology, and a Founding Fellow of the Academy of Cognitive Therapy.

William Fals-Stewart, PhD, is a Senior Research Scientist at the Research Institute on Addictions and an Associate Research Professor in the Department of Psychology at the State University of New York at Buffalo. Author of over 120 articles and chapters, his primary research interests include marital and family interventions for substance-abusing patients, longitudinal outcomes of alcohol- and drug-dependent patients, and neuropsychological assessment. His research has been funded by the National Institute on Drug Abuse, the National Institute on Alcohol Abuse and Alcoholism, and private foundations.

Alan E. Fruzzetti, PhD, is Associate Professor of Psychology and Director of the Dialectical Behavior Therapy (DBT) and Research Program at the University of Nevada at Reno. His research focuses on the interplay between psychopathology and couple and family interactions, and the development of effective treatments for these problems. Dr. Fruzzetti is Research Advisor and Member of the Board of Directors of the National Educational Alliance for Borderline Personality Disorder, maintains a clinical practice with individuals and families, and has provided extensive training in the United States, Europe, and Australia in DBT with individuals, couples, and families.

Armida R. Fruzzetti, MA, is Professor of Psychology at Truckee Meadows Community College in Reno, Nevada. She has trained professionals in the United States and Europe in clinical applications of dialectical behavior therapy with adolescents, adults, couples, and families. Her research focuses on the effects of validating and invalidating parental behaviors on children's behavior and development. She is fluent in both Spanish and English and works within the Hispanic community regarding mental health issues.

Maya Gupta, MS, is a doctoral candidate in clinical psychology at the University of Georgia. Her research interests center on depression, batterer typologies, and the link between cruelty to animals and interpersonal violence.

Gwen Hales, MS, is a doctoral candidate in clinical psychology at the Illinois Institute of Technology. Her research interests include pain management and the role of psychosocial factors in health.

Amy Holtzworth-Munroe, PhD, is Professor of Psychology at Indiana University, Bloomington. For over 15 years, she has investigated partner violence and, specifically, patterns and subtypes of male partner aggression. Her research has contributed to the development and evaluation of treatment groups for male batterers. She is a past Associate Editor of the *Journal of Consulting and Clinical Psychology* and *Cognitive Therapy and Research.*

Susan M. Johnson, EdD, is Professor in the Departments of Psychology and Psychiatry at the University of Ottawa, and also serves as Director of the Ottawa Couple and Family Institute. She is the leading developer and proponent of emotionally focused couple therapy, as described in her recent books, *Emotionally Focused Couple Therapy with Trauma Survivors* and *The Practice of Emotionally Focused Marital Therapy.* In 2000, the American Association for Marriage and Family Therapy honored Dr. Johnson with the Outstanding Contribution to the Field award.

Judy Makinen, MA, is a doctoral student in clinical psychology at the University of Ottawa. Her research interests include the process of resolving attachment-related injuries in couples. Currently she is in an internship at the Royal Ottawa Health Care Group.

Amy D. Marshall, BA, is a doctoral candidate in clinical psychology at Indiana University. Her research interests include husband-to-wife sexual aggression, dating violence, and the relationship between husband violence and men's ability to recognize facial expressions of emotion displayed by their partners.

Barry W. McCarthy, PhD, is Professor of Psychology at American University and a partner at the Washington Psychological Center, where he practices individual, couple, and sex therapy. He is a diplomate in clinical psychology and a certified sex and marital therapist. He has published widely on the treatment of sexual and relationship disorders, and is a frequent presenter of clinical workshops in this domain both nationally and internationally. With his wife, Emily, he has written numerous books on sexual and couple issues for the lay public, including *Sexual Awareness: Couple Sexuality for the Twenty-First Century* and *Rekindling Desire: A Step-by-Step Program to Help Low-Sex and No-Sex Marriages.*

Jeffrey C. Meehan, AB, is a doctoral candidate in clinical science and social cognitive neuroscience at Indiana University. His research interests include using biological and cognitive science models to study human social phenomena, especially as applied to intimate relationships.

David J. Miklowitz, PhD, is Professor of Psychology at the University of Colorado, Boulder, and specializes in psychosocial processes and interventions relevant to bipolar affective disorder. He has received a Distinguished Investigator Award from the National Alliance for Research on Schizophrenia and Depression and an Outstanding Research Publication Award from the American Association for Marriage and Family Therapy. His most recent book is *The Bipolar Disorder Survival Guide.*

Chad D. Morris, PhD, is an Instructor in the Department of Psychiatry at the University of Colorado Health Sciences Center, where he is also Director of the Program Evaluation and Administration Postdoctoral Fellowship.

Kim T. Mueser, PhD, is Professor in the Departments of Psychiatry and Community and Family Medicine at the Dartmouth Medical School in Hanover, New Hampshire. His clinical and research interests include the psychosocial treatment of severe mental illnesses, dual diagnosis, and posttraumatic stress disorder. He has published extensively and has presented numerous workshops on psychiatric rehabilitation. He is the coauthor of several books, including *Coping with Schizophrenia: A Guide for Families, Behavioral Family Therapy for Psychiatric Disorders,* and *Integrated Treatment for Dual Disorders: A Guide to Effective Practice.*

William O'Donohue, PhD, is the Nicholas Cummings Professor of Organized Behavioral Health Care Delivery at the University of Nevada at Reno. He is also a Professor in the Department of Psychology and an Adjunct Professor in both the Departments of Psychiatry and Philosophy. Dr. O'Donohue has published widely in the area of sexual behavior. His edited books include *Theories of Human Sexuality, Handbook of Sexual Dysfunction,* and *Sexual Harassment: Theory, Research, and Practice.*

Timothy J. O'Farrell, PhD, is Professor of Psychology in the Harvard Medical School Department of Psychiatry at the VA Boston Healthcare System in Brockton, Massachusetts, where he directs the Harvard Families and Addiction Program and the Counseling for Alcoholics' Marriages (CALM) Project. His clinical and research interests focus primarily on couple and family therapy in alcoholism and drug abuse treatment, as well as various aspects of substance abusers' family relationships, including partner violence. His books include *Treating Alcohol Problems: Marital and Family Interventions.*

Gail P. Osterman, MS, is a doctoral candidate in clinical psychology at the Illinois Institute of Technology. Her research interests include psychosocial oncology, use of the Internet in health populations, and personality styles.

Sara Honn Qualls, PhD, is Professor of Psychology at the University of Colorado at Colorado Springs, where she also serves as Director of the Center on Aging. She has published two books, *Psychology and the Aging Revolution* and *Aging and Mental Health.* Her research and writing focus on marital and family development in later life and clinical interventions for later-life couples and families. She is also a practicing clinical psychologist who helped establish the CU Aging Center, a community-based geriatric mental health training clinic.

Lisa G. Regev, MA, is a doctoral candidate in clinical psychology at the University of Nevada, Reno. She has collaborated with William O'Donohue to develop a semistructured interview and self-help treatment manual for couples suffering from sexual dysfunction.

Uzma Rehman, BA, is a doctoral candidate in the clinical science program at Indiana University. Her research interests include husband violence, marital communication, and cross-cultural differences in the linkage of communication behaviors and marital satisfaction.

Jill Savege Scharff, MD, is Clinical Professor of Psychiatry at Georgetown University, a teaching analyst at the Washington Psychoanalytic Institute, and codirector of the International Institute of Object Relations Therapy in Washington, DC. She has written numerous books on object relations therapy for individuals, couples, and families, as well as *Object Relations Therapy of Physical and Sexual Trauma* and *Self-Hatred in Psychoanalysis: Detoxifying the Persecutory Object.* She maintains a clinical practice in Chevy Chase, Maryland.

W. Joel Schneider, MS, is a doctoral candidate in clinical psychology at Texas A&M University and Instructor of Psychology at Illinois State University. His research interests include integrative approaches to therapy, group interventions with couples, and emerging techniques in test development and interpretation.

Tamara G. Sher, PhD, is Associate Professor of Clinical Psychology at Illinois Institute of Technology. She has written extensively in the couple and health literature and is the Principal Investigator of *Partners for Life,* a project funded by the National Heart, Lung and Blood Institute to investigate a couples approach to cardiac risk reduction. She is also the coeditor, with Karen Schmaling, of *The Psychology of Couples and Illness.*

Reema Singla, BA, is a doctoral candidate in clinical psychology at the Illinois Institute of Technology. Her research interests center on developing culturally relevant interventions with ethnic minority populations, specifically the Asian Indian community.

Douglas K. Snyder, PhD (see "About the Editors").

Susan Stanton, MA, is a doctoral candidate in clinical psychology at the University of North Carolina at Chapel Hill. Her current research interests include process and intervention research of social support in couples, particularly as related to individuals' physical and mental health problems.

Mia Sypeck, MA, is a doctoral candidate in clinical psychology at the American University in Washington, DC, and is currently affiliated with the Yale Center for Eating and Weight Disorders, as well as the Connecticut Mental Health Center, Department of Psychiatry, Yale University. Her research interests include the mediating effects of attachment on resiliency among child abuse survivors.

Kenneth G. Terkelsen, MD, is the Medical Director of Inpatient Services at Cape Cod and Islands Community Mental Health Center, which is the Commonwealth of Massachusetts' Department of Mental Health facility for the Cape and Islands. Before relocating to Cape Cod in 1999, he was Associate Professor of Clinical Psychiatry at the Joan and Sanford I. Weill Medical College of Cornell University and Director of Residency Training at the New York Presbyterian Hospital–Westchester Division. He was a recipient of the National Alliance for the Mentally Ill's Exemplary Psychiatrist Award in 1992.

Tracy Tilton, MA, is a doctoral candidate in clinical psychology at the Illinois Institute of Technology. Her clinical and research interests center on forensic psychology.

Lisa A. Uebelacker, PhD, is a postdoctoral fellow at Brown University Medical School and Butler Hospital in Providence, Rhode Island. She completed her doctoral studies at Yale University. Her research interests include family functioning and depression, brief family interventions, and combined treatments for depression.

Mark A. Whisman, PhD (see "About the Editors").

Robert M. Wills, MSW, MDiv, is an Adjunct Instructor in both the School of Social Work and Department of Psychiatry at Wayne State University in Detroit. He is also an ordained Episcopal priest, and maintains a clinical practice in Birmingham, Michigan. He has published several articles on couple and family therapy. In 1992, the American Association for Marriage and Family Therapy (AAMFT) honored him with its Outstanding Research Award for his 4-year follow-up study (along with Douglas Snyder), funded by the National Institute of Mental Health, comparing behavioral and insight-oriented approaches to couple therapy. Mr. Wills is former president of the Michigan Chapter of the AAMFT.

Preface

When conducting couple therapy, therapists encounter diverse couples presenting with a wide range of individual and relationship problems and histories. Among these couples there are some that are particularly difficult or challenging to treat. The usual intervention strategies appear less effective with these couples, and their therapists struggle with how to promote enduring positive changes in the individual partners and their relationships. What is it about these couples that makes couple therapy more difficult or challenging?

In 1992 the editors began working together on a coauthored chapter on evaluating and improving couple therapy (Whisman & Snyder, 1997). Preparing that chapter served as an impetus for deepening our understanding of common factors among couples who present a challenge for even the most seasoned therapist. We concluded that some of the most difficult couples to treat are those not only experiencing problems in their relationships but in which one or both partners are also experiencing emotional, behavioral, or health problems. Consistent with this conclusion, national surveys indicate that couple therapists report such "individual" problems not only as common but also as some of the most difficult problems they encounter in clinical practice (e.g., Northley, 2002; Whisman, Dixon, & Johnson, 1997).

Not surprisingly, individual therapists also struggle with clients whose emotional and behavioral difficulties are exacerbated or at least partially maintained by influences from their intimate relationships. Indeed, studies have shown that the presence of relationship problems is associated with poorer outcome for individually oriented treatments for a range of emotional and behavioral problems. Consequently, therapists who typically work only with individuals are likely to improve their success in therapy by incorporating couple interventions into their practice. For therapists unaccustomed to working directly with couples, however, incorporating couple interventions, either as an adjunct or an alternative to individual treatment for such clients, can be particularly daunting. For these therapists, guidelines regarding emotional and behavioral disorders for which specific couple interventions have been developed and empirically evaluated, including explicit assessment and treatment strategies for such couples, constitute a sorely needed resource.

This book integrates recent clinical, theoretical, and empirical developments in working with co-occurring relationship distress and emotional, behavioral, and health problems. In so doing, this text addresses a fundamental and pervasive challenge for therapists working with complex cases in which individual disorders interact with relationship distress. Specifically, we sought to produce a book that is clinically oriented, with specific guidelines for conceptualizing, evaluating, and treating emotional, behavioral, and health concerns in couple therapy. Few resources are available on this topic, and the existing literature has been restricted primarily to a subset of Axis I disorders. Consequently, in addition to assembling chapters on the major existing couple-based interventions for this subset of Axis I disorders, we sought to compile chapters that offer a conceptual framework and specific clinical procedures for addressing a broad range of emotional and behavioral disorders, including personality disorders and health problems, that challenge couple therapists but for which few or no guidelines exist. The techniques described in this volume generally represent empirically based interventions. In cases in which research is limited, promising preliminary techniques are provided. Although chapters are written with a clinical emphasis, each chapter also summarizes such empirical issues as the prevalence and comorbidity of individual disorders with couple distress, as well as any empirical findings regarding the efficacy of couple-based interventions for these disorders.

Consistent with these goals, the book is organized into four parts. The first part discusses empirical research on the co-occurrence of relationship problems and emotional, behavioral, and health problems, and proposes a conceptual model for the integrative treatment of co-occurring relationship and individual difficulties. The second part is devoted to couple interventions that have been empirically evaluated as treatments for specific emotional or behavioral problems. In some cases, couple therapy is presented as an independent treatment for these problems, whereas, in other cases, couple therapy is described as an adjunct to individual treatment. The third part offers specific guidelines for adapting couple therapy in working with couples struggling with emotional, behavioral, or health problems for which empirical research regarding couple therapy remains less fully developed. Finally, the book concludes with an integrative chapter addressing the implications of co-occurring relationship and individual problems for research, practice, and training in couple therapy.

To ensure continuity in style and organization across chapters, we asked contributing authors to adhere to a similar format. Each of the chapters begins with a framework for conceptualizing the specific disorder or problem it addresses, including a review of the defining features of the individual disorder and the existing research on the co-occurrence between the disorder and relationship difficulties. The focus of the chapters then moves to the clinical implications of the co-occurring disorder for couple therapy. Specifically, authors address methods for assessing and treating couples in which the individual disorder or problem occurs within the context of relationship problems. Authors were encouraged to delineate their approaches using behaviorally descriptive terms, rather than in language or jargon specific to a particular theoretical model, in order for the text to have broad appeal to therapists from diverse theoretical orientations and professional backgrounds. In addition, to help illustrate the core aspects of the approach, each chapter includes a case study that highlights the conceptual and treatment issues addressed in the chapter.

In designing this book, we sought to develop a text that would be beneficial for several different audiences. First, for *couple and family therapists,* the chapters in this book should prove beneficial in routine clinical practices in which co-occurring emotional, behavioral, and health problems are frequently encountered. Virtually every couple and family therapist confronts difficult cases where individual disorders interact with relationship distress and demand special consideration, forcing the therapist to modify his or her typical treatment approach. Information regarding assessment, conceptualization, and intervention for these co-occurring problems should improve the outcomes for couples who present with such difficulties. Second, *for the therapist who primarily works with individuals,* the chapters in this book should be helpful toward incorporating the impact of relationship problems in conceptualizing and treating persons who may not initially respond to individual-based treatments. Third, *for the scientist-researcher* investigating the comorbidity between relationship and individual functioning, the chapters in this book should assist in advancing research for understanding and treating co-occurring relationship and individual disorders. Finally, the chapters in this book offer clear implications *for training* both individual and couple therapists in recognizing and intervening with emotional and behavioral difficulties across multiple levels of the family system.

Each of the chapters in this volume reflects a wealth of information and wisdom for conceptualizing and treating couples in which one or both partners exhibit significant emotional, behavioral, or health problems. Therapists will benefit not only from acquiring the technical competence in administering specific interventions described in these chapters but also from gaining a firm understanding of the theoretical and empirical underpinnings that guide their implementation.

REFERENCES

Northley, W. F., Jr. (2002). Characteristics and clinical practices of marriage and family therapists: A national survey. *Journal of Marital and Family Therapy, 28,* 487–494.

Whisman, M. A., Dixon, A. E., & Johnson, B. (1997). Therapists' perspectives of couple problems and treatment issues in couple therapy. *Journal of Family Psychology, 11,* 361–366.

Whisman, M. A., & Snyder, D. K. (1997). Evaluating and improving the efficacy of conjoint marital therapy. In W. K. Halford & H. J. Markman (Eds.), *Clinical handbook of marriage and couples intervention* (pp. 679–693). New York: Wiley.

Contents

Empirical and Conceptual Issues in Managing Emotional, Behavioral, and Health Concerns in Couple Therapy

An Overview

Working with difficult couples requires that therapists recognize the recursive influences of individual and relationship problems, understand the impact of these factors on both the content and process of couple therapy, and develop a comprehensive therapeutic strategy integrating specific techniques tailored to both intrapersonal as well as interpersonal functioning. In the first chapter, Whisman and Uebelacker review compelling evidence concerning the high comorbidity between couple distress and emotional or behavioral disorders in one or both partners. Their review makes clear that couple distress relates to individual dysfunction across a broad spectrum of psychopathology and that this association between individual and relationship disorders is generally quite large. Based on these findings, they propose specific mechanisms by which individual disorders contribute to common rela-

1

tionship problems concerning communication, power struggles, unrealistic expectations, and the couple's sexual relationship.

Snyder, Schneider, and Castellani argue that no single treatment modality or theoretical approach fully addresses the broad spectrum of individual and relationship dysfunction that difficult couples present. Hence, working with difficult couples requires therapists to tailor interventions to individual differences by practicing integratively across diverse theoretical orientations, specific intervention modalities, and levels of individual and family functioning. In Chapter 2, these authors discuss clinical and conceptual issues in tailoring interventions to individual and relationship problems. They propose an organizational model for sequencing and pacing couple interventions by emphasizing technical integration within a theoretically pluralistic approach.

CHAPTER 1

Comorbidity of Relationship Distress and Mental and Physical Health Problems

MARK A. WHISMAN
LISA A. UEBELACKER

> To have and to hold from this day forward, for better for worse, for richer for poorer, in sickness and in health.
> —Book of Common Prayer

There is a large and growing literature that links problems in intimate relationships with the onset, co-occurrence, and course of mental and physical health problems in adults. Results from this line of research should come as no surprise, as satisfaction with intimate relationships has been identified as an important aspect of life satisfaction. In a recent study of life goals in young adult women and men, having a satisfying marriage or relationship was identified as the single most important goal in life (Roberts & Robins, 2000). Similarly, Cambell, Converse, and Rodgers (1976) found that people's feelings about their relationships have a larger impact on their overall life satisfaction than do their job, income, community, or physical health. It follows, therefore, that problems in intimate relationships are likely to both influence, and be influenced by, mental and physical health problems. Certainly, for the large number of couples who have made vows to stay together "in sickness and in health" and are confronted with co-occurring relationship and health problems, the close link between the two is very apparent.

In the first part of this chapter, we highlight research findings on the comorbidity between relationship distress and mental and physical health problems. The purpose of this review is to provide a broad overview of the association between relationship distress and health. The close connection between relationship distress and a broad spectrum of health problems provides the key rationale for the couple-based interventions discussed in the remainder of the book. Because relationship and health problems are closely related, consideration of their joint occurrence may be critical when designing and implementing effective treatment for a wide range of problems. In the second part of the chapter, we discuss how the presence of mental and physical health problems can complicate the practice of couple therapy. That is, we outline several ways in which health problems in one or both partners may require couple therapists to give special consideration to common topic areas that they routinely address when treating couples. This part of the chapter is meant to introduce the reader to issues that will be addressed, in various ways, in subsequent chapters devoted to therapies for specific problems. Given the size of the literature on relationship functioning and mental and physical health, the material covered in both sections of the chapter is intended to be illustrative rather than comprehensive in focus. More specific and detailed discussions of the associations and implications of the co-occurrence of relationship distress and specific health problems can be found in the remaining chapters of this volume.

THE ASSOCIATION BETWEEN RELATIONSHIP FUNCTIONING AND HEALTH

Relationship Functioning and Mental Health

We begin our discussion with a brief theoretical overview of the ways in which relationship functioning and mental health may influence each other. First, relationship distress can increase the probability of onset and prolong the course of mental health problems. For instance, one common model for conceptualizing mental health problems is the diathesis (i.e., vulnerability)–stress model, which proposes that mental health problems arise when a vulnerable person experiences stressful events. Considered from this perspective, poor relationship functioning (i.e., interpersonal stress) increases the likelihood of already vulnerable individuals developing and/or maintaining mental health problems. Second, the presence of mental health problems can also contribute to increases in relationship distress. For example, mental health problems can result in emotional and financial burdens, and disruptions in family routine, family leisure activities, and family interactions (Chakrabarti, Kulhara, & Verma, 1993). Taken together, these models suggest that relationship distress (and other aspects of relationship functioning, such as communication) mutually influence one another in a bidirectional and reciprocal fashion.

There have been two primary research paradigms used in evaluating the association between relationship functioning and mental health. In the first paradigm, the relationship functioning of people seeking treatment for a particular mental health problem is compared with people in treatment for some other problem or, more commonly, people not in treatment. Although providing important information on the association between relationship functioning and mental health, particularly for making decisions regarding appropriate intervention for people in treatment, the results from these types of studies are limited in their generalizability. Epidemiological studies suggest that only approximately 20% of people with a recent or active psychiatric disorder obtain professional help (Kessler et al., 1994). Therefore, a second paradigm for studying the association between relationship functioning and mental health has been to evaluate their co-occurrence in community samples, including representative epidemiological samples.

In this chapter, we highlight some of the empirical findings regarding the association between relationship distress and specific psychiatric disorders; more detailed information is provided in the individual chapters in this volume. Before doing so, however, we provide an overview of the methods and findings from a large epidemiological study that obtained a representative sample of adults from the community. Whisman (1999) evaluated the association between marital distress and 12-month prevalence rates of 13 psychiatric disorders using data from the National Comorbidity Survey. This epidemiological sample included 2,538 married persons between the ages of 15 and 54 drawn from across the United States. Assuming that approximately 20% of the population is distressed—a percentage that is consistent both with prior research involving community samples (e.g., Ren, 1997) and with theoretical discussions about cutoff scores for identifying clinically significant levels of distress (Jacobson & Truax, 1991)—Table 1.1 shows the association between marital distress and psychiatric disorders, expressed in terms of odds ratios. Thus, the values in this table indicate the odds of a maritally distressed spouse having the psychiatric disorder or class of disorders in comparison to spouses that are not maritally distressed. Several points can be made regarding the information provided in this table. First, maritally distressed people are more likely to have psychiatric disorders than nondistressed people. For example, in comparison to nondistressed individuals, distressed individuals are 3 times more likely to have a mood disorder, 2.5 times more likely to have an anxiety disorder, and 2 times more likely to have a substance use disorder. Second, marital distress is associated with each class of disorder and with each specific disorder that was evaluated, with the exception of bipolar disorder; this exception was likely due to the low prevalence and resulting low statistical power for bipolar disorder. In other words, the association between marital distress and psychiatric disorders is not limited to a select group of disorders. Third, the magnitudes of the associations between marital distress and disorders were generally quite large.

It may seem tautological to report that relationship distress is associated with mental health problems, insofar as clinically significant impairment or distress in social, occupational, or other important areas of functioning is required for making the diagnosis of a mental disorder (American Psychiatric Association, 1994). This issue was partially addressed in an epidemiological study by Whisman, Sheldon, and Goering (2000). In this study, the association between marital distress and

TABLE 1.1. Association between Marital Distress and Psychiatric Disorders

Disorder	Percentage with disorder		Wald χ^2	Odds ratio	95% CI
	Distressed	Nondistressed			
Mood disorder	15.5	6.9	72.29**	3.1	2.4–4.0
Major depression	14.5	6.2	71.11**	3.2	2.4–4.1
Bipolar disorder	1.4	0.9	3.36	2.0	1.0–4.0
Dysthymia	4.5	1.2	41.25**	5.7	3.3–9.6
Anxiety disorder	28.3	14.8	80.97**	2.5	2.1–3.1
Panic disorder	3.9	1.5	25.25**	3.5	2.2–5.8
Agoraphobia	4.3	2.0	8.60*	2.1	1.3–3.5
Social phobia	10.7	5.9	26.34**	2.2	1.6–2.9
Simple phobia	12.2	7.7	22.19**	1.9	1.5–2.5
GAD	5.6	2.5	29.82**	3.2	2.1–4.8
PTSD	7.4	2.1	36.54**	3.8	2.5–5.8
Substance use disorder	14.8	7.3	22.52**	2.0	1.5–2.6
Alcohol abuse/ dependence	11.8	6.4	12.68**	1.8	1.3–2.4
Drug abuse/ dependence	5.3	2.0	9.29*	2.2	1.3–3.6

Note. CI, confidence interval; GAD, generalized anxiety disorder; PTSD, posttraumatic stress disorder.
* $p < .005$; ** $p < .001$.

nine psychiatric disorders was evaluated using data from the Mental Health Supplement to the Ontario Health Survey, an epidemiological sample that included 4,933 spouses between the ages of 18 and 64 from Ontario, Canada. Specifically, the association between psychiatric disorders and marital distress was evaluated while controlling for distress in relationships with relatives and close friends. When controlling for this more general relationship distress, marital distress was still associated with six specific disorders (i.e., major depression, social and simple phobia, panic disorder, generalized anxiety disorder, and alcohol dependence/abuse). In comparison, not getting along with relatives and friends was generally unrelated to psychiatric disorders when the quality of the other social relationships was statistically controlled. Thus, it appears that the presence of mental health problems is associated with greater marital distress, above and beyond general distress in other close relationships. We turn now to the findings for specific psychiatric disorders and classes of disorders.

Mood Disorders

The theoretical importance of interpersonal functioning for understanding depression has a long history. For example, Bowlby (1969) proposed that individuals are vulnerable to depression when attachment bonds are disrupted or threatened. Interpersonal psychotherapy (Klerman, Weissman, Rounsaville, & Chevron, 1984) was developed as a treatment for depression based on theoretical developments and empirical findings regarding the interpersonal functioning of depressed individuals. It certainly seems reasonable that problems in intimate relationships could have a substantial negative impact on one's mood, appetite, sleep, and other functioning. On the other hand, it is also likely that the symptoms of depression (such as lack of interest, fatigue, hopelessness) may result in fewer mutually enjoyable activities, more interpersonal distance, and lower satisfaction for the depressed person and his or her partner.

The association between marital distress and depression has been well documented (for a review, see Whisman, 2001a). In a recent meta-analysis of existing studies evaluating the association between self-report measures of marital distress and depressive symptoms, Whisman (2001a) reported a mean correlation of .42 for women (based on 3,745 participants from 26 studies) and .37 for men (based on 2,700 participants from 21 studies). Furthermore, compared to nondepressed married persons, marital distress is greater among individuals with major depression who seek treatment. In a recent meta-analysis of 10 existing studies, Whisman (2001a) reported a mean correlation between marital distress and major depression of .66. In addition, there is evidence that marital distress predates, and therefore is potentially causally related to, the onset of major depression. Whisman and Bruce (1999) found that spouses who were unhappy with their marriage were approximately three times more likely than happily married spouses to develop an episode of major depression over a 12-month period. In addition, the attributable risk for marital distress on major depression was estimated to be approximately 30%. The attributable risk refers to the maximum percentage of cases that could be eliminated if exposure to the risk factor was prevented. Thus, these findings suggest that nearly 30% of cases of major depression among married individuals could be prevented if marital distress was successfully prevented or treated. Furthermore, specific "humiliating" marital events, such as discovery of a partner's infidelity or threats of separation and divorce, may increase the risk for major depression above and beyond the risk conferred by relationship distress alone, perhaps because they result in the person feeling devalued (Cano & O'Leary, 2000).

Substance Use Disorders

Because of the behavioral problems associated with the acquisition and consumption of substances of abuse, it is not surprising that substance use disorders can pose serious ongoing problems for couples, as indicated by greater relationship distress and greater relationship instability. Furthermore, some persons may use substances as a way to escape from relationship problems; repeated use of this coping strategy may lead to abuse or dependence over time.

Research suggests that one-third of male partners of couples who request couple therapy will report significant problems with alcohol use, and many more of these couples will report that alcohol use is a source of conflict (Halford & Osgarby, 1993). Similarly, O'Farrell and Birchler (1987) found that alcoholic couples reported greater marital distress and had more thoughts about separation or divorce than nondistressed couples. Couples in which one or both members are abusing drugs also report high levels of marital distress (Fals-Stewart, Birchler, & O'Farrell, 1999). Furthermore, there is evidence for a longitudinal association between substance abuse and relationship distress. Marital functioning predicts the likelihood of relapse and time to relapse in alcoholic patients in treatment (Maisto, O'Farrell, Connors, McKay, & Pelcovits, 1988; O'Farrell, Hooley, Fals-Stewart, & Cutter, 1998). Similarly, problematic drinking predicts increases in marital distress and the likelihood of divorce or separation a year later (Leonard & Roberts, 1998). Of note, a study that followed male alcoholics for 10 years after initial treatment reported that rate of divorce among relapsed alcoholics was 39% (vs. 9% in nonrelapsed alcoholics and a community control group; Moos, Finney, & Cronkite, 1990).

A serious danger of alcohol abuse is its association with partner physical abuse. Male alcohol problems may increase the likelihood of male-to-female physical abuse in relationships (e.g., Leonard & Blane, 1992). Certain aspects of these alcohol problems, such as binge drinking and greater severity and earlier onset of alcoholism, tend to confer even higher risk for men's relationship aggression (Murphy & O'Farrell, 1994).

Interestingly, whether one or both partners have a substance use problem may have different repercussions for the relationship. When both partners show the same dysfunctional pattern of substance use, relationship distress tends to be lower than when only one partner exhibits a particular pattern (Fals-Stewart et al., 1999; Mudar, Leonard, & Soltysinski, 2001). In fact, in dual drug abuse relationships, the longer partners are abstinent, the less stable is their marriage. This is in contrast to single-partner drug abuse relationships, in which length of abstinence is positively related to stability of relationship (Fals-Stewart et al., 1999).

Anxiety Disorders

The class of anxiety disorders includes a heterogeneous range of problems with anxiety. Although they differ somewhat in their course and treatment, the etiological factors that give rise to various anxiety disorders may be applicable to more than one disorder. For example, both biologically based (e.g., Cloninger, 1986) and cognitively based (e.g., Beck & Emery, 1985) models of anxiety emphasize the importance of hypervigilance to potentially dangerous situations as forming one of the core components of anxiety. Given the importance of interpersonal relationships, it seems logical that actual or perceived threat of relationship problems, relationship dissolution, or both would be associated with increased anxiety. On the other hand, once present, different anxiety disorders may impact couple functioning in different ways. For example, persons with obsessive–compulsive disorder (OCD) may require frequent reassurance from a partner regarding the content of their obsessions, or may create elaborate rituals that involve the partner. Individuals with severe agoraphobia, who are unable to leave their homes, may require assistance from significant others to meet basic needs (e.g., shopping for groceries). The emotional numbing associated with posttraumatic stress disorder (PTSD) may make it difficult to feel close to friends, family, and relationship partners. In the following review, we focus in detail on agoraphobia, OCD, and PTSD because much of the research on anxiety and relationship functioning has focused on these problems. However, relationship distress has also been associated with other anxiety disorders as well. For example, McLeod (1994) found that 12-month prevalence of generalized anxiety disorder (GAD) was associated with greater marital distress, and Markowitz, Weissman, Ouellette, Lish, and Klerman (1989) reported that marital distress was associated with a sevenfold increased odds of having panic disorder.

Agoraphobia. Writers from various theoretical perspectives have long been interested in describing the close relationships of individuals (especially women) with agoraphobia. Bowlby (1973) viewed agoraphobia as a manifestation of anxious attachment, and therefore, by definition, interpersonal in nature. From a behavioral perspective, social reinforcement has been a key in understanding the maintenance of agoraphobic symptoms. Thus, agoraphobic behavior may elicit caring responses from a partner, resulting in reinforcement of the agoraphobia. Despite the theoretical connection between anxiety and relationships, in a review of the literature on marital distress and agoraphobia, Emmelkamp and Gerlsma (1994) concluded that "the marriages of individuals with agoraphobia are not much different from that of normal individuals" (p. 502). This conclusion, however, may be overly conservative, given that the reported effect sizes (Cohen's *d*) ranged from 0.10 to 2.73, with all but one study having effect sizes in the medium or large range. Other studies have found that, although agoraphobic couples may be more distressed than non-psychiatric couples, they may not be as distressed as other psychiatric patients (Arrindell & Emmelkamp, 1986).

Obsessive–Compulsive Disorder. OCD can cause numerous problems for families and partners. Calvocoressi et al. (1999) reported that as many as 90% of persons with OCD live with family members (parents or spouses) who accommodate to their symptoms. This occurs despite the fact many of these family members believe that the OCD-related requests are unreasonable, and experience distress or hostility when accommodating the symptoms. Approximately 30% of family members reported providing reassurance on a daily basis that obsessions were unfounded; 30% also changed their own behavior (i.e., did not say or do certain things) because of their loved one's OCD symptoms, also on a daily basis. Available evidence suggests that the level of relationship distress in treatment-seeking individuals with OCD is high (Riggs, Hiss, & Foa, 1992). Although there are few studies specifically addressing the question, as many as 50% of the individuals with OCD met conventional criteria for relationship distress (Riggs et al., 1992).

Posttraumatic Stress Disorder.   Given that symptoms of PTSD include emotional numbing and feelings of detachment, it is not surprising that PTSD is associated with relationship distress. A substantial body of research on PTSD and relationship distress has been conducted with male Vietnam veterans and their female partners. Many of these studies compare veterans with PTSD to those without it. As many as 70% of veterans with PTSD may have clinically significant levels of relationship distress (vs. 30% of veterans without PTSD; Riggs, Byrne, Weathers, & Litz, 1998). Veterans with PTSD have taken more steps toward separation or divorce, have more difficulties with intimacy (Riggs et al., 1998), have lower levels of self-disclosure and expressiveness (e.g., talking about the activities of the day) with a romantic partner, and exhibit more physical aggression (Carroll, Rueger, Foy, & Donahoe, 1985). Their partners tend to be more demoralized, less satisfied with their lives, and more physically aggressive than the partners of veterans without PTSD (Jordan, Marmar, Fairbank, & Schlenger, 1992).

For many individuals, the event or events that trigger PTSD are closely linked to their experience of intimate relationships. Based on national representative surveys, it is estimated that each year, one out of every eight men will be physically aggressive toward his wife, and between 1.5–2 million women will be severely assaulted by their husbands (Straus & Gelles, 1986). Of abused women, a survey of available research suggests that 31–84% will develop PTSD (Cascardi, O'Leary, & Schlee, 1999).

Personality Disorders

Compared to the research on Axis I disorders, there is relatively little research on Axis II disorders. This is somewhat surprising, given that personality disorders are often conceptualized as disorders of interpersonal behaviors. It would seem, therefore, that there would be high comorbidity between relationship distress and the occurrence of personality disorders. Indeed, the limited research findings support such an association. For example, Reich, Yates, and Nduaguba (1989) found that married adults with personality disorders reported more relationship difficulties than adults without personality disorders. Furthermore, this association seems to be stronger than the association between relationship distress and Axis I disorders. In a sample of inpatients and outpatients, Truant (1994) reported that individuals with personality disorders (most of whom also had an Axis I disorder) reported greater relationship distress than individuals with only Axis I disorders. Given that there are only a limited number of studies that have evaluated the importance of relationship distress for personality disorders, this is clearly an area that is in need of additional empirical evaluation.

Relationship Distress and Physical Health

Early research on the association between relationships and physical health often evaluated the impact of marital status (i.e., married, divorced, widowed, never married). Results from these studies indicate that married people are healthier than nonmarried people (e.g., Verbrugge, 1979). More recently, however, researchers have recognized that perceived physical health is associated not only with marital status, but also with relationship quality. For example, in a study evaluating global health perceptions among over 12,000 American adults, Ren (1997) found that perceived health was related to relationship distress in married and cohabiting participants. The association between relationship functioning and physical health is not, however, limited to perceptions of health but is also related to objective physical health status or physiological data. For example, Carels, Szczepanski, Blumenthal, and Sherwood (1998) found that relationship distress was associated with higher systolic blood pressure and heart rate responses to a problem-solving interaction task.

Relationship functioning is associated not only with subjective and objective indices of physical health, but also with adjustment to physical health problems. For example, in a study on psychological adjustment of adults with cancer, Rodrique and Park (1996) found that people with high relationship distress reported more depression and anxiety, a less positive health care orientation, and more illness induced family difficulties. Thus, it appears that when people have a major physical illness, and they are dissatisfied with their relationships, they are more likely to have greater difficulty coping with the illness. Furthermore, quality of relationship functioning has been found to predict mortality. For example, in a 15-year longitudinal study, Hibbard and Pope (1993) found that for married women, equality in decision making and companionship in marriage were protective against death.

In a recent review, Kiecolt-Glaser and Newton (2001) conclude that there is convincing evidence from research conducted in the past decade, particularly marital interaction research, indicating that marital relationships affect health outcomes. They present a conceptual model for organizing the existing research, in which they conclude that negative dimensions of relationship functioning have indirect effects on health, through the pathways of depression and health habits. For example, relationship conflict may lead to difficulties in quitting smoking, getting enough exercise, or eating in a healthy fashion, which, in turn, has negative health consequences. Furthermore, they conclude that relationship functioning, particularly negative communication patterns, has direct effects on cardiovascular, endocrine, immune, neurosensory, and other physiological mechanisms that may, in turn, affect health.

Relationship Distress and Treatment Outcome for Mental and Physical Health Problems

In addition to evaluating the cross-sectional and longitudinal association between relationship functioning and mental and physical health problems, investigators have evaluated the association that relationship distress has with outcome to treatments for such problems. Specifically, several studies show that marital distress is associated with a slower recovery (Goering, Lancee, & Freeman, 1992) and a greater likelihood of relapse (e.g., Hooley & Teasdale, 1989; Whisman, 2001b) for depression. As previously mentioned, relationship functioning also predicts the likelihood of relapse and time to relapse in alcoholic patients in treatment (Maisto et al., 1988; O'Farrell et al., 1998). Research has also shown that relationship distress is associated with poorer outcome to individual treatment for married or cohabiting people with GAD (Durham, Allan, & Hackett, 1997), although the association between distress and outcome to treatments for other types of anxiety disorders is less conclusive (Emmelkamp & Gerlsma, 1994).

One particular aspect of relationship functioning that is an important predictor of short- and long-term outcome to health problems is expressed emotion (EE). Results from several studies have shown that high EE, which refers to high levels of criticism, hostility, or emotional overinvolvement, is related to poorer recovery and higher rates of relapse for a variety of mental health problems. A recent meta-analysis of existing studies found a reliable and robust association between high EE and relapse in schizophrenia, mood disorders (unipolar depression and bipolar disorder), and eating disorders (Butzlaff & Hooley, 1998). Furthermore, as reviewed by Wearden, Tarrier, Barrowclaugh, Zastowny, and Rahill (2000), there is an increasing number of studies that have found an association between high EE and poor outcome to a variety of physical health problems, including diabetes, asthma, epilepsy, and rheumatoid arthritis.

Taken together, the existing research suggests that people who are unhappy with their intimate relationships and have poor relationship functioning are not only more likely to have a mental or physical health problem, they are also less likely to respond to treatment for such a problem. As such, these findings support the use of couple therapy, singly or in combination with other interventions, in the treatment of

health problems. Indeed, studies have found that couple therapy is effective in treating a variety of mental health problems. In a review of
this literature, Baucom, Shoham, Mueser, Daiuto, and Stickle (1998)
concluded that couple therapy has successfully been applied in the
treatment of depression, anxiety disorders, sexual dysfunctions, and alcoholism and problem drinking. We refer the reader to the Baucom et
al. (1998) paper and to relevant chapters of this book for more specific
information regarding these studies.

Having provided a brief overview of the research on the association
between relationship distress and the onset, course, and treatment of
mental and physical health problems, we turn now to the influence of
mental and physical health problems on the practice of couple therapy.

THE IMPACT OF HEALTH PROBLEMS ON THE PRACTICE OF COUPLE THERAPY

In reviewing the literature on couple therapy for mental health problems, Baucom et al. (1998) conclude that couple therapy is most often
provided as part of a multicomponent treatment package, and less commonly as the only treatment provided. Whether provided by itself or in
combination with other interventions, couple therapy in which one or
both partners has a mental or physical health problem is often more
challenging and more complicated than when both partners do not
have health problems. As a heuristic for considering how the presence
of mental or physical health problems might make the delivery of couple therapy more challenging, we consider the kinds of issues that couple therapists commonly address in conducting couple therapy. Whisman, Dixon, and Johnson (1997) conducted a survey of practicing
couple therapists in the United States regarding the problem areas and
therapeutic needs they encountered in couple therapy. The five most
common problems that therapists reported dealing with in their practices were, in decreasing order, communication, power struggles, unrealistic expectations (of the relationship or of the partner), sex, and
problem solving. These results suggest that many therapists would anticipate that a couple presenting for therapy is experiencing problems in
one or more of these areas, and that these areas would be likely targets
for intervention.

In the paragraphs that follow, we discuss how the presence of mental or physical health problems might be related to each of these areas
that couple therapists commonly treat. Couple therapy with these couples may be more challenging than would be anticipated for partners
without health problems. Consideration of the challenges in working

with people with health problems is not meant to be discouraging but rather to highlight issues to bear in mind when treating certain types of couples in order to improve outcome. As with the previous section of this chapter, this information is to be viewed as illustrative in nature; details regarding couple interventions for specific mental and physical health problems are provided in the other chapters of this volume. This discussion will focus on the first four of the five common problems reported by Whisman et al. (1997). The fifth problem—problem solving—is subsumed under the section on communication.

Communication

Therapists in the Whisman et al. (1997) study identified communication as the most common problem addressed in couple therapy. Communication difficulties, in turn, are associated with a range of mental health problems. Psychotic disorders, by definition, may involve problems with communication, because disorganized speech is one of five core symptoms of schizophrenia (American Psychiatric Association, 1994). More subtle dysfunctional communication patterns (i.e., social skills deficits) have been associated with the presence of other psychological disorders, most notably major depression and substance use disorders.

Communication researchers often disaggregate the myriad of partners' communications with one another into two major categories. The first category of communication focuses on partners' conflict or problem-solving interactions. Based on early research indicating that the way in which couples solve relationship problems was strongly associated with relationship distress (Gottman, 1979), mental health researchers have tended to focus on how couples communicate when they are trying to solve a problem in their relationship. In observational coding of problem-solving interactions, major depression has been associated with decreased positive behavior and increased negative behavior, including "depressive" behavior (e.g., self-derogation, depressive affect) (e.g., Biglan et al., 1985; Johnson & Jacob, 1997; Schmaling & Jacobson, 1990). Substance use disorders have been associated with less positive communication, more struggles for control, avoidance of taking responsibility, and verbal abusiveness (e.g., Fals-Stewart & Birchler, 1998; O'Farrell & Birchler, 1987). Agoraphobia, too, has been associated with greater criticism and less positive problem-solving interaction (Chambless et al., 2002).

Communication patterns have also been shown to be associated with physical health outcomes. For example, negative communication behavior has been associated with alterations in both endocrine

(Malarky, Kiecolt-Glaser, Pearl, & Glaser, 1994) and immune functioning (Kiecolt-Glaser, Malarky, Chee, & Newton, 1993) following problem-solving interactions. These studies are particularly interesting in that they showed that negative behavior is associated with biological systems among happily married couples who do not have any known mental or physical problems. In addition, hostile behavior during problem-solving interaction tasks has been associated with increased blood pressure among community couples (e.g., Morell & Apple, 1990) and among couples in which one partner is suffering from hypertension (Ewart, Taylor, Kraemer, & Agras, 1991).

As suggested by this brief review, research has shown that the presence of mental and physical health problems is associated with poorer communication during problem-solving interactions. Therefore, poor problem-solving skills are likely in couples with health problems. Furthermore, for individuals or couples with health problems, difficulties with problem solving may be global rather than limited to the relationship. General deficits in general problem solving have been implicated in the onset and course of depression (Nezu, 1987) and other mental health problems such as PTSD (Nezu & Carnevale, 1987), and predict distress in people with physical health problems such as cancer (Nezu et al., 1999). Clinically, this means that it may be more challenging and time-consuming to teach couples problem-solving skills because the clinician may not be able to point to successful models of problem solving in other parts of the couples' lives. However, the extra effort may be well worth it insofar as teaching couples effective problem-solving strategies (see Jacobson & Margolin, 1979) may be effective in improving individual physical and mental health conditions, as well as improving relationship distress.

The second major category of communication focuses on partners sharing information and providing support for one another. As previously noted, this has not been the focus of most empirical research. However, recent research suggests that partners' supportive behaviors can be reliably coded and are associated with longitudinal changes in relationship satisfaction, over that which can be accounted for by problem-solving communication (Pasch & Bradbury, 1998). Although we are not aware of any published research evaluating observations of supportive interactions among couples in which one partner has a mental or physical health problem, it seems likely that couples would exhibit problems in this area, insofar as people with mental and physical health problems often report low levels of general social support.

When working with a couple, one or both partners of which has a health problem, a clinician would be well advised to consider the limitations that health problems might place on communication, including both problem solving and supportive communication. For example, problems with concentration may result in partners being unable to maintain a lengthy conversation. In these kinds of situations, couples may need to modify their expectations regarding communication (e.g., expectations that partners should be available to talk with one another at any time or for any length of time), as well as their actual communication patterns (e.g., partners may decide to have shorter conversations).

Second, clinicians should be sensitive to communication patterns that may be contributing to the health problem. For example, given the association between expressed emotion and mental and physical health outcomes, clinicians will want to carefully assess criticism and intrusive communication and to work with couples on reducing these types of communication. Partners of people with health problems may be critical of the person if they believe that the person's behavior is intentional and under their control. Consequently, they may become less critical if they change their attributions for the person's behavior. This could be accomplished through providing couples with information about the effects of the health problem on behavior, including communication. Thus, behavior that could be seen as interpersonally manipulative, such as crying, acting odd, or repeatedly seeking reassurance from the partner, may be reframed as symptomatic of the underlying health problem. Finally, couples could be taught problem-solving skills in order to introduce and define problems in a noncritical fashion.

The perspective that communication behaviors associated with mental or physical health problems could increase the complexity of conducting couple therapy has received indirect support from a recent study on the difficulty implementing family therapy for bipolar patients (Tompson, Rea, Goldstein, Miklowitz, & Weisman, 2000). It was found that relatives' critical behavior toward patients before treatment was associated with independent observers' ratings of overall treatment difficulty and therapists' perceptions of problems during treatment. Thus, these types of communication problems may pose both the biggest challenges as well as the biggest payoffs for therapists working with couples with comorbid relationship and health problems.

Power Struggles

Power struggles were the second most commonly treated problem reported by therapists in the Whisman et al. (1997) study. Similar to communication, there is some, albeit limited, research showing that power struggles in relationships may also be important for understanding mental health problems. Studies have found that depression is associated with greater inequality in, and distress with, how partners make decisions in their relationships (e.g., Whisman & Jacobson, 1989); inequality and distress with decision making has long been considered to measure the power distribution of a couple. Power inequality has also been associated with outcomes other than depression. For example, Babcock, Waltz, Jacobson, and Gottman (1993) found that physical aggression was associated with greater power inequality.

Although limited, these findings suggest that the relationships of couples in which one or both partners has a mental health problem may be characterized by greater power inequality than the relationships of couples in which neither partner has a mental health problem. If people do not believe that they have much influence or power in a relationship, then they may be more likely to feel helpless or hopeless about making important changes in that relationship. Such helplessness and hopelessness may, in turn, increase the likelihood or severity of health problems. Helping the person with less power become more empowered may serve to increase optimism and perceived ability to make changes in the relationship. This increased optimism may be associated with decreases in health problems, and increases in positive health behaviors (e.g., exercise). However, given that power inequality may be greater in couples with health problems, this is likely to be more difficult to achieve. Furthermore, couples may resist modifying their relationship, saying that the power inequality has been necessary in order to compensate for the behavior in the person with a health problem. For example, one person might argue that she has to be in charge of balancing the checkbook, because the partner is depressed, cannot concentrate, and makes more mistakes. Therefore, treatment of power inequality in the relationship, and treatment of individual mental health problems, may need to occur simultaneously.

Unrealistic Expectations

Unrealistic expectations of the partner or relationship were the third most commonly treated problem reported by therapists in the Whisman et al. (1977) study. How might the presence of physical or mental health problems make it more difficult to treat these types of expectations? It seems likely that the occurrence of health problems could impact the degree to which one holds unrealistic expectations, the types of unrealistic expectations one holds, or both.

First, health problems could impact the degree of endorsement of unrealistic expectations. According to cognitive models of relationship distress and treatment (Dattilo & Padesky, 1990), many of the same types of cognitive processes that are associated with mental health problems are also associated with relationship distress. For example, among the most common distortions associated with both relationship difficulties and mental health problems are dichotomous thinking (viewing situations in terms of categories vs. continua), mind reading (believing one knows what others are thinking or feeling), and magnification–minimization (magnifying the negative or minimizing the positive in evaluations of experience). Consequently, a particularly strong endorsement of those beliefs that represent these cognitive distortions might result in both relationship distress and mental health problems. Although there has been no research evaluating whether both relationship distress and psychiatric disorders are associated with these types of cognitive processes, there has been some limited research evaluating whether mental health problems are associated with general relationship beliefs. For example, a recent study by Uebelacker and Whisman (2002) compared depressed and nondepressed women, and found that clinically depressed women reported greater endorsement of several dysfunctional relationship beliefs, including the beliefs that disagreement is destructive to a relationship and that mind reading is expected in relationships. Furthermore, other researchers have reported that greater levels of depressive symptoms are associated with greater endorsement of dysfunctional attributional style—attributing negative partner behavior to stable, global, and partner-based causes (e.g., Fincham & Bradbury, 1993). To the extent that mental health problems are associated with greater endorsement of dysfunctional relationship cognitions, including unrealistic beliefs, then the presence of such problems could make the practice of couple therapy more difficult. These strongly endorsed beliefs are likely to be difficult to modify. However, modifying such belief systems is likely to influence outcome in both relationship and health domains.

A second way in which the occurrence of mental health problems could impact unrealistic expectations concerns the type or range of unrealistic expectations. According to Beck's (1983) cognitive model of psychopathology, the core beliefs associated with mental disorders (i.e., the most central ideas about the self) can be categorized into one of two realms. The first realm concerns the belief that one is personally helpless (e.g., powerless, vulnerable) and does not measure up in terms of achievement (e.g., failure, inferior), whereas the second realm concerns the belief that one is unlovable (e.g., unworthy, undesirable). To the extent that this theory is true and people with mental health problems have one or both of these beliefs, then these core beliefs could significantly impact the practice of couple therapy. For instance, if a person strongly endorsed the core belief of being helpless, he or she could have problems following through with a clinician's recommendations or homework assignments, believing that these changes could not successfully be accomplished. One clinical implication of this notion would be to recommend that therapists working with clients with mental health problems begin with smaller initial assignments (i.e., graded task assignments), as well as ones that are more easily accomplished (e.g., increasing the frequency of caring behaviors). Similarly, the clinician could directly ask the couple if they have any concerns about being able to follow through with recommendations or homework assignments.

A person who strongly endorsed the core belief of being unlovable may also have a difficult time making changes in the relationship as well. However, change may be difficult for a very different reason, namely, the belief that making changes will not matter because the partner will ultimately reject them. It may be helpful, when working with individuals who strongly endorse this belief, to encourage them to withhold judgment about the outcome until after the changes have been made. Furthermore, people who see themselves as unlovable may be more likely to be submissive to their partner's requests, and have a difficult time expressing their own needs and desires in the relationship, believing that they are not worthy of requesting anything from their partner. They may be also more likely to continually seek reassurance from their partner that he or she will not leave. Both of these patterns of behavior are likely to contribute to greater relationship distress, and suggest further areas of intervention with couples that present with comorbid relationship distress and mental health problems.

Thus, in addition to working with the couple on relationship cognitions, the couple therapist working with a person with a mental health problem may also want to consider some individual sessions focusing on individual belief systems, particularly as they impact the relationship.

Sex

Sex was the fourth most commonly treated problem reported by therapists in the Whisman et al. (1977) study. Not only are sexual problems more likely to be found among people who are dissatisfied with their relationship, sexual problems are also common among couples in which one or more partners have a mental health problem. For example, a decrease or loss of libido is a common symptom of depression, and compared to those who are not depressed, women who are depressed more strongly endorse the belief that one must be a perfect sexual partner (Uebelacker & Whisman, 2002). In addition, researchers have documented a higher prevalence of sexual problems among male alcoholics

(O'Farrell, 1990) than in the general population. Sexual dysfunction is related to chronic problem drinking in women as well (Wilsnack, 1991). Similarly, anxiety disorders have been associated with sexual problems. For example, OCD and panic disorder are associated with high rates of sexual dysfunction in women (Minnen & Kampman, 2000), and significant sexual difficulties may be present in up to 80% of veterans being treated for PTSD (Letourneau, Schewe, & Frueh, 1997). Sexual dissatisfaction and sexual disorders are a common side effect of physical health problems, such as diabetes or stroke. Sexual problems are also associated with many of the medications prescribed in the treatment of health problems, such as antidepressant medications (Ferguson, 2001). Taken together, these results suggest that sexual problems may be more likely and more severe in couples in which one or both partners has a mental or physical health problem.

One implication of these findings for the practice of couple therapy is that therapists would be well advised to consider the impact that mental and physical health problems and the medications used to treat these problems can have on sexual functioning. Basic psychoeducation about the impact of illness on sexual functioning may be extremely helpful. This is particularly important for spouses who blame their partner for problems in sexual functioning, or who interpret such problems as due to lack of interest or due to problems in the relationship. Such information may aid couples to adjust their expectations regarding sexuality in the relationship.

CONCLUSION

There is a large and expanding literature that links relationship functioning with the onset, course, and treatment of mental and physical health problems. Examples of these types of findings have been reviewed in this chapter. In addition, there is growing research suggesting that couple therapy, singly or as part of multicomponent treatment programs, is effective in the treatment of mental health problems. Although providing couple therapy for people with health problems has been shown to be beneficial, the presence of mental and physical health problems may be more challenging than couple treatment in which neither partner has a health problem. In particular, we have proposed several ways in which health problems may make the practice of couple therapy more challenging through their influence on commonly treated areas of functioning, and we have offered some examples of how to address these challenges. Careful consideration for how the presence of mental or physical health problems may impact on the functioning of each partner, as well as on their relationship, may lead to more focused treatment and better outcomes for people with mental or physical health problems. Subsequent chapters in this volume provide more detailed suggestions about how to successfully treat these disorders in the context of couple therapy.

REFERENCES

American Psychiatric Association. (1994). *Diagnostic and statistical manual of mental disorders* (4th ed.). Washington, DC: Author.

Arrindell, W. A., & Emmelkamp, P. M. G. (1986). Marital adjustment, intimacy and needs in female agoraphobics and their partners: A controlled study. *British Journal of Psychiatry, 149,* 592–602.

Babcock, J. C., Waltz, J., Jacobson, N. S., & Gottman, J. M. (1993). Power and violence: The relation between communication patterns, power discrepancies, and domestic violence. *Journal of Consulting and Clinical Psychology, 61,* 40–50.

Baucom, D. H., Shoham, V., Mueser, K. T., Daiuto, A. D., & Stickle, T. R. (1998). Empirically supported couple and family interventions for marital distress and adult mental health problems. *Journal of Consulting and Clinical Psychology, 66,* 53–88.

Beck, A. T. (1983). Cognitive therapy of depression: New perspectives. In J. E. Barrett (Ed.), *Treatment of depression: Old controversies and new perspectives* (pp. 265–290). New York: Raven.

Beck, A. T., & Emery, G. (1985). *Anxiety disorders and phobias: A cognitive perspective.* New York: Basic Books.

Biglan, A., Hops, H., Sherman, L., Friedman, L. S., Arthur, J., & Osteen, V. (1985). Problem-solving interactions of depressed women and their husbands. *Behavior Therapy, 16,* 431–451.

Bowlby, J. (1969). *Attachment and loss: Vol. 1. Attachment.* New York: Basic Books.

Bowlby, J. (1973). *Attachment and loss: Vol. 2. Separation.* New York: Basic Books.

Butzlaff, R. L., & Hooley, J. M. (1998). Expressed emotion and psychiatric relapse: A meta-analysis. *Archives of General Psychiatry, 55,* 547–552.

Calvocoressi, L., Mazure, C. M., Kasl, S. V., Skolnick, J., Fisk, D., Vegso, S. J., Van Noppen, B. L., & Price, L. H. (1999). Family accommodation of obsessive–compulsive symptoms: Instrument development and assessment of family behavior. *Journal of Nervous and Mental Disease, 187,* 636–642.

Campbell, A., Converse, P. E., & Rodgers, W. L. (1976). *The quality of American life.* New York: Russell Sage Foundation.

Cano, A., & O'Leary, K. D. (2000). Infidelity and separations precipitate major depressive episodes and symptoms of nonspecific depression and anxiety. *Journal of Consulting and Clinical Psychology, 68,* 774–781.

Carels, R. A., Szczepanski, R., Blumenthal, J. A., & Sherwood, A. (1998). Blood pressure reactivity and marital distress in employed women. *Psychosomatic Medicine, 60,* 639–643.

Carroll, E. M., Rueger, D. B., Foy, D. W., & Donahoe, C. P. (1985). Vietnam combat veterans with posttraumatic stress disorder: Analysis of marital and cohabiting adjustment. *Journal of Abnormal Psychology, 94*, 329–337.

Cascardi, M., O'Leary, K. D., & Schlee, K. A. (1999). Co-occurrence and correlates of posttraumatic stress disorder and major depression in physically abused women. *Journal of Family Violence, 14*, 227–249.

Chakrabarti, S., Kulhara, P., & Verma, S. K. (1993). The pattern of burden in families of neurotic patients. *Social Psychiatry and Psychiatric Epidemiology, 28*, 172–177.

Chambless, D. L., Fauerbach, J. A., Floyd, F. J., Wilson, K. A., Remen, A. L., & Renneberg, B. (2002). Marital interaction of agoraphobic women: A controlled, behavioral observation study. *Journal of Abnormal Psychology, 111*, 502–512.

Cloninger, C. R. (1986). A unified biosocial theory of personality and its role in the development of anxiety states. *Psychiatric Developments, 3*, 167–226.

Dattilo, F. M., & Padesky, C. A. (1990). *Cognitive therapy with couples.* Sarasota, FL: Professional Resource Exchange.

Durham, R. C., Allan, T., & Hackett, C. A. (1997). On predicting improvement and relapse in generalized anxiety disorder following psychotherapy. *British Journal of Clinical Psychology, 36*, 101–119.

Emmelkamp, P. M. G., & Gerlsma, C. (1994). Marital functioning and the anxiety disorders. *Behavior Therapy, 25*, 407–429.

Ewart, C. K., Taylor, C. B., Kraemer, H. C., & Agras, W. S. (1991). High blood pressure and marital discord: Not being nasty matters more than being nice. *Health Psychology, 10*, 155–163.

Fals-Stewart, W., & Birchler, G. R. (1998). Marital interactions of drug-abusing patients and their partners: Comparisons with distressed couples and relationship to drug-using behavior. *Psychology of Addictive Behaviors, 12*, 28–38.

Fals-Stewart, W., Birchler, G. R., & O'Farrell, T. J. (1999). Drug-abusing patients and their intimate partners: Dyadic adjustment, relationship stability, and substance use. *Journal of Abnormal Psychology, 108*, 11–23.

Ferguson, J. M. (2001). The effects of antidepressants on sexual functioning in depressed patients: A review. *Journal of Clinical Psychiatry, 62*, 22–34.

Fincham, F. D., & Bradbury, T. N. (1993). Marital satisfaction, depression, and attributions: A longitudinal analysis. *Journal of Personality and Social Psychology, 64*, 442–452.

Goering, P. N., Lancee, W. J., & Freeman, J. J. (1992). Marital support and recovery from depression. *British Journal of Psychiatry, 160*, 76–82.

Gottman, J. M. (1979). *Marital interaction: Experimental investigations.* New York: Academic Press.

Halford, W. K., & Osgarby, S. M. (1993). Alcohol abuse in clients presenting with marital problems. *Journal of Family Psychology, 6*, 245–254.

Hibbard, J. H., & Pope, C. R. (1993). The quality of social roles as predictors of morbidity and mortality. *Social Science and Medicine, 36*, 217–225.

Hooley, J. M., & Teasdale, J. D. (1989). Predictors of relapse in unipolar depressives: Expressed emotion, marital distress, and perceived criticism. *Journal of Abnormal Psychology, 98*, 229–235.

Jacobson, N. S., & Margolin, G. (1979). *Marital therapy: Strategies based on social learning and behavior exchange principles.* New York: Brunner/Mazel.

Jacobson, N. S., & Truax, P. (1991). Clinical significance: A statistical approach to defining meaningful change in psychotherapy research. *Journal of Consulting and Clinical Psychology, 59,* 12–19.

Johnson, S. L., & Jacob, T. (1997). Marital interactions of depressed men and women. *Journal of Consulting and Clinical Psychology, 65,* 15–23.

Jordan, B. K., Marmar, C. R., Fairbank, J. A., & Schlenger, W. E. (1992). Problems in families of male Vietnam veterans with posttraumatic stress disorder. *Journal of Consulting and Clinical Psychology, 60,* 916–926.

Kessler, R. C., McGonagle, K. A., Zhao, S., Nelson, C. B., Hughes, M., Eshleman, S., Wittchen, H.-U., & Kendler, K. S. (1994). Lifetime and 12-month prevalence of DSM-III-R psychiatric disorders in the United States: Results from the National Comorbidity Survey. *Archives of General Psychiatry, 51,* 8–19.

Kiecolt-Glaser, J. K., Malarky, W. B., Chee, M., & Newton, T. (1993). Negative behavior during marital conflict is associated with immunological downregulation. *Psychosomatic Medicine, 55,* 395–409.

Kiecolt-Glaser, J. K., & Newton, T. L. (2001). Marriage and health: His and hers. *Psychological Bulletin, 12,* 472–503.

Klerman, G. L., Weissman, M. M., Rounsaville, B. J., & Chevron, E. (1984). *Interpersonal psychotherapy of depression.* New York: Basic Books.

Leonard, K., & Blane, H. (1992). Alcohol and marital aggression in a national sample of young men. *Journal of Interpersonal Violence, 7,* 19–30.

Leonard, K. E., & Roberts, L. J. (1998). Marital aggression, quality and stability in the first year of marriage: Findings from the Buffalo Newlywed Study. In T. N. Bradbury (Ed.), *The developmental course of marital dysfunction* (pp. 44–73). New York: Cambridge University Press.

Letourneau, E. J., Schewe, P. A., & Frueh, B. C. (1997). Preliminary evaluation of sexual problems in combat veterans with PTSD. *Journal of Traumatic Stress, 10,* 125–132.

Maisto, S. A., O'Farrell, T. J., Connors, G. J., McKay, J. R., & Pelcovits, M. (1988). Alcoholics' attributions of factors affecting their relapse to drinking and reasons for terminating relapse episodes. *Addictive Behaviors, 13,* 79–82.

Malarky, W., Kiecolt-Glaser, J. K., Pearl, D., & Glaser, R. (1994). Hostile behavior during marital conflict alters pituitary and adrenal hormones. *Psychosomatic Medicine, 56,* 41–51.

Markowitz, J. S., Weissman, M. M., Ouellette, R., Lish, J. D., & Klerman, G. L. (1989). Quality of life in panic disorder. *Archives of General Psychiatry, 46,* 984–992.

McLeod, J. D. (1994). Anxiety disorders and marital quality. *Journal of Abnormal Psychology, 103,* 767–776.

Minnen, A. V., & Kampman, M. (2000). The interaction between anxiety and sexual functioning: A controlled study of sexual functioning in women with anxiety disorders. *Sexual and Relationship Therapy, 15,* 47–57.

Moos, R. H., Finney, J. W., & Cronkite, R. C. (1990). *Alcoholism treatment: Context, process, and outcome.* New York: Oxford University Press.

Morell, M. A., & Apple, R. F. (1990). Affect expression, marital satisfaction, and stress reactivity among premenopausal women during a conflict marital discussion. *Psychology of Women Quarterly, 14,* 387–402.

Mudar, P., Leonard, K. E., & Soltysinski, K. (2001). Discrepant substance use and marital functioning in newlywed couples. *Journal of Consulting and Clinical Psychology, 69,* 130–134.

Murphy, C. M., & O'Farrell, T. J. (1994). Factors associated with marital aggression in male alcoholics. *Journal of Family Psychology, 8,* 321–335.

Nezu, A. M. (1987). A problem-solving formulation of depression: A literature review and proposal of a pluralistic model. *Clinical Psychology Review, 7,* 121–144.

Nezu, A. M., & Carnevale, G. J. (1987). Interpersonal problem solving and coping reactions of Vietnam veterans with posttraumatic stress disorder. *Journal of Abnormal Psychology, 96,* 155–157.

Nezu, C. M., Nezu, A. M., Friedman, S. H., Houts, P. S., DelliCarpini, L., Bildner, C., & Faddis, S. (1999). Cancer and psychological distress: Two investigations regarding the role of social problem-solving. *Journal of Psychosocial Oncology, 16,* 27–40.

O'Farrell, T. J. (1990). Sexual functioning of male alcoholics. In R. L. Collins, K. E. Leonard, & J. S. Searles (Eds.), *Alcohol and the family: Research and clinical perspectives* (pp. 244–271). New York: Guilford Press.

O'Farrell, T. J., & Birchler, G. R. (1987). Marital relationships of alcoholic, conflicted, and nonconflicted couples. *Journal of Marital and Family Therapy, 13,* 259–274.

O'Farrell, T. J., Hooley, J., Fals-Stewart, W., & Cutter, H. S. G. (1998). Expressed emotion and relapse in alcoholic patients. *Journal of Consulting and Clinical Psychology, 66,* 744–752.

Pasch, L. A., & Bradbury, T. N. (1998). Social support, conflict, and the development of marital dysfunction. *Journal of Consulting and Clinical Psychology, 66,* 219–230.

Reich, J., Yates, W., & Nduaguba, M. (1989). Prevalence of DSM-III personality disorders in the community. *Social Psychiatry and Psychiatric Epidemiology, 24,* 12–16.

Ren, X. S. (1997). Marital status and quality of relationships: The impact on health perception. *Social Science and Medicine, 44,* 241–249.

Riggs, D. S., Byrne, C. A., Weathers, F. W., & Litz, B. T. (1998). The quality of the intimate relationships of male Vietnam veterans: Problems associated with posttraumatic stress disorder. *Journal of Traumatic Stress, 11,* 87–101.

Riggs, D. S., Hiss, H., & Foa, E. B. (1992). Marital distress and the treatment of obsessive compulsive disorder. *Behavior Therapy, 23,* 585–597.

Roberts, B. W., & Robins, R. W. (2000). Broad dispositions, broad aspirations: The intersection of personality traits and major life goals. *Personality and Social Psychology Bulletin, 26,* 1284–1296.

Rodrigue, J. R., & Park, T. L. (1996). General and illness-specific adjustment to cancer: Relationship to marital status and marital quality. *Journal of Psychosomatic Research, 40,* 29–36.

Schmaling, K. B., & Jacobson, N. S. (1990). Marital interaction and depression. *Journal of Abnormal Psychology, 99,* 229–236.

Straus, M. A., & Gelles, R. J. (1986). Societal change and change in family violence from 1975 to 1985 as revealed by two national surveys. *Journal of Marriage and the Family, 48,* 465–479.

Tompson, M. C., Rea, M. M., Goldstein, M. J., Miklowitz, D. J., & Weisman, A. G. (2000). Difficulty in implementing a family intervention for bipolar disorder: The predictive role of patient and family attributes. *Family Process, 39,* 105–120.

Truant, G. S. (1994). Personality diagnosis and childhood care associated with adult marital quality. Canadian *Journal of Psychiatry, 39,* 269–276.

Uebelacker, L. A., & Whisman, M. A. (2002). *Relationship beliefs, attributions, and partner behaviors among depressed married women.* Manuscript submitted for publication.

Verbrugge, L. (1979). Marital status and health. *Journal of Marriage and the Family, 41,* 267–285.

Wearden, A. J., Tarrier, N., Barrowclough, C., Zastowny, T. R., & Rahill, A. A. (2000). A review of expressed emotion research in health care. *Clinical Psychology Review, 20,* 633–666.

Whisman, M. A. (1999). Marital dissatisfaction and psychiatric disorders: Results from the National Comorbidity Survey. *Journal of Abnormal Psychology, 108,* 701–706.

Whisman, M. A. (2001a). The association between marital dissatisfaction and depression. In S. R. H. Beach (Ed.), *Marital and family processes in depression: A scientific foundation for clinical practice* (pp. 3–24). Washington, DC: American Psychological Association.

Whisman, M. A. (2001b). Marital adjustment and outcome following treatments for depression. *Journal of Consulting and Clinical Psychology, 69,* 125–129.

Whisman, M. A., & Bruce, M. L. (1999). Marital distress and incidence of major depressive episode in a community sample. *Journal of Abnormal Psychology, 108,* 674–678.

Whisman, M. A., Dixon, A. E., & Johnson, B. (1997). Therapists' perspectives of couple problems and treatment issues in couple therapy. *Journal of Family Psychology, 11,* 361–366.

Whisman, M. A., & Jacobson, N. S. (1989). Depression, marital satisfaction, and marital and personality measures of sex roles. *Journal of Marital and Family Therapy, 15*(2), 177–186.

Whisman, M. A., Sheldon, C. T., & Goering, P. (2000). Psychiatric disorders and dissatisfaction with social relationships: Does type of relationship matter? *Journal of Abnormal Psychology, 109,* 803–808.

Wilsnack, S. C. (1991). Sexuality and women's drinking: Findings from a U.S. national study. *Alcohol Health and Research World, 15,* 147–150.

CHAPTER 2

Tailoring Couple Therapy to Individual Differences

A Conceptual Approach

DOUGLAS K. SNYDER
W. JOEL SCHNEIDER
ANGELA M. CASTELLANI

W orking with difficult couples requires thinking and practicing "outside the box." No single treatment modality or theoretical approach fully addresses the full spectrum of individual and relationship
dysfunction that difficult couples frequently present. Thus, the more
difficult the couple, the greater the need for therapists to draw on increasingly diverse intervention strategies to address individual and relationship problems. However, without an overarching conceptual framework for integrating specific techniques from diverse theoretical
approaches and tailoring these to individual and couple differences,
therapeutic interventions are likely to be disjointed, contradictory, and
ultimately ineffective.

Considerable advances have been achieved in adapting existing
therapies or developing new treatments for a variety of emotional, behavioral, and health problems that couples frequently present. The
chapters that follow comprise the most current empirical and theoretical developments for working with difficult couples. These chapters
cover a wide spectrum of theoretical approaches and treatment modalities, written by authors in diverse settings and with assorted back-

grounds including psychology, psychiatry, and social work. The theoretical foundations, empirical findings, and clinical wisdom underlying these chapters provide rich offerings in terms of specific techniques for treating difficult couples. However, to take advantage of these contributions, readers will need two attributes: (1) flexibility in considering concepts and techniques with which they may be either unfamiliar, inexperienced, or vaguely uncomfortable; and (2) an organizing conceptual framework for thinking about how to integrate new constructs and specific interventions into their existing therapeutic repertoire. The intent of this chapter is to facilitate the latter.

Rarely do couples come to us as therapists with simple, encapsulated complaints amenable to brief interventions that, after a few sessions, restore the couple to individual and relationship health. Too often, couples avoid seeking professional assistance until initial differences or disappointments fester over a protracted period into generalized disillusionment and deeply engrained patterns of negative interaction. By one account, couples wait an average of 6 years once they start having problems before seeking outside assistance (Gottman & Gottman, 1999). Moreover, as the previous chapter makes clear, relationship problems frequently interact with substantial emotional, behavioral, or health problems in one or both partners (Whisman & Uebelacker, Chapter 1, this volume). Even among couples in the community, research suggests that relationship conflict both contributes to, and is exacerbated by, disorders of mood, anxiety, substance abuse, physical aggression, sexual dysfunctions, personality disorders, and physical illness. Among couples entering therapy, the comorbidity of relationship problems with individual emotional or behavioral deficits often seems the norm rather than the exception.

Even to the experienced couple therapist, the term "difficult couple" may appear redundant. What distinguishes difficult from nondifficult couples? Is it the intensity and disinhibition of hostility exchanged between partners within sessions, or the apparent immutability of dysfunctional patterns of interaction reenacted over many years? Is it the deep roots of maladaptive relationship patterns in partners' early developmental experiences, or their vulnerability to acute stressors beyond their control in their current personal or professional lives? Are couples more difficult to treat when individual and relationship dysfunctions interact recursively to reinforce and maintain each other? Each of these factors may distinguish more difficult from less difficult couples. And as experienced couple therapists know too well, several of these complicating factors often coexist.

Working with difficult couples requires therapists to tailor interventions to individual differences by practicing integratively across diverse theoretical orientations, specific intervention modalities, and levels of individual and family functioning. It requires "an inclusive and empirical approach in which the valuable contributions of pure-form therapies are collegially acknowledged and their respective strengths collaboratively enlisted" (Goldfried & Norcross, 1995, p. 269). Pursuing integrative couple therapy does not mean applying assorted interventions in trial-and-error fashion to determine what works for a particular couple; nor does it involve developing a new agglomerative approach and applying it uniformly to all couples. Rather, integrative practice entails (1) matching specific interventions to individual and relationship characteristics from both inclusionary and exclusionary perspectives, (2) synthetically linking interventions within an overarching organizational framework, and (3) sequencing and pacing interventions in a manner consistent with both guiding theoretical and specific clinical case formulations.

Regretfully, clinical training sometimes fails to provide therapists with either the theoretical breadth or technical competence essential to integrative practice (Norcross & Beutler, 2000). Clinicians trained primarily in individual interventions sometimes stumble into couple therapy when their client makes clear the importance of attending to etiological factors underlying presenting complaints embedded in the client's primary relationship—only to discover that their training leaves them poorly equipped for understanding or managing the process of couple interventions. Similarly, therapists trained primarily in couple or family interventions sometimes feel ill prepared to address significant individual psychopathology contributing to or interacting with relationship concerns—in part because traditional systemic formulations have often marginalized or ignored the etiological role of individual pathology in family system functioning (Brunner, 1998).

Our goal in this chapter is to provide a structural framework for conceptualizing relationship difficulties and tailoring couple therapy to individual differences from an integrative approach. The concepts presented here should assist readers in making use of conceptual approaches and specific intervention strategies described in subsequent chapters in this book. The chapter is organized into three sections. First, issues of matching interventions to individual and relationship characteristics are considered. Couple therapy will be most effective when couples are matched to treatments for which they possess prerequisite attributes and are excluded from treatments for which they are particularly ill suited. Second, we differentiate among eclectic, pluralistic, and integrative practice and propose a model linking each to overall effectiveness as a function of a couple's complexity. Specifically, we argue that therapeutic success results from an optimal, intermediate level of technical integration within a theoretically pluralistic approach, but that this function is moderated by the level of case complexity. Finally, we describe an organizational model for sequencing and pacing couple interventions. The model argues for using initial structural and strategic interventions to contain crises and strengthen the couple's relationship, followed with behavioral techniques for promoting essential relationship skills, and then incorporating cognitive and psychodynamic approaches as appropriate to address intrapersonal factors linked to relationship functioning.

MATCHING COUPLES TO TREATMENT

At the simplest level, tailoring treatment to individual differences involves matching clients to therapeutic approaches designed specifically to remediate individual and relationship deficits and build on existing strengths. Matching couples to treatment rests on the premise that individuals or relationships exhibiting particular attributes may respond more favorably to one treatment or set of interventions than to an alternative approach (Beutler & Clarkin, 1990). For example, evidence suggests that couples in which one partner exhibits major depression may benefit most from a combination of social learning and cognitive interventions emphasizing increases in positive exchanges, enhanced decision-making and emotional expressiveness skills, and partners' improved understanding of depression and its correlates in facilitating realistic relationship expectations (Beach & Gupta, Chapter 4, this volume). By comparison, couples with pervasive and intense negativity, high levels of mistrust, and limited awareness or understanding of emotions may initially be ill suited for therapeutic approaches encouraging introspection, developmental exploration, and vulnerable self-disclosures (Snyder & Schneider, 2002).

Couples vary dramatically in terms of presenting issues, marital and family structure, individual dynamics and psychopathology, and psychosocial stressors or support. So, too, approaches to couple therapy vary in terms of underlying theoretical assumptions, degree of structure, level of system functioning targeted by particular techniques, the specific content of interventions, and documented effectiveness (Gurman & Jacobson, 2002). Because the functional sources of couples' distress vary so dramatically, the critical mediators or mechanisms of change should also be expected to vary—as should the therapeutic strategies intended to facilitate positive change.

Although the challenge of matching treatments to clients has been examined to a modest degree in individual therapy, less consideration has been devoted to treatment matching in couple therapy. Two factors limit progress in this area. First, although considerable evidence has been garnered supporting the overall efficacy of cognitive-behavioral approaches to couple distress, relatively few studies have examined non-behavioral strategies (Baucom, Shoham, Mueser, Daiuto, & Stickle, 1998; Dunn & Schwebel, 1995). Exceptions include research on emotionally focused couple therapy (Johnson, Hunsley, Greenberg, & Schindler, 1999) and an insight-oriented approach examining recurrent maladaptive relationship patterns (Snyder & Wills, 1989). Even fewer studies have compared alternative approaches in controlled trials with random assignment of couples to condition, and only a small number have examined therapy outcome beyond 2 years posttreatment (Christensen & Heavey, 1999). The relative dearth of comparative couple therapy studies examining long-term outcome restricts treatment selection on an empirical basis. Treatment matching is precluded when (1) insufficient data are available regarding the efficacy of two or more approaches, or (2) the available data fail to demonstrate reliable differences in treatment outcome across different conditions.

A second factor limiting treatment matching in couple therapy involves the limited findings regarding aptitude-by-treatment interaction (ATI) effects. Briefly, ATI effects occur when individual or couple characteristics influence or moderate therapy outcome. Replicated findings in this area are relatively few and largely confined to intuitive indicators. For example, couples responding more favorably to treatment are those characterized by higher levels of positive feelings, stronger commitment, lower levels of overt conflict, fewer psychosocial stressors, and partners relatively free of individual emotional or behavioral dysfunction (Snyder, Cozzi, & Mangrum, 2002). More importantly, the utility of these findings for treatment matching is low because the interaction of these moderators with treatment modality remains virtually unknown (Whisman & Snyder, 1997).

The importance of ATI effects in treatment matching is depicted in Figure 2.1. In each alternative matching model, assignment of couples to condition presumes two or more treatments with documented efficacy. Treatments are initially considered on the basis of their efficacy in addressing *targeted* characteristics of the person or couple, that is, aspects of individual or relationship functioning which (1) are present at an insufficient level or rate, as in positive emotional expressiveness, or (2) are present at an excessive level or rate, as in verbal or physical aggression. Each model also distinguishes between inclusionary and exclusionary characteristics. Inclusionary characteristics are those individual or relationship attributes deemed either essential or advantageous for a favorable response to that treatment. For example, commitment

No-Gain Model	Treatment A	Treatment B
Inclusionary	Essential or Advantageous Characteristics A, B, C	Essential or Advantageous Characteristics A, B, C
Exclusionary	Harmful or Detrimental Characteristics X, Y, Z	Harmful or Detrimental Characteristics X, Y, Z

Ideal Model	Treatment A	Treatment B
Inclusionary	Essential or Advantageous Characteristics A, B, C	Essential or Advantageous Characteristics X, Y, Z
Exclusionary	Harmful or Detrimental Characteristics X, Y, Z	Harmful or Detrimental Characteristics A, B, C

Probable Model	Treatment A	Treatment B
Inclusionary	Essential or Advantageous Characteristics A, B	Essential or Advantageous Characteristics A, B, C, D
Exclusionary	Harmful or Detrimental Characteristics W, X	Harmful or Detrimental Characteristics W, X, Y, Z

FIGURE 2.1. Alternative treatment matching models in no-gain, ideal, and probable matching conditions. In the "probable-model" matching condition, couples exhibiting attributes A, B, C, and D and *not* characteristics W, X, Y, or Z would be assigned to the more restrictive but also more effective Treatment B.

to the relationship or the capacity to defer self-gratification for the sake of the other's well-being may be regarded as inclusionary characteristics in couple therapy. By contrast, exclusionary characteristics are those attributes deemed either harmful or detrimental to a treatment's outcome. For example, high levels of overt hostility or partners' lack of introspection may be regarded as exclusionary for one or more approaches to couple treatment.

In the first, "no-gain," model, both the essential or advantageous characteristics for inclusion in treatment and the harmful or detrimental characteristics for exclusion from treatment are identical across two alternative treatments A and B. Because no distinguishing individual or relationship attributes have been shown to be more or less favorable to one approach relative to the other, couples would be assigned to (1) that treatment demonstrated to be most effective overall, or (2) if treatments are equally effective, then to that treatment which is least expensive or that in which the therapist has greatest expertise. The no-gain model is also the default model when no data are available regarding differential effectiveness across either treatment modality or couple characteristics.

In the "ideal" model for treatment matching, known moderators of therapeutic outcome interact completely with treatment modality—such that essential or favorable characteristics for one approach are detrimental or unfavorable for the other, and vice versa. Following from this model, couples possessing some combination of either individual or relationship attributes A, B, and C—and *not* possessing any of attributes X, Y, or Z—would be assigned to treatment A. Similarly, couples possessing some combination of attributes X, Y, and Z—and *not* possessing any of attributes A, B, or C—would be assigned to treatment B. In the ideal model, treatments A and B are both presumed to be effective, although not necessarily equally so.

For several reasons, this "ideal" matching scenario rarely if ever exists. First, the interaction of essential and detrimental characteristics with treatment condition is unlikely to be complete; instead, one or more essential (or detrimental) characteristics for one treatment may also be essential (or detrimental) for the other. Second, it is unlikely that treatments themselves are as distinct as this model suggests. Although treatments may be distinguishable by their unique specific interventions, they likely also share a variety of active but nonspecific components (Wills, Faitler, & Snyder, 1987). Third, even if treatment conditions existed that followed the ideal model (i.e., treatments that were nonoverlapping and interacted completely with essential and detrimental moderators of outcome), couples might be anticipated to possess both essential and detrimental attributes for each condition (e.g., characteristics A, B, and X).

A more "probable model" depicted in Figure 2.1 involves alternative therapy approaches in which treatment B is more effective than treatment A, but is also more restrictive in that it has more prerequisite essential characteristics as well as more exclusionary disadvantageous or detrimental ones. Following this model, couples exhibiting attributes A or B, and *not* possessing attributes C, D, W, or X would be assigned to the less effective but also less restrictive treatment A. By comparison, couples exhibiting attributes A, B, C, and D and not characteristics W, X, Y, or Z would be assigned to the more restrictive but also more effective treatment B.

How may consideration of these matching models inform clinical practice? Familiarity with treatments' demonstrated effectiveness, relative costs and levels of restrictiveness, and potential interaction with partner or couple characteristics provides a potential foundation for tailoring couple therapy to differences in individual and relationship functioning. Does the empirical literature provide any suggestions of treatment differences in both effectiveness and restrictiveness? Although findings in this regard are limited both in number and in size and reliability of effect, they provide some basis for tentative guidelines. For example, there is growing evidence that traditional behavioral couple therapy (TBCT), although potentially least restrictive in inclusionary and exclusionary characteristics, at times may be less effective than alternative approaches. For example, Johnson and Greenberg (1985) found emotionally focused couple therapy (EFCT) to produce a better outcome at both termination and 2-month follow-up compared to a behavioral approach emphasizing communication and problem-solving skills training. In their study comparing TBCT with insight-oriented couple therapy (IOCT), Snyder and Wills (1989) observed comparable effectiveness for TBCT and IOCT both at termination and at 6 months posttreatment; however, at 4-year follow-up, 38% of couples in the TBCT condition had divorced, compared to only 3% receiving IOCT (Snyder, Wills, & Grady-Fletcher, 1991). More recently, Jacobson and colleagues (Jacobson, Christensen, Prince, Cordova, & Eldridge, 2000) compared TBCT with an integrative behavioral approach (IBCT) combining behavior-change techniques with strategies aimed at promoting emotional acceptance; preliminary data suggested greater effectiveness for the IBCT condition at termination.

However, each of these studies also suggested potential moderator effects that may interact with treatment condition. Johnson and Talitman (1997) found that favorable response to EFCT was predicted by a positive therapeutic alliance and women's trust in their partner's caring. Snyder, Mangrum, and Wills (1993) found that couples were more likely to be divorced or maritally distressed 4 years after completing either TBCT or IOCT if partners' intake measures reflected high levels of negative marital affect, poor problem-solving skills, low psychological resilience, high levels of depression , or low emotional responsiveness; however, the low rate of divorce for IOCT couples at 4-year follow-up precluded examining interaction effects of moderators with treatment condition in long-term outcome. The most recent evidence for interaction effects comes from preliminary findings by Christensen and colleagues in their study comparing TBCT with IBCT, indicating that highly distressed couples gained more rapidly in early stages of treatment in the traditional behavioral condition, but appeared to gain less overall in the longer term than couples receiving the integrative therapy (Atkins & Christensen, 2001). Overall, these findings suggest that couples characterized by high levels of relationship distress or partners exhibiting higher levels of defensiveness, greater impulsivity, or diminished capacity for introspection may respond less favorably to more restrictive emotionally focused, insight-oriented, or acceptance-based interventions than to a less restrictive traditional behavioral approach. Although these characteristics by themselves may not comprise an emotional or behavioral disorder, they may serve as common characteristics or indicators of more serious conditions warranting formal diagnosis.

Treatment approaches described in subsequent chapters of this volume also imply specific treatment matching guidelines. For example, impaired cognitive processes accompanying a bipolar or schizophrenia-spectrum disorder clearly argue for exclusion from insight-oriented interventions and, instead, inclusion in psychoeducational approaches emphasizing medication compliance, strategies for minimizing the disorder's adverse impact, and relapse prevention. Couple interventions for treatment of individual disorders (e.g., dysthymia, agoraphobia, or alcohol abuse)—whether from a traditional conjoint strategy or partner-assisted approach—clearly require a degree of collaboration between partners that may be precluded by severe or pervasive negativity. Similarly, emotionally focused approaches may be compromised by persistent emotional dysregulation stemming from childhood sexual abuse or other traumatic events and require initial stabilization or containment of couple interactions using more structured techniques.

Unfortunately, couples often present with multiple difficulties that render matching to treatment particularly difficult. For example, physical aggression between partners may warrant inclusion in treatment interventions for violence such as those described by Holtzworth-Munroe and colleagues (Holtzworth-Munroe, Marshall, Meehan, & Rehman, Chapter 9, this volume). If a partner's aggression results from behavioral disinhibition precipitated by excessive use of alcohol, the pre-

ferred approach might instead involve treatment strategies for substance abuse outlined by Fals-Stewart, Birchler, and O'Farrell (Chapter
7, this volume). However, comorbid aggression and substance abuse
may be exclusionary characteristics for both treatment approaches. In
that case, how should the couple therapist proceed?

Because couples often demonstrate attributes that either lend
themselves to a particular approach (e.g., high levels of psychological
mindedness conducive to interpretive techniques) or demand a specific
intervention (e.g., features of agoraphobia warranting partner-assisted
interventions tailored to that diagnosis)—but *also* demonstrate concurrent detrimental attributes that detract from or preclude use of that approach (e.g., high negativity or low commitment)—therapists frequently confront situations in which no well-defined treatment has
documented efficacy. On such occasions, rather than asking, "Which
treatment is best?" or "Which treatment for which couple?" the therapist must address questions of "Which elements from which treatments
will address this couple's interwoven and competing needs? What theoretical or other organizing framework can be drawn on for tailoring interventions and integrating these diverse techniques into a comprehensive treatment strategy?" It is to these issues that we direct our attention
next.

DISTINGUISHING AMONG ECLECTICISM, PLURALISM, AND INTEGRATION

At a level of complexity beyond matching couples to existing treatments,
tailoring couple therapy to differences in individual and relationship
functioning may proceed by selecting specific interventions from two or
more treatment strategies described in subsequent chapters of this book.
Such selection may borrow from diverse treatments within the same theoretical orientation (e.g., combining cognitive-behavioral couple interventions for depression with those for alcohol abuse for couples in which
both issues are presenting concerns), or combining treatment components from different theoretical modalities (e.g., incorporating behavioral de-escalation strategies for couples exhibiting emotional dysregulation but subsequently exploring the developmental origins of affective
arousal using more insight-oriented techniques).

The borrowing of specific intervention techniques across theoretical approaches or treatment modalities comprises a common strategy
for tailoring therapy to individual differences. Indeed, therapists' alle-
giance to "pure-form" therapies has diminished over the past few
decades, in part as a function of economic pressures for short-term

therapies, meta-analyses often showing equivalent outcomes across various approaches to treatment, and the delineation of "common factors" among systems of psychotherapy (Norcross & Newman, 1992). A majority of therapists now identify themselves as either "eclectic" or "integrative," with the latter term preferred by a margin of nearly 2:1 (Norcross, Prochaska, & Farber, 1993). Similarly, the most common theoretical orientation identified in a recent survey of couple therapists was "eclectic" (28%), with an additional 10% not identifying any primary orientation (Whisman, Dixon, & Johnson, 1997). However, distinctions between eclecticism and integration, and their differences from "pluralism," are not consistent in the literature—nor do they seem clear among practitioners espousing any of the three. In our consideration, we define each of the terms as follows:

- *Eclecticism.* Eclecticism is an approach characterized by selecting specific techniques or theoretical constructs from diverse theoretical systems or schools of psychotherapy. Eclecticism may occur at two levels. *Technical eclecticism* involves borrowing specific techniques or interventions from multiple, competing therapeutic approaches separate from the theoretical constructs that underlie those techniques (Lazarus, 1992). For example, a couple therapist could use "reframing" techniques consistent with both strategic or cognitive restructuring approaches while practicing primarily from a psychodynamic perspective, without incorporating broader theoretical tenets of either family systems or cognitive-behavioral theory. By comparison, *theoretical eclecticism* entails adopting specific constructs from diverse theoretical systems without necessarily ascribing to any of the theories themselves, and without integrating these constructs into a novel theoretical system of their own (Messer, 1992). For example, a therapist could endorse both "projective identification" and "modeling" as useful constructs for understanding the effects of early developmental experiences on subsequent adult relationship patterns, yet practice primarily using structural and strategic interventions from systems theory.

- *Pluralism.* Pluralism is a perspective that recognizes the validity of multiple systems of epistemology, theory, and practice and that draws on these as intact units (as distinct from eclecticism), although not necessarily concurrently or from an integrated perspective. Pluralism is similar to constructs of "empirical pragmatism" (Goldfried & Norcross, 1995), "systematic treatment selection" (Beutler & Clarkin, 1990), and "prescriptive eclecticism" characterized "by drawing on effective methods from across theoretical camps (eclecticism), by matching those methods to particular cases on the basis of psychological science and clinical wisdom (prescriptionism), and by adhering to an explicit and orderly model of treatment selection" (Norcross & Beutler, 2000, p. 248). Pluralism may be demonstrated in two ways: concurrently across cases or serially within a case. Concurrent pluralism would be evident from treatment matching in which couples are assigned to alternative therapies based on inclusionary and exclusionary characteristics, and the same therapist practices in a theoretically consistent but distinct manner under alternative treatment conditions. By comparison, serial pluralism would occur when a therapist begins treatment for a given case using both theoretical constructs and techniques derived from one approach, but subsequently shifts to constructs and interventions derived from a different approach (Snyder, 1999). Serial pluralism most likely proceeds across stages of treatment or—at a minimum, across consecutive sessions—as opposed to changes in theoretical stance within in a session.

• *Integration.* Integration is the blending of theoretical constructs or therapeutic techniques into a unified system or whole. Analogous to eclecticism, integration may occur at two levels. *Technical integration* involves borrowing specific interventions from multiple treatment approaches in a manner directed by an overarching and organizing theoretical framework or clinical case conceptualization. Similarly, *theoretical integration* entails incorporating specific constructs from diverse theoretical approaches but blending these in a rational, internally consistent, and synthetic manner. Both technical and theoretical integration are distinguished from their eclectic counterparts by the number and explanatory power of linkages among interventions or their theoretical substrates. Theoretical integration may develop from either assimilative or accommodative processes (Messer, 1992). In assimilative integration, theoretical constructs from one approach are explained by the theoretical tenets of some alternative approach. By comparison, accommodative integration involves blending of constructs in a synergistic manner so as to generate some new construct or theory not derivable from either original approach separate from the other.

Similar to Norcross (1985), we regard integrationists as a subset of eclectics in that the former draw on both theories and techniques from diverse approaches, but from a smaller universe than eclectics because contemporary integrative theories typically synthesize only a small number of theoretical perspectives while leaving many others unaddressed (Lebow, 1997). Similarly, we consider eclectics as a subset of pluralists. Although eclectics could potentially select from the entire universe of principles and techniques across theoretical modalities, in practice most clinicians adopting an eclectic approach draw on the few theoretical perspectives encountered in their previous training experiences (Norcross & Beutler, 2000). The more broadly trained therapists are

theoretically and the more diverse the systems or schools of psychotherapy they consider potentially valid, the more varied the techniques they
are likely to adopt in practice.

It is important to distinguish among eclecticism, integration, and
pluralism at the intervention versus the theoretical level. For example,
one could practice eclectically within an integrative conceptual framework by drawing selectively on techniques congruent with that theory
and excluding other interventions. Alternatively, one could practice integratively by synthetically incorporating diverse interventions for a
given client, but without an overarching theoretical model guiding
treatment selection across clients.

What are the potential benefits and risks of borrowing techniques
from diverse theoretical or treatment modalities when attempting to
tailor couple therapy to differences in individual and relationship functioning? We would predict that the relationship of eclecticism to treatment outcome is curvilinear, and that this relationship is further moderated both by degree of integration (i.e., the extent to which
techniques or theoretical tenets from diverse treatment approaches are
linked by an overarching organizational or conceptual framework) and
by level of case complexity (see Figure 2.2). At some intermediate range
of eclecticism, treatment outcome is optimized by the therapist's ability
to draw on diverse interventions targeting unique attributes of clients'
individual or relationship functioning that lie outside the domain of

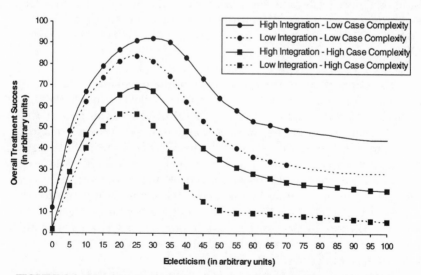

FIGURE 2.2. Hypothesized relations among eclecticism, integration, case complexity, and overall treatment success. The moderating effect of integration on
the curvilinear relation between eclecticism and treatment success is hypothesized to be greater for highly complex couples than for less complex cases.

any one system or school of psychotherapy. For example, advocates of various integrative models of psychotherapy have emphasized the strengths of psychodynamic approaches for identifying enduring problematic interpersonal themes, the benefits of experiential techniques for promoting emotional awareness, gains from cognitive interventions targeting dysfunctional beliefs and attributional processes, and advantages of behavioral strategies for promoting new patterns of behavior (Bongar & Beutler, 1995; Norcross & Goldfried, 1992). Practicing exclusively from a single theoretical approach potentially restricts the individual complaints or relationship processes on which the therapist is likely to have a significant impact.

However, we would also argue that extensive use of techniques from diverse therapeutic approaches, particularly in the absence of any organizing or integrative framework, potentially compromises treatment effectiveness. The negative impact of high levels of eclecticism may derive either from (1) the unsystematic, chaotic, or contradictory use of specific interventions; or (2) the dismantling of interventions within treatment approaches that rely on the synergistic effects of specific components that lose their effectiveness when administered in isolation from one another. Paradoxically, the more difficult the couple, the more likely the therapist may be to draw on increasingly diverse intervention strategies to address multiple individual and relationship problems, and the less likely these interventions are to be integrated within a theoretically coherent system. The combined effects of low integration and high case complexity are depicted in Figure 2.2 by the bottom, most leptokurtic (peaked) curve that reflects (1) lowest overall treatment success, and (2) rapidly diminishing effectiveness as interventions become increasingly eclectic.

The implications of these assertions for the practicing couple therapist can be summarized as follows: (1) When tailoring couple therapy to individual differences, a moderate level of eclecticism affords the best outcome; (2) a higher level of integration provides some protection against the weakening effects of high levels of eclecticism; (3) highly complex couples are more difficult to treat and will likely have lower overall positive therapeutic response; and (4) the moderating effect of integration on the relation between eclecticism and treatment success is greater for highly complex couples than for less complex cases. Stated more simply, integration is always important, but it is particularly critical for couples with more complicated, interactive deficits in both individual and relationship functioning.

Because a pluralistic approach is less constrained than theoretically integrative approaches forced to reconcile competing constructs, it benefits from greater opportunity to accommodate diverse theoretical perspectives. By its systematic inclusion of multiple approaches across the theoretical spectrum, a pluralistic approach also promotes greater attention to diverse constructs and interventions than shown by the typical eclectic clinician. At the same time, theoretical pluralism may avert haphazard, disjointed, or contradictory interventions resulting from expedient borrowing of diverse principles or techniques without regard for their potential inconsistency or adverse interaction. In the following section we advocate a pluralistic model for selecting, sequencing, and pacing interventions across theoretical approaches when working with difficult couples.

INTEGRATING TECHNIQUES WITHIN A
SEQUENTIAL PLURALISTIC APPROACH

How can therapists optimally draw on the diverse theoretical approaches and specific interventions presented in the following chapters when treating couples with complex emotional, behavioral, or health problems? We advocate an approach to tailoring couple therapy to individual differences that promotes technical integration within a theoretically pluralistic model. In terms of techniques, the approach is integrative rather than eclectic in that (1) specific interventions are linked to one another within any given stage of therapy by the theoretical model most relevant to treatment at that time, and (2) interventions across treatment stages are organized by a broader organizational framework that proposes a sequential progression of theoretical models from a pluralistic perspective. Our model is theoretically pluralistic rather than integrative in that it asserts the validity of multiple theoretical approaches to couple therapy and draws on each of these as relatively intact units. We make no attempts to translate constructs from one theory into those of another. Nor do we claim by this organizational framework to have created a new theoretical system of couple therapy. Rather, ours is a pluralistic model in which we argue that different theoretical approaches to couple therapy have their greatest applicability during distinct phases of treatment, and that these phases generally follow a modal serial progression (Snyder, 1999).

Our model is depicted in Figure 2.3 and proposes six levels of intervention. The most fundamental step in couple therapy involves developing a collaborative alliance between partners and between each partner and the therapist (Gurman, 1981; Jacobson & Margolin, 1979). The collaborative alliance begins with establishing an atmosphere of therapist competence by engaging in relevant assessment and modeling appropriate communication behaviors. It requires establishing an atmosphere of safety by limiting partners' negative exchanges and clarifying policies governing such issues as confidentiality. Finally, the collabo-

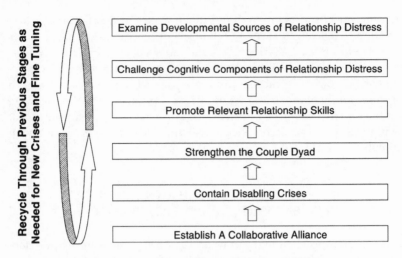

Primary Therapeutic Task

FIGURE 2.3. A sequential, pluralistic approach to couple therapy. The model depicts progression from (1) lower-order interventions aimed at establishing a collaborative alliance and crisis containment, through (2) positive-exchange and skills-building techniques, to (3) higher-order interventions targeting cognitive and developmental sources of relationship distress. Couple therapy may include recycling through earlier stages as required by emergent crises or erosion of individual or relationship skills.

rative alliance is strengthened by offering a clear formulation of the couple's difficulties, outlining treatment objectives and basic strategies, and defining all participants' respective roles.

As fundamental as this stage is to virtually any theoretical approach to therapy, achieving a collaborative alliance with difficult couples can be particularly challenging. In some cases, the alliance is compromised by the partner exhibiting higher levels of individual pathology. This may result from anticipated blame from the other (as in substance-abusing partners), difficulty mobilizing individual resources necessary for conjoint treatment (as in individuals with bipolar disorder or progressive dementia), or features of the disorder itself that preclude a trusting and collaborative stance (as in paranoid disorders). In other cases, the alliance is compromised by the healthier individual's reluctance to become involved in treatment of their partner's disorder. This reluctance may stem from resentments that preclude offering support (e.g., individuals who feel victimized by their partner's chronic substance abuse), concerns about having their own inadequacies exposed (as in conjoint treatment of sexual dysfunctions), or fear of being assigned a causal role in their partner's disorder (e.g., partners of individuals attributing their depression to relationship distress). Finally, in still other cases, a collaborative alliance may be rendered difficult to achieve because both partners view the other as the primary source of relationship problems and regard themselves as beyond reproach (as when working with narcissistic couples). Although the chapters in this volume vary both in theoretical perspective and specific clinical focus, each wrestles with the challenges of establishing a collaborative alliance with difficult couples.

The second level of intervention proposed in our model involves addressing disabling relationship crises. Occasionally such crises emerge in otherwise healthy couples who experience illness or death of a family member, an unplanned or terminated pregnancy, unexpected job loss or financial hardship, and similar events (see Wills, Chapter 17, this volume). More often, relationship crises among couples presenting for therapy occur against a backdrop of communication deficits and an impoverished or insecure emotional context. A common crisis involves physical aggression by one or both partners against the other; another crisis involves emotional or sexual infidelity. Other crises requiring immediate attention involve major psychopathology and substance abuse disorders.

From the perspective of a sequential pluralistic approach, partners' willingness to engage in higher-order interventions aimed at promoting vulnerable self-disclosure first requires both emotional and physical safety. Similarly, the ability to engage in effective decision-making strategies presumes a cognitive capacity not impaired by substance abuse or psychotic processes. And sustained efforts of any magnitude in couple therapy require levels of both emotional and physical energy not compromised by a major psychiatric disorder or medical illness. Some of the chapters comprising this volume themselves adopt a sequential approach for addressing specific crises (e.g., stabilizing major pathology with medication prior to interventions emphasizing communication and relationship enhancement; see Miklowitz & Morris, Chapter 5; Mueser & Brunette, Chapter 6; and Terkelsen, Chapter 11, this volume). Others can be viewed collectively as facilitating a sequential approach for containing initial crises before addressing more sensitive individual or relationship concerns—for example, addressing issues of physical aggression prior to partner-assisted interventions for substance abuse, or drawing on structured interventions to minimize recurrent cycles of affective dysregulation accompanying a borderline personality disorder prior to emotionally focused or interpretive interventions examining early childhood trauma that may play an important etiological role in these disruptive exchanges.

At the third and fourth levels of intervention, our model distinguishes between interventions undertaken by the therapist directly to strengthen the couple dyad, and those intended to promote specific skills enabling couples to strengthen and sustain their relationship on their own. Strengthening a couple's relationship sometimes requires systems-based interventions promoting a hierarchical organization emphasizing parents' responsibility and influence relative to their children's, and establishing appropriate boundaries with respect to families of origin (Nichols & Minuchin, 1999). Other couples are difficult to treat because they exhibit overwhelming negativity and an erosion of positive exchanges that leaves their relationship more vulnerable to subsequent challenges and conflicts. Such couples typically require positive exchange agreements negotiated to a large degree by the therapist from a social learning perspective before assisting the couple to develop behavior-exchange and communication skills of their own (Weiss & Halford, 1996).

With only a modicum of strengthening interventions by the therapist, well-functioning couples can sometimes mobilize previously acquired but dormant communication skills. However, other couples may require assistance in developing relationship skills to modify dysfunctional patterns of interacting and replace them with new ones. Sustaining a satisfying relationship requires a broad range of interpersonal skills. Primary among these are communication skills including emotional expressiveness, empathic listening, conflict resolution, and effective decision making. However, the essential skills for a satisfying relationship extend beyond communication and include skills in parenting, handling of finances, time management, and physical intimacy. In many domains effective communication presumes a prerequisite knowledge base—something that partners often lack and that must be provided by the therapist from a psychoeducational model or through adjunct resources identified by the therapist. Several chapters in this volume address intervening with couples for whom knowledge about a specific disorder or developmental challenge may be limited or absent—as for couples confronting major psychopathology, physical illness, or cognitive decline related to aging (e.g., see Osterman, Sher, Hales, Canar, Singla, & Tilton, Chapter 15, and Qualls, Chapter 16, this volume).

The final two levels of intervention in our pluralistic model emphasize intrapersonal components of relationship distress. Although nearly all couples struggle with the need to articulate relationship expectations and challenge unrealistic standards or assumptions, these struggles are rendered far more difficult when normative expectations are disrupted by the onset of major mental or physical illness, or when partners' understanding of relationship processes are distorted by the absence of appropriate models earlier in their development. Separate from relationship beliefs or expectations, a common impediment to behavior change involves misconceptions and other interpretive errors that individuals may have regarding both their own and their partner's behavior. Not only do such cognitive mediators contribute to negative affect, but they also result in behavioral strategies that frequently maintain or exacerbate relationship distress. A couple's resistance to interventions aimed directly at strengthening their relationship or promoting relevant skills can often be diminished by examining and restructuring cognitive processes interfering with behavior change efforts (Epstein & Baucom, 2002).

However, not all psychological processes relevant to couples' interactions lend themselves to traditional cognitive interventions. Of particular importance are previous relationship injuries resulting in sustained interpersonal vulnerabilities and related defensive strategies interfering with emotional intimacy, many of which operate beyond partners' conscious awareness. Such sources of relationship distress may be examined by a range of psychodynamic or other interpretive approaches to couple therapy emphasizing recurrent maladaptive relationship patterns stemming from previous interpersonal experiences (Snyder & Schneider, 2002). Interpretive approaches vary in the extent to which they emphasize the unconscious nature of these relational patterns and the developmental period during which these maladaptive patterns were acquired. However, interpretive approaches to couple therapy share a common focus on previous relationships, their affective components, and ways in which coping strategies vital to prior relationships represent distortions or inappropriate solutions for emotional intimacy and satisfaction in the current relationship.

For example, emotionally focused couple therapy (EFCT) views distressed relationships as comprising "insecure bonds in which essentially healthy attachment needs are unable to be met due to rigid interaction patterns that block emotional engagement" (Johnson & Greenberg, 1995, p. 121). Hence, EFCT strives to "access information that couples have selectively excluded from processing, sustain attention to this new information, and facilitate couples' abilities to incorporate and use this information in moving toward more accurate, integrated working models of self and partner" (Kobak, Ruckdeschel, & Hazan, 1994, pp. 60–61). Similarly, in the insight-oriented couple therapy described by Snyder and Wills (1989), previous relationships, their affective components, and strategies for emotional gratification and anxiety containment are reconstructed with a focus on identifying for each partner consistencies in their interpersonal conflicts and maladaptive coping styles across relationships. This new understanding and exploration serve to reduce partners' anxiety and defensive strategies and permit them to develop alternative, healthier relationship patterns.

Our pluralistic model suggests two important caveats regarding the interpretation of developmental sources of relationship distress when working with difficult couples. First, the model makes explicit that interpretive techniques should only be considered after initial crises have been contained and the couple possesses both specific communication skills and a sufficiently positive relationship for examining developmental issues in a constructive manner. Couples are not able to examine developmental sources of distress when contending with immediate crises from individual psychopathology, physical illness, or severe psychosocial stressors. Moreover, individuals are not willing to examine intrapersonal components of relationship distress when they cannot trust their partner's commitment to participating in this process from an empathic or at least neutral posture. Hence, examining developmental sources of relationship distress demands a prerequisite foundation of physical and emotional security, partners' trust in the therapeutic process, the couple's ability to respond empathically to feelings of vulnerability exposed by their partner, and an introspective stance initially prompted by examining dysfunctional relationship expectancies and attributions residing at a more conscious level.

Second, our pluralistic model suggests that interpretive techniques may be unnecessary with couples for whom relationship difficulties are largely resolved by lower-order interventions earlier in the treatment hierarchy. Although one might argue that all couples could benefit from greater awareness of intrapersonal components to relationship dynamics, either pragmatic constraints or personal preference may argue for more time-limited therapy emphasizing structural or behavioral interventions. Even among the most difficult couples, developmental contributions to current relationship problems may fade in comparison to situational exigencies that overwhelm otherwise adequate individual and relationship resources.

However, long-term follow-up of couple therapy confined to traditional behavioral interventions suggests a risk of relapse among a substantial portion of couples initially responding favorably to this treatment. Hence, the potential benefits from examining developmental sources of relationship distress increase when (1) one or both partners exhibit a previous history of compromised relationships or interpersonal trauma, or (2) partners demonstrate good interpersonal skills when interacting with persons outside their own relationship, but their communication with each other shows recurrent disruption by exaggerated emotional responses that suggest distortions of objective relationship content in the moment.

CONCLUSIONS

Couples can be difficult to treat for multiple reasons. These include acute psychosocial stressors, intense and pervasive hostility, recursive interactions between individual psychopathology and relationship distress, and maladaptive relationship patterns deeply rooted in partners' early developmental experiences. Often several of these complicating factors coexist. Consequently, effective treatment of difficult couples requires therapists to conceptualize and practice integratively across diverse theoretical orientations, specific intervention modalities, and levels of individual and family functioning.

To a considerable degree, both the clinical and empirical literature has offered only limited guidance for tailoring interventions to characteristics of individual partners and their relationship. Empirically supported treatments for individual disorders using either conjoint couple therapy or partner-assisted interventions have begun to emerge—particularly for a subset of Axis I disorders; however, other than diagnostic criteria for these disorders themselves, inclusionary and exclusionary criteria for selecting these treatments often remain unspecified. Moreover, because controlled trials of couple therapy for specific disorders often apply multiple exclusionary criteria to reduce individual differences within treatment conditions, their findings may not generalize to practice settings in which comorbid disorders prove to be the norm rather than the exception.

The treatment-matching paradigms described in this chapter offer a way of thinking about tailoring interventions with difficult couples. As evidence accumulates regarding differential therapeutic outcome, adverse response indicators restricting a given treatment's application, and aptitude-by-treatment interactions, therapists will face both increased opportunity and obligation to select treatment modalities tailored to couples' specific strengths and liabilities. However, until both essential and detrimental couple characteristics for various treatments are known—including comorbid relationship and individual dysfunction across multiple Axis I and Axis II disorders—therapists will continue to confront the challenge of selecting specific interventions from diverse approaches and organizing these in a conceptually coherent and clinically effective manner.

Difficult couples often require thinking outside the parameters of any one theoretical perspective. The more difficult the couple, the greater the need to draw on increasingly diverse intervention strategies to address multiple individual and relationship problems. However, the risk of technical eclecticism is that, in the absence of an overarching organizational framework, diverse techniques may be applied in an unsystematic, chaotic, or inconsistent manner. We contend that, to date, no single theoretical approach to couple therapy adequately addresses the multiple components of individual and relationship dysfunction that difficult couples present. Although a number of integrative theoretical models have been proposed, these vary in both their conceptual breadth and technical specificity; moreover, each has a delimited range of individual and relationship issues for which it is particularly well suited, while leaving other aspects of couples' functioning largely unaddressed. The more comprehensive a theoretical model strives to be, often the less explicit it becomes in addressing specific couple attributes or directing specific interventions. Moreover, a frequent shortcoming of integrative approaches is their failure to articulate the specific sequence in which various interventions incorporated from diverse theoretical modalities should be implemented (Lebow, 1997).

Until a comprehensive integrative theoretical model emerges, we advocate technical integration within a sequential, pluralistic approach. In principle, no theoretical model is excluded from this approach—presuming empirical evidence of its effectiveness. Instead, when working from this pluralistic approach, therapists can draw on specific interventions from alternative theoretical models as they apply to partners' individual and relationship needs at any specific stage of couple therapy. Our pluralistic model proposes using initial structural and strategic interventions to contain crises and strengthen the couple's relationship, followed with behavioral techniques for promoting essential relationship skills, and then incorporating cognitive and psychodynamic approaches as appropriate to address intrapersonal factors linked to relationship functioning.

From this perspective, moderators influencing both the selection and pacing of interventions would include (1) partners' commitment to conjoint therapy and views toward their own roles in relationship problems; (2) acute psychosocial stressors or individual crises precluding sustained attention to relationship issues; (3) family organization regarding patterns of influence and emotional attachment; (4) partners' effectiveness in enlisting support but limiting intrusion from individuals outside their relationship; (5) intensity and pervasiveness of hostility; (6) levels and resiliency of emotional warmth and positive regard; (7) communication skills involving emotional expressiveness, listening, and decision making; (8) additional relationship skills in such domains as parenting, money management, and physical intimacy; (9) disruption of relationship functioning by unrealistic assumptions or standards, faulty attributions, or related cognitive processes; and (10) recurrent maladaptive relationship patterns rooted in early developmental experiences or operating beyond immediate awareness.

Both individually and collectively, the chapters in this volume reflect a wealth of information and wisdom for working with couples with emotional, behavioral, or health problems. Therapists will benefit from acquiring both technical competence in administering the specific interventions described in these chapters, as well as a firm understanding of the theoretical and empirical underpinnings that guide their implementation.

REFERENCES

Atkins, D. C., & Christensen, A. (2001, November). Main outcome findings from active treatment: Self-report of marital quality. In K. Sutherland (Chair), *The effects of marital therapy: Posttreatment results of a dual-site clinical trial.* Symposium presented at the meeting of the Association for Advancement of Behavior Therapy, Philadelphia.

Baucom, D. H., Shoham, V., Mueser, K. T., Daiuto, A. D., & Stickle, T. R. (1998). Empirically supported couple and family interventions for marital distress and adult mental health problems. *Journal of Consulting and Clinical Psychology, 66,* 53–88.

Beutler, L. E., & Clarkin, J. (1990). *Systematic treatment selection: Toward targeted therapeutic interventions.* New York: Brunner/Mazel.

Bongar, B., & Beutler, L. E. (1995). *Comprehensive textbook of psychotherapy: Theory and practice.* New York: Oxford University Press.

Brunner, E. J. (1998). Family interaction and family psychopathology. In L. L'Abate (Ed.), *Family psychopathology: The relational roots of dysfunctional behavior* (pp. 75–93). New York: Guilford Press.

Christensen, A., & Heavey, C. L. (1999). Interventions for couples. *Annual Review of Psychology, 50,* 165–190.

Dunn, R. L., & Schwebel, A. I. (1995). Meta-analytic review of marital therapy outcome research. *Journal of Family Psychology, 9,* 58–68.

Epstein, N., & Baucom, D. H. (2002). *Treating couples in context: Innovations in cognitive-behavioral therapy.* Washington, DC: American Psychological Association.

Goldfried, M. R., & Norcross, J. C. (1995). Integrative and eclectic therapies in historical perspective. In B. Bongar & L. E. Beutler (Eds.), *Comprehensive textbook of psychotherapy: Theory and practice* (pp. 254–273). New York: Oxford University Press.

Gottman, J. M., & Gottman, J. S. (1999). The marriage survival kit: A research-based marital therapy. In R. Berger & M. T. Hannah (Eds.), *Preventive approaches in couples therapy* (pp. 304–330). Philadelphia: Brunner/Mazel.

Gurman, A. S. (1981). Integrative marital therapy: Toward the development of an interpersonal approach. In S. H. Budman (Ed.), *Forms of brief therapy* (pp. 415–457). New York: Guilford Press.

Gurman, A. S., & Jacobson, N. S. (2002). *Clinical handbook of couple therapy* (3rd ed). New York: Guilford Press.

Jacobson, N. S., Christensen, A., Prince, S. E., Cordova, J., & Eldridge, K. (2000). Integrative behavioral couple therapy: An acceptance-based, promising new treatment for couple discord. *Journal of Consulting and Clinical Psychology, 68,* 351–355.

Jacobson, N. S., & Margolin, G. (1979). *Marital therapy: Strategies based on social learning and behavioral exchange principles.* New York: Brunner/Mazel.

Johnson, S. M., & Greenberg, L. S. (1985). Differential effects of experiential and problem-solving interventions in resolving marital conflict. *Journal of Consulting and Clinical Psychology, 53,* 175–184.

Johnson, S. M., & Greenberg, L. S. (1995). The emotionally focused approach to problems in adult attachment. In N. S. Jacobson & A. S. Gurman (Eds.), *Clinical handbook of couple therapy* (pp. 121–141). New York: Guilford Press.

Johnson, S. M., Hunsley, J., Greenberg, L., & Schindler, D. (1999). Emotionally focused couples therapy: Status and challenges. *Clinical Psychology: Science and Practice, 6,* 67–79.

Johnson, S. M., & Talitman, E. (1997). Predictors of success in emotionally focused marital therapy. *Journal of Marital and Family Therapy, 23,* 135–152.

Kobak, R., Ruckdeschel, K., & Hazan, C. (1994). From symptom to signal: An attachment view of emotion in marital therapy. In S. M. Johnson & L. S. Greenberg (Eds.), *The heart of the matter: Perspectives on emotion in marital therapy* (pp. 46–71). New York: Brunner/Mazel.

Lazarus, A. A. (1992). Multimodal therapy: Technical eclecticism with minimal integration. In J. C. Norcross & M. R. Goldfried (Eds.), *Handbook of psychotherapy integration* (pp. 231–263). New York: Basic Books.

Lebow, J. L. (1997). The integrative revolution in couple and family therapy. *Family Process, 36,* 1–17.

Messer, S. B. (1992). A critical examination of belief structures in integrative and eclectic psychotherapy. In J. C. Norcross & M. R. Goldfried (Eds.), *Handbook of psychotherapy integration* (pp. 130–165). New York: Basic Books.

Nichols, M. P., & Minuchin, S. (1999). Short-term structural family therapy with couples. In J. M. Donovan (Ed.), *Short-term couple therapy* (pp. 124–143). New York: Guilford Press.

Norcross, J. C. (1985). Eclecticism: Definitions, manifestations and practitioners. *International Journal of Eclectic Psychotherapy, 4,* 19–32.

Norcross, J. C., & Beutler, L. E. (2000). A prescriptive eclectic approach to psychotherapy training. *Journal of Psychotherapy Integration, 10,* 247–261.

Norcross, J. C., & Goldfried, M. R. (1992). *Handbook of psychotherapy integration.* New York: Basic Books.

Norcross, J. C., & Newman, C. F. (1992). Psychotherapy integration: Setting the context. In J. C. Norcross & M. R. Goldfried (Eds.), *Handbook of psychotherapy integration* (pp. 3–45). New York: Basic Books.

Norcross, J. C., Prochaska, J. O., & Farber, J. A. (1993). Psychologists conducting psychotherapy: New findings and historical comparisons on the psychotherapy division membership. *Psychotherapy, 30,* 692–697.

Snyder, D. K. (1999). Affective reconstruction in the context of a pluralistic approach to couple therapy. *Clinical Psychology: Science and Practice, 6,* 348–365.

Snyder, D. K., Cozzi, J. J., & Mangrum, L. F. (2002). Conceptual issues in assessing couples and families. In H. A. Liddle, D. A. Santisteban, R. F. Levant, & J. H. Bray (Eds.), *Family psychology: Science-based interventions* (pp. 69–87). Washington, DC: American Psychological Association.

Snyder, D. K., Mangrum, L. F., Wills, R. M. (1993). Predicting couples' response to marital therapy: A comparison of short- and long-term predictors. *Journal of Consulting and Clinical Psychology, 61,* 61–69.

Snyder, D. K., & Schneider, W. J. (2002). Affective reconstruction: A pluralistic, developmental approach. In A. S. Gurman & N. S. Jacobson (Eds.), *Clinical handbook of couple therapy* (3rd ed., pp. 151–179). New York: Guilford Press.

Snyder, D. K., & Wills, R. M. (1989). Behavioral versus insight-oriented marital therapy: Effects on individual and interspousal functioning. *Journal of Consulting and Clinical Psychology, 57,* 39–46.

Snyder, D. K., Wills, R. M., Grady-Fletcher, A. (1991). Long-term effectiveness of behavioral versus insight-oriented marital therapy: A 4-year follow-up study. *Journal of Consulting and Clinical Psychology, 59,* 138–141.

Weiss, R. L., & Halford, W. K. (1996). Managing marital therapy: Helping partners change. In V. B. Van Hasselt & M. Hersen (Eds.), *Sourcebook of psychological treatment manuals for adult disorders* (pp. 489–537). New York: Plenum.

Whisman, M. A., Dixon, A. E., & Johnson, B. (1997). Therapists' perspectives of couple problems and treatment issues in couple therapy. *Journal of Family Psychology, 11,* 361–366.

Whisman, M. A., & Snyder, D. K. (1997). Evaluating and improving the efficacy of conjoint couple therapy. In W. K. Halford & H. J. Markman (Eds.), *Clinical handbook of marriage and couples interventions* (pp. 679–693). New York: Wiley.

Wills, R. M., Faitler, S. M., & Snyder, D. K. (1987). Distinctiveness of behavioral versus insight-oriented marital therapy: An empirical analysis. *Journal of Consulting and Clinical Psychology, 55,* 685–690.

PART II

Couple-Based Treatments for Emotional and Behavioral Disorders

The chapters in this section emphasize couple-based interventions targeting specific mental health problems for which empirical studies regarding efficacy have already been conducted. As Baucom, Stanton, and Epstein note in their chapter on anxiety disorders, these couple interventions generally fall into one of three classes: (1) disorder-specific interventions, in which relationship issues are addressed to the extent that they impact, or are impacted by, the partner's disorder; (2) partner-assisted interventions, in which the partner acts as a surrogate therapist, coaching the individual to complete homework assignments and providing support; and (3) general couple therapy addressing specific domains of relationship functioning that contribute to or exacerbate the emotional or behavioral problems exhibited by one or both partners.

There are few couples for whom some level of anxiety or depressed affect does not interact with relationship distress—whether from apprehension about their relationship's future or their own individual well-being, or discouragement about the potential for relationship change or the loss of intimacy previously shared. The chapters by Baucom and colleagues on anxiety disorders, and by Beach and Gupta on depression, offer guidance for selecting among and sequencing specific couple-based interventions for individuals and their partners struggling with reciprocal effects of these emotional disorders and relationship difficulties.

Less frequently encountered, and more challenging both for couples and their therapists, are occasions when one partner develops a major mental illness that significantly disrupts cognitive processes or results in psychotic symptoms. Both the chapters by Miklowitz and Morris on bipolar disorders and by Mueser and Brunette on schizophrenia-spectrum disorders build on previous advances in assisting families of individuals with major mental illness from a behavioral approach. Each chapter emphasizes the importance of a comprehensive system-based model not only for assisting the individual suffering the disorder but also for minimizing the deleterious effects and mobilizing the support of their partner and other family members.

The treatment of various impulse-related disorders within a couple context has sometimes been met with both theoretical and sociopolitical controversy. Nowhere has this been clearer than in treatment strategies for substance abuse and partner aggression. In their chapter on alcohol- and other substance-abuse disorders, Fals-Stewart, Birchler, and O'Farrell emphasize the compatibility of couple-based interventions with both disease- and family-system models of addictions. The research they summarize indicating that untreated relationship problems predict poorer individual response to alcohol and drug abuse treatment should sober any clinician who persists in emphasizing individual-based treatment to the neglect of relationship interventions. Critical to discussion of any emotional or behavioral disorder, but particularly relevant to treatment of partner aggression using couple-based interventions, are issues of individual differences in the frequency, intensity, and patterning of the disorder. In their chapter on partner aggression, Holtzworth-Munroe, Marshall, Meehan, and Rehman emphasize the distinction between severe physical aggression and common couple violence characterized by more moderate and frequently bidirectional aggression. Although more than half of couples entering therapy have experienced physical aggression in their relationship, couple therapists frequently report feeling ill-prepared to adequately assess and intervene in this problem. The authors of this chapter offer explicit guidelines for screening for aggression, evaluating the couple for appropriateness of conjoint treatment, and disrupting partner violence and both the individual and relationship processes that contribute to or perpetuate it.

In contrast to impulse disorders, sexual disorders have historically been viewed as comprising relationship as well as individual problems. As in other domains, relationship difficulties may contribute to, exacerbate, or result from individual sexual disorders. Depending on the functional relations among individual and relational processes for a given couple, the optimal treatment may involve a unique blending of individual, partner-assisted, or more traditional couple-based interventions. In their chapter on sexual dysfunctions, Regev, O'Donohue, and Avina provide a rich conceptual model and explicit guidelines for addressing psychological, physiological, and relational factors that interact with sexual difficulties and are critical to their remediation.

CHAPTER 3

Anxiety Disorders

DONALD H. BAUCOM
SUSAN STANTON
NORMAN B. EPSTEIN

THE EMPIRICAL LINK BETWEEN RELATIONSHIP
DISTRESS AND ANXIETY DISORDERS

All humans are equipped with an internal signal that alerts them to the
presence of danger. Physiological arousal in the form of a racing heart,
sweating, nervous stomach, or difficulty breathing warns people about
dangers ranging from an imminent attack to a bad decision. Anxiety,
this innate, adaptive response to perceived danger, triggers the well-
documented fight-or-flight reaction, in which people choose either to
flee the source of danger or engage in behaviors to combat it. Although
anxiety commonly serves a valuable function through which people
protect themselves, it may become overlearned or occur at inappropriate times such that it interferes with people's lives. These excessive feelings of arousal may comprise a diagnosable anxiety disorder or a subclinical chronic state of distress and worry. In either case, living with
this maladaptive anxiety often causes severe distress for the individual
and his or her partner. This chapter focuses on the ways in which anxiety can disrupt a couple's relationship, and how couple-based interventions can alleviate an individual's anxiety symptoms and contribute to
healthy relationship functioning.

Anxiety disorders cover a spectrum of diagnosable conditions with
some common features, including physiological arousal to a feared stimulus, distorted thoughts about the consequences of the feared condi-

tions, and avoidance or rituals intended to reduce the anxiety. A person who confronts a feared stimulus may experience sweating, racing heart, upset stomach, shakiness, disorientation, and shortness of breath. As the individual attempts to cope with the increased arousal, his or her mind may be flooded with thoughts about catastrophic immediate or future events and the importance of preventing them. Often, the person will avoid the object or situation that evokes the fear, sometimes by thinking about other topics or by staying in "safe" places. Some individuals engage in rituals that they believe will prevent the imagined negative consequences. Even when the ritualistic behavior does not make sense to the individual, he or she feels compelled to carry it out in order to decrease the anxiety. The particular constellation of symptoms that an individual experiences determines whether the anxiety disorder is categorized as obsessive–compulsive disorder (OCD), generalized anxiety disorder (GAD), panic disorder with or without agoraphobia (PD, PDA), a social or simple phobia, or posttraumatic stress disorder (PTSD). These disorders have in common excessive anxiety about an objectively nonthreatening object or situation, and the individual's tendency to respond with disruptive rumination, avoidance, or rituals.

Epidemiology

Excessive anxiety is one of the most frequent mental health problems in the U.S. population. Barlow, O'Brien, and Last (1984) reported that anxiety is the fifth most common presenting complaint to primary care physicians. In the National Comorbidity Survey (NCS), which uses DSM-III-R criteria, the lifetime prevalence rate of any anxiety disorder is 24.9 %, with a range of 3.5 % for panic disorder to 13.3 % for social phobia (Kessler et al., 1994). Results from the Epidemiologic Catchment Area study (ECA), which uses DSM-III criteria, place 1-month prevalence rates for any anxiety disorder at 7.3%, with a range of 0.5 % for panic disorder to 6.2% for phobias (Regier, Narrow, & Rae, 1990). People who reported symptoms of anxiety disorders are more likely to be divorced or separated than people who do not report such symptoms (Regier et al., 1990).

The degree of comorbidity between particular anxiety disorders and relationship distress presents a complicated picture. Several investigators have explored this issue, using different methodologies and statistical strategies (e.g., Arnow, Taylor, Agras, & Telch, 1985; Arrindell, Emmelkamp, & Sanderman, 1986; McLeod, 1994). These different strategies have made it difficult to derive agreed-upon rates of comorbidity. In the most comprehensive examination of epidemiological data to date, Whisman (1999) found significant associations between self-reports of anxiety disorders and self-reported marital dissatisfaction in data collected for the National Comorbidity Survey. He indicated that a major shortcoming of research on the comorbidity of marital satisfaction and particular anxiety disorders has been the failure to control for the presence of comorbid disorders. When Whisman (1999) examined marital dissatisfaction in individuals with particular anxiety disorders, while controlling for the presence of other psychiatric disorders, he only found a unique effect for PTSD in women, which he attributed to the possibility that the women's male partners were the perpetrators of the traumatic events responsible for the PTSD responses. Apparently, many couples function well when one person experiences a single anxiety disorder. Whisman (1999) concluded that marital dissatisfaction is associated with anxiety in individuals who experience more than one anxiety or depressive disorder. Thus, a specific anxiety disorder appears to be important in relationship functioning when it is part of a larger picture of an individual's psychological symptoms that likely pose significant stress for the relationship. Alternatively, the observed association between broad-based disorders and relationship distress might be due to problematic relationships that create stress for the individual and result in a broader range of symptoms. Consequently, when working with a couple in which one person has an anxiety disorder, the clinician should assess how these anxiety symptoms fit into a broader context of individual and relationship functioning.

The Cycle of Anxiety Disorders and Relationship Distress

After noting an association between relationship dissatisfaction and anxiety disorders, researchers have sought to understand the bases of this relationship and the implications for couple-based interventions. The two issues receiving the most attention are the extent to which relationship problems contribute to the development and maintenance of anxiety disorders, and the extent to which anxiety disorders create distress in couples' relationships. Although these two directions of influence are likely to operate concurrently, clinicians can conduct a more thorough assessment by considering them independently before integrating the data in the conceptualization of a couple's difficulties and a treatment plan.

The Impact of a Couple's Relationship on an Individual's Anxiety Disorder

Relationship distress, as well as other life stressors such as physical illness, childbirth, financial difficulties, and other relationship difficulties, often precede the development of panic disorder with agoraphobia and OCD (e.g., Calvocoressi et al., 1995). In addition to creating partners' concerns about the well-being and stability of their close relationship, relationship distress may cause heightened physiological arousal. Individuals who are vulnerable to developing anxiety disorders may make overly negative interpretations of this arousal as dangerous or intolerable and may attempt to cope with it in maladaptive ways. For example, one woman had become increasingly distressed as she experienced her husband as excessively controlling. He interrogated her about any contacts with friends, discouraged her from working outside the home, and frequently criticized her. She often thought about leaving him but felt trapped because it appeared that she could not support herself financially. One day as she was driving to the grocery store and had fleeting thoughts about her marriage she suddenly experienced her first panic attack. Due to its unexpected onset and the fact that she interpreted it as a possibly dangerous problem with her heart, she immediately sought medical attention, and thereafter avoided driving alone.

Relationship adjustment also might play a role in an individual's response to treatment for anxiety. For example, although married people with GAD were more likely to improve on anxiety measures than single people with GAD, the likelihood of improvement within the married group decreased as marital tension increased (Durham, Allan, & Hackett, 1997). Similarly, reviews of studies on agoraphobia have found that higher global relationship satisfaction at pretreatment predicts a better response to treatment (e.g., Daiuto, Baucom, Epstein, & Dutton, 1998). Thus, living in an environment marked by *general* relationship distress might contribute to the development of anxiety disorders and interfere with optimal treatment outcome.

The Impact of an Individual's Anxiety Disorder on the Couple's Relationship

Studies have provided inconsistent findings about whether improvement in anxiety symptoms harms or benefits relationship quality. Some researchers have found that remittance of agoraphobic symptoms was associated with decreased relationship satisfaction in patients or their partners (e.g., Arrindell et al., 1986). Arguing that agoraphobia creates closeness and dependency, some researchers have suggested that husbands of agoraphobic women may have their own dependency needs met by their wives' lack of autonomy. Consequently, these husbands either would leave the relationship when their partner's dependency lessened due to therapy, or they would undermine treatment gains in order to keep their wives at home and to prevent their own inadequacies from being revealed (Fry, 1962; Goldstein & Chambless, 1978). Barlow et al. (1984) proposed that improvement in anxiety symptoms leads to decreased relationship satisfaction for partners when changes occur quickly and partners lack the ability to adjust to new roles in their relationship. Abrupt increases in the agoraphobic individuals' autonomy and independence may startle their partners, suggesting that negotiation of new roles may be important in the prevention of decreased relationship satisfaction and the maintenance of treatment gains. Thus, improvement in anxiety symptoms may not increase relationship satisfaction if underlying issues or patterns affected by the disorders are not addressed.

Despite the suggested functional role of agoraphobic symptoms in some relationships, the predominance of research has shown no deterioration in relationship quality following treatment of agoraphobic or obsessive–compulsive symptoms. Instead, couples tend to maintain or increase their level of satisfaction as symptoms decrease (e.g., Emmelkamp et al., 1992; Monterio, Marks, & Ramm, 1985). Avoidance behaviors, the primary symptom of anxiety disorders, can affect close relationships adversely by restricting the couple's environment, shifting roles, accommodating the couple's interaction patterns to the needs of the anxious individual, and creating conflict. As symptoms of anxiety prevent individuals from working, going places, making decisions, living comfortably in their homes, sleeping, and engaging in social situations, the couple's relationship also suffers. Positive couple behaviors, such as attending social activities, disappear as the anxious individual's avoidance behaviors increase (see also Friedman, 1990).

At the same time that positive interactions decrease, negative interactions may increase as arguments erupt about the renegotiation of roles in the relationship. Not only do nonanxious partners accommodate to anxiety by assuming duties (e.g., going out shopping) that now frighten their partners, they also may participate in avoidance or ritualistic behaviors in an attempt to alleviate their partner's anxiety or to stop arguments. For example, the wife of a man with OCD spent an hour every evening washing towels and reorganizing the linen closet because her husband would become furious if the towels were out of order. Although she had initially refused to perform this ritual, she accommodated to his compulsion in order to maintain peace. Studies suggest that between 40 and 88% of relatives accommodate to a family member's obsessive–compulsive symptoms, and that such accommodation results in poorer family functioning as well as the maintenance of anxiety symptoms (Calvocoressi et al., 1995; Steketee, 1997). As nonanxious partners fail to see improvement in the other's anxiety, particularly after making sacrifices in order to help the anxious person, they may experience mounting frustration, resentment, and guilt. Criticism, hostile behavior, conflict, or emotional distancing may contribute to a negative environment that is unhealthy for the relationship as well as for improvement in the individual's anxiety disorder (Steketee, 1997).

In addition to interfering directly with a couple's behavioral patterns, an anxiety disorder may contribute to relationship distress by eliciting negative emotions in both partners. Literature on depression has reported that living with a depressed person commonly produces depression and other negative emotions in significant others, and that depressed individuals tend to feel irritation and frustration toward family members (Coyne et al., 1987). Similarly, an anxiety disorder may foster an atmosphere of tension and stress between members of a couple. Nonanxious partners may empathize with their anxious partners at first, only to grow weary of the impact that the symptoms have on their daily life. In order to gain relief for their own distress, they may either distance themselves physically or psychologically, or criticize their partners for anxiety-related symptoms. A further consequence of the persistent atmosphere of tension is the nonanxious individual's cognitive appraisal of the anxious partner, in particular a loss of respect for their partners as competent and capable people. Although nonanxious individuals may be understanding initially, they may fail to see why their partners continue to perceive threats in objects and situations that are not dangerous. Some individuals may not understand anxiety disorders and perceive that their partners have "lost their minds." For example, the husband of a woman with social phobia expressed worry that his wife was paranoid because she perceived the neighbors as threatening. In other situations, nonanxious partners may experience the anxious person's preoccupation with anxiety-provoking stimuli as detracting from the satisfaction of their own needs in the relationship. In our clinical experiences, partners of individuals with anxiety disorders have complained that the person's fears or obsessions dominate their conversations. When relationship issues do arise, the heightened arousal from the anxious partners' fears may escalate relationship conflicts. In turn, the anxious individual may become increasingly frustrated or angry if their nonanxious partner appears to lack empathy for the distress involved in their anxiety disorder. For example, a woman with GAD became angry each time her husband teased her about being "a worrywart" in front of their children and friends.

Conclusion

Anxiety disorders potentially disrupt couple functioning subtly through the alteration of interaction patterns, or more dramatically by increasing tension and arguments, restricting relationship activities, or decreasing attention paid to the needs of nonanxious partners. Conversely, the quality of couples' relationships may affect the course of anxiety disorders. Overall, relationship dissatisfaction may serve as a stressor that heightens individuals' arousal, thereby exacerbating anxiety symptoms and the rituals or avoidance responses used in attempts to reduce the symptoms. Even if the couple does not have a distressed relationship overall, specific interaction patterns between the partners can contribute to, or interfere with, gains in treatment of the anxiety disorder. Thus, combining efficacious aspects of couple therapy with treatments for anxiety disorders has the potential to aid couples in addressing these complicated individual and relationship concerns.

TREATMENT

Principles of Treating Anxiety Disorders

Exposure and Response Prevention

The most widely researched efficacious individual treatment for anxiety disorders is exposure and response prevention (ERP; see DeRubeis & Crits-Cristoph, 1998). Exposure and response prevention attempts to break an overlearned cycle between the thoughts and feelings of anxiety, and avoidance behaviors. Typically, individuals with anxiety overestimate the probability of a feared event occurring, experience anxiety in the presence of cues for those feared events, and then seek to escape subjective feelings of anxiety through avoidance behaviors. These avoidance behaviors temporarily lower anxiety and thus maintain the association between feared consequences and harmless stimuli. ERP is designed to break the cycle of anxiety and avoidance behavior by having people face the consequences they fear and prevent themselves from engaging in anxiety-reduction behaviors. The rationale behind these treatment principles is that people can become habituated to the experience of anxiety, observe that the anticipated dire consequences do not materialize, and associate new affective and cognitive experiences with the anxiety-provoking stimuli. In addition, people unlearn the association between avoidance behaviors and reduced anxiety, as well as gain a sense of mastery over unpredictable situations (see also Craske & Barlow, 2001).

In developing a realistic exposure exercise, the clinician first should obtain detailed descriptions of the anxiety-provoking stimuli, the client's automatic thoughts about the feared consequences of the situation, and avoidance behaviors used to reduce anxiety. Next, the clinician asks the client to monitor the intensity and content of his or her anxiety and coping responses after an anxious episode. Clients and therapists then generate an exposure hierarchy of least anxiety-provoking to most anxiety-provoking stimuli based on the client's reported level of subjective units of distress (SUDS), on a 1–100 scale, in each situation. Finally, clients carry out the exposure in the actual anxious situations (i.e., public restroom, home, store) or in therapy sessions by imagining themselves in the situations. When confronting the stimuli, clients refrain from enacting any avoidance behaviors and instead allow themselves to experience the anxiety. Clients take note of their SUDS rating continually (e.g., every 5 minutes), ending the exposure when their anxiety has dropped sufficiently. Generally, clients are instructed to repeat each exposure situation until their anxiety is low, at which point they move to a situation higher on the hierarchy (see Foa & Franklin, 2001, or Craske & Barlow, 2001, for a complete description of ERP).

Other Therapeutic Approaches: Cognitive Restructuring and Relaxation Training

Cognitive restructuring and relaxation training are efficacious treatments for anxiety disorders, and may be especially helpful as adjuncts to ERP (DeRubeis & Crits-Cristoph, 1998). Relaxation training teaches clients how to relax muscle groups progressively and to retrain their breathing in order to cope with the physical sensations of anxiety (see Bernstein & Borkovec, 1973, for a description of these procedures). During formal exposure sessions, however, clients should refrain from using relaxation techniques that might prevent them from habituating to anxious feelings.

Cognitive restructuring techniques target thoughts that clients experience when anticipating or confronting anxiety-provoking stimuli. Clinicians should attend to two major types of cognitive errors made by clients with anxiety disorders: the overestimation of the chances of feared negative events occurring and the tendency to view the events as intolerable and beyond their ability to cope (Brown, O'Leary, & Barlow, 2001). This approach asks clients to challenge these automatic thoughts by examining the likelihood that their feared consequences will occur, generating alternative outcomes of the situation, and considering the meaning of the feared consequence in their lives. In the search for the meaning of the feared consequence, therapists attempt to guide clients to the core schemas that are driving their excessive fears, such as the belief that they are responsible for ensuring others' safety, or the belief that they are incompetent and likely to fail in life.

The therapist then attempts to help clients modify these underlying beliefs, to reduce the cycle of negative automatic thoughts and feelings of anxiety (see Beck & Emery, 1985, for a further description of these cognitive techniques).

Assessment

In developing a thorough treatment plan for couples with comorbid anxiety disorders and relationship distress, assessment should proceed from three perspectives: the history of the individual's anxiety disorder, the way in which the relationship and anxiety disorder interact, and overall couple functioning.

Individual History

As in any assessment of individual psychiatric history, clinicians should gather information relevant to the onset, course, and past treatment of the anxiety. Any information that the client can recall concerning life circumstances associated with increases or decreases in anxiety symptoms may be helpful in identifying the conditions that elicit and reinforce anxiety symptoms and coping responses such as avoidance. For example, the woman described earlier, who experienced her first panic attack while driving and thinking about her controlling husband, was able to identify patterns in their relationship that increased both her unhappiness and her sense of hopelessness about "ever escaping this suffocating life." Her personal history also revealed that her parents had been controlling when she was a child, and she grew up with little confidence in her ability to function autonomously.

Clinicians also may wish to contact past or present therapists with the client's consent to learn about the relative success of psychotherapy approaches and medication. As noted in the discussion of exposure and response prevention, this treatment also requires a detailed understanding of the situational and internal triggers of anxiety, as well as the client's behavioral responses. Consequently, cognitive-behavioral therapists recommend asking the client to use a self-monitoring form and questionnaires to assess instances of the particular anxiety disorder between sessions, to provide information for the development of appropriate exposure exercises, cognitive restructuring, and other interventions.

Symptom–System Fit

When examining the role of anxiety in the client's life, clinicians should attend particularly to the ways that anxiety symptoms affect the couple's relationship and that the relationship affects anxiety symptoms. Rohrbaugh, Shoham, Spungen, and Steinglass (1985) describe this step as an assessment of the "symptom–system fit." In anxiety disorders, couples often rearrange their relationship to accommodate to the person's avoidance behaviors. This accommodation may be subtle or extreme, from partners' participation in rituals to their avoidance of places or activities, from their constant reassurances to their assumption of tasks or responsibilities. As might be anticipated, this accommodation often occurs within couples who are happy with their relationship. The partner of the anxious person might be distressed at seeing the person whom he or she loves become anxious, and therefore adapts his or her behavior to lessen the anxiety, for example, taking on tasks that make the partner anxious. The couple's deliberate or unknowing accommodation of their relationship to anxiety creates a system that may fit with the symptoms to maintain the cycle of anxiety and avoidance.

Other couples may present with a poor symptom–system fit, in which nonanxious partners refuse to accommodate to anxiety or resent the ways in which anxiety symptoms have altered the relationship. These couples are likely to display high conflict concerning the individual's anxiety. Although we advise couples not to accommodate to anxiety symptoms, some partners have not negotiated this refusal to accommodate in a healthy way. For example, one man who feared contamination from gasoline fumes faced belittling remarks from his wife whenever he requested that she place her clothes in a plastic bag after she put gasoline in the car. In other cases, a nonanxious partner initially attempts to resist accommodation but gives in after hearing repeated pleas from the anxious person to alleviate his or her anxiety. One woman who had GAD asked her partner if he thought their son was safe at school and when outside playing with friends in their neighborhood. At first her husband told her that he would not respond to her groundless fears, but he later yelled at her that everything was fine, phoning the school, and going outside to monitor the son's activities in the neighborhood in order to reduce her nagging behavior. Such negative reactions by partners to the individual's anxiety disorder both increase relationship distress and fail to alleviate anxiety symptoms.

General Couple Functioning

In some couples, one person's anxiety disorder may not be the primary presenting complaint. Routine assessment of couple functioning may include consideration of the couple's communication skills, a gauge of the level of positive and negative interactions in the relationship, the examination of unmet needs, and an understanding of partners' standards, assumptions, attributions, and expectancies for the relationship (see Epstein & Baucom, 2002, for a description of these procedures). Couples may experience distress from general relationship issues, such as arguments over in-laws or disagreements about finances. Whereas these issues might be unrelated to anxiety, in some cases clinicians might determine that an anxiety disorder does play a role in the couple's conflict. For example, an individual with OCD may avoid going to the in-laws' house because of contamination fears, or someone with social phobia is unemployed due to an inability to work in an office, which leads to conflict about financial constraints. Even if the members of a couple fail to present one person's anxiety as a major concern, the anxiety symptoms and the person's ways of coping with them might create a more negative emotional atmosphere that lowers the threshold for arguments on most issues. As noted earlier, overall relationship distress also might increase tension for partners who are susceptible to anxiety.

Finally, clinicians should include a thorough individual history of the nonanxious partner in order to determine how the partner's personality, psychopathology, past relationships, or motives helped to create the system in which the anxiety disorder exists. For example, a man whose first wife left him was especially solicitous whenever his second wife experienced panic symptoms, thereby contributing to her avoidance pattern.

Types of Couple-Based Interventions for Anxiety Disorders

Baucom, Shoham, Mueser, Daiuto, and Stickle (1998) have identified three different types of couple-based interventions that can be used when one person has individual psychological problems such as anxiety disorders. The three approaches vary along a continuum of increased attention to the couple's relationship in treating the individual's disorder. All three approaches can be integrated into the treatment plan for a given couple, as illustrated in this chapter's case example.

Partner-Assisted Interventions

The approach most commonly used in previous studies on the treatment of anxiety with a partner is partner-assisted interventions (PAIs). In PAIs, the partner acts as a surrogate therapist, coaching the individual to complete homework assignments and providing support. Given that the dominant paradigm for treating anxiety disorders is exposure and response prevention, partner-assisted interventions have emphasized partners' participating in exposure exercises and encouraging alternatives to avoidance responses. In addition, the therapist provides both members of the couple with psychoeducation about the nature of the anxiety-avoidance cycle. However, little attention is paid to partner behaviors or couple functioning that may elicit or maintain the individual's anxiety. The focus of PAIs is on the client's anxiety disorder and individual functioning.

One potential drawback to partner-assisted interventions is that they may create an unbalanced couple treatment, with the anxious individual in the role of the "identified patient," such that one or both partners blame that individual's personal problems for any relationship difficulties. Thus, the wife of a man with GAD discounted any concerns he expressed about their relationship, attributing them to his excessive worry rather than taking personal responsibility for considering her role in the negative patterns that her husband saw in their relationship. Consequently, couple therapists need to assess the influences of both the individual's anxiety and couple interaction patterns in determining the negative experiences that the anxious person reports. In addition, broadening the focus in therapy to identify the anxious individual's strengths and contributions to the relationship can help prevent him or her from being a "second-class citizen" in the relationship.

Disorder-Specific Interventions

In order to address "symptom–system fit," Baucom et al. (1998) recommend targeting the ways in which the couple's relationship maintains the anxiety-avoidance cycle. In these disorder-specific interventions, the focus of treatment remains the individual's anxiety disorder, but couple relationship issues are introduced to the extent that they impact the disorder or are impacted by the disorder. Couple issues that do not directly maintain the anxiety are not included in a disorder-specific intervention. For example, if one person avoids shopping because of anxiety, the therapist might encourage the couple to reduce the nonanxious partner's tendency to take over most of the shopping, so that the anxious person does not continue to engage in avoidance. The couple's relationship is the focus of attention, but only in terms of how it relates to the anxiety. Discussing parenting concerns that are unrelated to the anxiety disorder would not be a disorder-specific intervention. The philosophy behind disorder-specific interventions is that individual improvement on anxiety symptoms might not persist if the couple system has not adjusted in a way to maintain treatment gains.

General Couple Therapy

Baucom et al. (1998) indicate that among couples with global distress in their relationships, couple therapy addressing various domains of relationship functioning serves to reduce chronic stress that may precipitate or exacerbate an individual's anxiety symptoms. For example, one man's GAD began during a period of arguing with his partner about financial pressures. His thoughts became dominated by worries that the couple would become bankrupt and lose their house, which then spread to worries about the stability of the relationship itself. When the couple learned to discuss finances calmly and make decisions about their income and expenses, the man's worry decreased dramatically. However, the couple therapist approached communication about finances as a broad relationship issue rather than framing it as an interaction pattern that maintained the man's GAD.

In addition to reducing levels of stress, general couple therapy might be necessary before engaging in partner-assisted or disorder-specific interventions when relationship distress precludes partners' abilities to work together. Using cognitive-behavioral couple therapy techniques such as reducing negative interactions, increasing positive interactions, teaching communication skills, or restoring trust may be necessary before beginning to address anxiety symptoms (see Epstein & Baucom, 2002, for a treatment manual for cognitive-behavioral couple therapy). In some cases, therapy might assist the couple in reaching a stable level at which anxiety treatments such as exposure and response prevention can be introduced. Consistent with these notions, Arnow et al. (1985) demonstrated that teaching couples communication skills improved outcomes for anxiety disorders treated by ERP.

Incorporating the Three Approaches

In deciding when and how to incorporate each of these approaches to couple-based treatment for anxiety disorders, the clinician should attend to the couple's presenting complaints, their level of insight into the individual's anxiety, and their capacity to provide support to each other. Couples who do not identify anxiety issues as a primary complaint may wish to focus on general relationship issues at the beginning of therapy, with the therapist gently introducing partner-assisted and disorder-specific interventions as the primary relationship complaints improve. As treatment goals shift to addressing the individual's anxiety disorder, therapists must present the symptom–system fit between anxiety and couple functioning. Such a contextual approach minimizes blaming the anxious partner for relationship problems. Some couples may recognize the interaction between the individual's anxiety disorder and patterns in their relationship, opening the door for disorder-specific interventions. In other cases, couples do not recognize an individual's symptoms as an anxiety disorder, in which case psychoeducation about anxiety would help to prepare them for partner-assisted or disorder-specific interventions. Finally, couples vary in the extent to which the members remain competent at providing emotional and instrumental support for each other in the face of relationship distress. Partner-assisted interventions are likely to succeed only when the nonanxious partner has the capacity to assist with exposure exercises without being hostile or intrusive. When anxiety and relationship distress coexist, clinicians initially should conceptualize how the three intervention approaches may benefit the individual's anxiety disorder and the couple's relationship.

Conclusions

Efficacious treatments for anxiety disorders, such as exposure and response prevention, cognitive restructuring, and relaxation training, can be introduced into couple-based interventions in three ways. Partner-assisted interventions use the partner as a surrogate therapist to assist with exposure exercises and provide support without targeting the couple's ongoing relationship. Disorder-specific interventions focus on ways in which couple functioning maintains anxiety symptoms, as well as ways in which the anxiety influences couple functioning. General couple therapy seeks to reduce overall relationship distress that may contribute to the anxiety disorder. These different approaches to couple-based interventions can be applied to any anxiety disorder. The next section demonstrates how to tailor these principles to a particular anxiety disorder, focusing on panic disorder with agoraphobia.

An Illustration of Treatment of an Anxiety Disorder: Panic Disorder with Agoraphobia

In order to clarify how couple-based interventions are used in clinical practice, we provide a case illustration of a couple experiencing relationship difficulties, complicated by the wife's panic disorder with agoraphobia (PDA). The clinician needs to understand broad domains of relationship functioning that are influenced by, and influence, agoraphobia and panic disorder in planning partner-assisted and disorder-specific interventions. Whereas these complications in relationship functioning are not universally present in cases of PDA, an awareness of frequent relationship factors can help to guide the clinician in developing appropriate treatment plans.

An agoraphobic individual experiences a lack of safety and efficacy in interacting with the outside world—in particular, a fear that he or she will experience highly aversive, frightening panic attacks in situations where assistance is unavailable. In many instances, persons with agoraphobia turn to their partners to provide a sense of safety. This means that the partner often accompanies the agoraphobic individual on outings, provides reassurance, and attempts to make the outside world seem safe. Whereas these efforts by the partner often are well intentioned, they inadvertently reinforce the agoraphobic individual's avoidance of major aspects of the environment and promote dependence on the partner.

Consequently, a major emphasis of the intervention is to help the agoraphobic individual interact with the world in a more autonomous fashion. In many instances, this means shifting the couple's relationship such that an end goal is for the partner not to accompany the agoraphobic individual on many ventures into the outside world. Whereas this can help alleviate the avoidance, it runs the risk of making the partners feel distant and even alienated from each other, because they previously learned to demonstrate caring and closeness through the nonanxious partner's involvement with the individual's anxiety and agoraphobic avoidance. Our previous research indicates that for couples in general, partners' facilitation of each other's autonomy and relatedness are two independent dimensions, both of which contribute to relationship satisfaction (Rankin-Esquer, Burnett, Baucom, & Epstein, 1997). The same study indicated that women particularly welcome their male partners' attempts at supporting their autonomy, so long as they also experience a sense of closeness with their partners. Extrapolating from these findings to the area of agoraphobia suggests that it is important to help the couple maintain a sense of closeness and caring so that the wives (whether they are the anxious or nonanxious partner) do not feel abandoned or unloved as they interact more autonomously from their male partners on a daily basis. Similarly, our clinical experience suggests that men may feel unneeded if the daily level of involvement with their partner is decreased significantly in the process of treatment for PDA.

In order to promote an increased sense of autonomy for the agoraphobic individual, the couple may need to renegotiate roles within the relationship concerning interactions with the outside world. For example, the partner of the agoraphobic often has assumed responsibilities, such as shopping or driving the children, that create anxiety for the agoraphobic. As a result, treatment involves helping the couple discuss the importance of redistributing these responsibilities to increase the agoraphobic individual's ability to function autonomously in the outside environment.

As the agoraphobic individual becomes less avoidant, the couple faces new interpersonal opportunities. Whereas the couple might have declined invitations for a variety of events such as crowded gatherings, the couple now can expand their social interactions. Not only might this enrich the couple's relationship, but it also serves as continuing exposure and helps to maintain treatment gains. In addition to increased interactions with friends and extended families, couples can reintroduce activities, such as vacation travel, that they had abandoned due to the agoraphobic individual's avoidance. Discussing such opportunities for increased enjoyment as a couple along with consolidated treatment gains is an important part of the intervention.

In summary, consideration of relationship issues is essential as partners work together to overcome the individual's agoraphobic avoidance. These include increasing mutual understanding of the internal and interpersonal factors affecting anxiety, developing a healthy sense of autonomy while maintaining a caring and intimate relationship, renegotiating roles and responsibilities in ways that continually expose the agoraphobic person to the outside world, and exploring the couple's newly derived opportunities for interacting with other individuals and the environment. These generally are disorder-specific interventions because they attempt to alter the couple's relationship in domains that are focal to panic disorder with agoraphobia. Such interventions are integrated with partner-assisted strategies for exposure and, when needed, more general relationship interventions to address areas of distress that are not central to panic and agoraphobia. The case example that follows demonstrates how these interventions can be used in a realistic and thoughtful manner to assist the couple.

Case Illustration

Mark and Mandy sought couple therapy for a variety of relationship difficulties. They were experiencing financial difficulties since Mandy had quit working 2 years earlier. They also were at odds over whether to have children soon. Both were in their late 20s, and Mandy was ready to become a parent. Although Mark wanted children, he was reluctant to begin their family now, given their financial concerns, relationship difficulties, and his worries about Mandy's individual functioning.

Both Mandy and Mark were intelligent, articulate, and had obtained graduate degrees. Mandy had begun a successful career, but over time, her anxiety had increased at work, and she had quit her job.

After 6 months on her first professional job, she began to experience panic attacks when project deadlines loomed closer. She consulted their family physician, who identified her symptoms as anxiety and pre-scribed an antianxiety medication to be used as needed, but Mandy found the medication to be ineffective in preventing or ameliorating panic attacks. She found the panic symptoms to be unbearable and began missing work, eventually quitting before she was fired. Within several months, her avoidance had spread such that it had become diffi-cult for her to drive far from home. As she stayed closer to home, Mark took over most of the shopping and accompanied her on almost all of her outings, even holding her arm when they went to the mall. If her anxiety increased, they immediately returned home. Her self-esteem and sense of efficacy plummeted. Her sense of failure and embarrass-ment professionally made her reluctant to interact with friends, and she soon became avoidant of social interactions. Although Mark resented the increased financial burden and loss of pleasure from his new role of sole breadwinner, his relaxed manner prevented him from asserting himself in the face of Mandy's strong personality. He noted that his dis-agreements with Mandy appeared to worsen her anxiety, which left him with guilt feelings.

Mandy and Mark's couple therapist provided them with a concep-tualization and treatment plan that emphasized two broad domains. First, the couple was experiencing relationship difficulties that were common to many young couples. These included communication prob-lems, difficulty with negotiating differences in individual styles and pri-orities, complex decisions such as whether to begin a family, and stress from living on restricted earnings. Second, the therapist noted how Mandy's panic and agoraphobia contributed to relationship difficulties by restricting their financial options, social interactions, and role re-sponsibilities. Furthermore, the therapist discussed the ways in which agoraphobia is reinforced by avoidance and how the couple's interac-tion patterns and division of responsibilities inadvertently helped to maintain the avoidance. The therapist was careful not to blame Mandy for the relationship difficulties. Instead, the therapist noted how both individuals in a couple often have specific vulnerabilities that affect their relationship, and a major goal in a close relationship is for part-ners to work effectively to support each other, address such vulnerabili-ties, and proceed in a manner that is adaptive for both individuals and the relationship.

Communication skills training served as an important first step in treatment because it facilitated discussions about general relationship issues and Mandy's panic and agoraphobia. Also, in order not to em-phasize Mandy's anxiety as the central focus of couple therapy, the therapist initially focused upon dyadic concerns not central to anxiety. Using interventions common to cognitive-behavioral couple therapy (Baucom & Epstein, 1990; Epstein & Baucom, 2002), the therapist helped Mandy and Mark learn to express their thoughts and feelings in a constructive manner. Mark learned to express negative feelings about the relationship and some aspects of Mandy's behavior. For Mandy, the emphasis was on helping her listen to Mark's perspective and accept their differences. In addition, the therapist taught the couple decision-making or problem-solving strategies that they could apply to a wide range of concerns in their relationship.

Because many of the couple's concerns were related to Mandy's anxiety, the therapy focused on helping them work together to lessen her panic and agoraphobia. The therapist began by explaining the cycle of physiological arousal, anxiety, catastrophic attributions, and avoidance. As Mandy experienced more arousal, she interpreted anxiety as a dangerous sign that she was going crazy or having a heart attack. As a result, she had developed avoidance strategies to minimize the physiological arousal or other anticipated negative consequences. The therapist noted that Mandy's occasional use of antianxiety medication also might be serving as a means of avoiding aversive symptoms, and in consultation with her physician the therapist recommended that she discontinue it. The treatment then involved *interoceptive exposure* in which the therapist and couple worked together to generate high levels of physiological arousal for Mandy to tolerate rather than avoid. In the therapy sessions, the therapist demonstrated to the couple how to generate arousal by such strategies as spinning in a chair, hyperventilating, breathing through a small straw, and so forth (Craske, Barlow, & Meadows, 2000). Both Mark and Mandy experienced these interoceptive exercises to give Mark an understanding of Mandy's panic. Then, during the sessions, Mark led Mandy though the exercises, encouraging her to experience the arousal and reinforcing her progress. For homework, the couple practiced these exercises several times a week, with Mark coaching Mandy to accept her arousal.

As Mandy became less threatened by symptoms of physiological arousal, the therapy progressed to *partner-assisted in vivo exposure* to help Mandy approach anxiety-provoking situations in the outside world. First, with Mark's input, Mandy selected three domains where she wanted to decrease her avoidance: driving her car by herself; shopping in the mall and in grocery stores without assistance; and engaging in social interactions with friends and groups away from home. For each of these three domains, the couple developed an exposure hierarchy for the specific situations that Mandy would confront. For example, with regard to shopping, a minimally anxiety-provoking setting for Mandy was to stand just inside the front of the local hardware store within easy view of the door and windows until her anxiety decreased. Near the top of her hierarchy was shopping in a crowded mall by herself while Mark was out of town.

In this partner-assisted strategy, Mark accompanied Mandy on her early exposure outings. Mark participated with Mandy in four stages of these exposure outings: preparing for a stressor prior to the outing, confronting the stressor, coping with feelings of being overwhelmed by the stressor, and evaluating the exposure experience after it was completed. The couple prepared for the day's exposure by clarifying the exercise, discussing each person's feelings about it, and anticipating potential difficulties during the exposure. While confronting the stressor, Mandy was encouraged to express her feelings to Mark rather than avoiding unpleasant feelings. His role was to listen, be empathic, compliment her for handling the situation, and help her remain focused on her feelings rather than distracting her. If Mandy and Mark felt that she needed to remove herself from the setting, they were to take a brief timeout rather than returning home, and then resume the exposure. After returning home, the couple was to discuss the exposure outing, describe their reactions to the experience, provide reinforcement for each other's efforts, and offer suggestions for changes in future outings. To develop Mandy's autonomy in approaching the outside world, Mark's participation in the exposure outings was decreased. Mandy could choose to discuss her planned exposure outings with Mark if she wished, and his role was to continue complimenting her for her efforts and her problem-solving skills. Thus, she continued to feel his support while she learned to confront anxiety-provoking situations alone.

Over 3 months, Mandy made considerable progress in all three domains. Perhaps the greatest challenge that the couple experienced was Mark's difficulty in seeing Mandy experience high levels of anxiety. On several occasions during their exposure outings together, he attempted to distract her, comfort her, and agreed when she suggested that they return home prematurely. The therapist provided strong encouragement and education to help Mark recognize that by providing immediate relief, he was helping to maintain Mandy's anxiety on a long-term basis.

As Mandy made progress in her exposure outings, treatment shifted to disorder-specific interventions to help the couple restructure aspects of their relationship focal to agoraphobia. The couple renegotiated chores and responsibilities, such that continued exposure would be built into Mandy's natural daily activities. She agreed to take on outside responsibilities, such as grocery shopping, running errands, and car maintenance. In order to prevent the redistribution of labor from feeling like a punishment to Mandy, the couple negotiated how Mark would assume increased household responsibilities, such as doing the laundry, cleaning up around the house, and mowing the lawn. As a result, the couple had a sense that they both were contributing to the necessary routine maintenance tasks, with Mandy increasing her interaction outside of the home and Mark contributing more within the home.

Mandy and Mark agreed that his support for her during moments of anxiety demonstrated his love and caring, providing a basis of closeness and intimacy for them. Because Mark was being taught not to lower Mandy's anxiety and to encourage her to go on outings by herself, the couple needed to develop and enhance alternative ways of caring for each other that did not focus on her symptoms. They decided to go out on a date together each week, they discussed their enjoyment of sitting together in front of the television, and they planned to show more physical affection to each other.

Over time, the couple renegotiated their roles and responsibilities in a way that maximized Mandy's progress, developed ways of showing love and concern that did not focus on her anxiety, and initiated a social life with friends. The therapist then discussed how relationship distress can be a general stressor that might exacerbate Mandy's anxiety symptoms. Therefore, the couple and therapist focused next on additional areas of concern in their relationship. For example, the couple returned to the issue of whether to have children, and if so, when. Both Mark and Mandy felt better about her ability to assume the role of mother, but they agreed that they wanted her to stay home while the children were young. In order to consolidate her treatment gains, the couple decided to postpone having children while Mandy continued to become more involved in outside activities. Because Mandy had more self-confidence, her returning to work was a possibility. Having found the procedures of an exposure hierarchy valuable, they decided that Mandy initially would seek a part-time job that was not too demanding. As she became comfortable with this involvement, she would consider returning to full-time work in her professional area. The therapist gave the couple positive feedback about their use of good communication and decision-making skills in resolving this important relationship issue. Subsequently, the therapist coached them in doing the same with other areas in which conflicts had the potential to increase tension and possibly fuel Mandy's anxiety.

After 6 months of weekly sessions, the sessions were spaced out so that the couple could take increased responsibility for their progress. Often people with anxiety difficulties seek safety signals in their lives, and it was important that the couple not become inappropriately dependent on the therapist in helping address Mandy's anxiety. By the time of termination 3 months later, the couple had made considerable progress in addressing general relationship concerns and decreasing Mandy's panic and agoraphobia. The couple was still aware that there were times when Mandy felt anxious and preferred to avoid stressful situations. They became effective at discussing these feelings and desires openly, acknowledging the importance of pushing forward in spite of the anxiety. Consequently, they learned to minimize the anxiety and to cope with it effectively when it did occur.

Adapting Treatment to Other Anxiety Disorders

The major components of the treatment plans for a broad range of anxiety disorders are forms of exposure and response prevention with some cognitive restructuring, and in some cases, training in anxiety management strategies such as relaxation (Barlow, 2002; Suinn, 1990). Within this overall plan, the interventions for each anxiety disorder are tailored to address the particular types of symptoms that are predominant, based on empirical evidence of their efficacy. For example, the case study illustrated how panic disorder with agoraphobia requires special attention to the reengagement of the agoraphobic with the outside world in an autonomous fashion, and the individual's increased ability to tolerate anxiety symptoms. Couple therapists may apply these principles in treating the individual's anxiety within the couple context in three ways: partner-assisted interventions, disorder-specific interventions, and general couple therapy. Below are some additional treatment considerations for each anxiety disorder that couple therapists may wish to consider in implementing their treatment plans.

Obsessive–Compulsive Disorder

The hallmark of OCD is the presence of irrational obsessions followed by ritualistic compulsions. Although the content of obsessions and compulsions vary, they commonly fall into a few major categories: contamination fears, followed by washing rituals; fears of harming oneself and others or being harmed, followed by checking rituals; and fears of wasting objects, followed by hoarding behaviors. These thoughts and behaviors follow the same pattern as in other anxiety disorders: Obsessions create anxiety, which leads to ritualistic avoidance behaviors to escape the anxiety.

OCD requires special consideration by couple therapists because the ritualistic avoidance behaviors are active rather than passive. Because rituals are noticeable to the partner, they frequently create conflict or alter the couple's relationship. At times, the partner might feel pressured to participate in rituals. Refusing to participate can lead to arguments as the individual with OCD pushes the other person to help relieve anxiety. For example, one couple argued about the husband's refusal to keep his belongings in a four 4 × 4 foot "contamination zone" in the house. When he left his belongings in other areas of the house, his wife became angry and anxious, engaging in elaborate cleaning rituals to relieve her anxiety. A partner may participate in rituals to relieve the other person's anxiety or avoid conflict, only to find that doing so restricts the couple's life. Furthermore, this symptom–system fit only serves to reinforce the person's OCD symptoms, leading to frustration and possible resentment if the partner does not see improvement in the individual's anxiety and rituals. Thus, a wife participated in her husband's ritual of extensively checking whether their stove and all other appliances were off or unplugged before they could leave the house, because she believed that he would be reassured that his fears of fire danger were unfounded. However, the reduction in anxiety that resulted from the checking actually reinforced the ritual, and the wife soon became resentful as the time spent in checking usually made the couple late for appointments and social engagements.

Even when an individual with OCD does not ask the partner to participate in rituals, conflict can ensue as the individual with OCD appears to doubt the partner's competency in certain tasks. For example, one wife interpreted her husband's ritualistic cleaning of the kitchen after she had cleaned it as a sign that he did not believe she was capable of performing this task. Because she did not understand the function of the cleaning in reducing his anxiety, she became hurt and angry at his lack of trust in her abilities. When she expressed her upset, the tension in the couple's relationship increased her husband's anxiety and ritualistic behavior.

Obsessions also can elicit negative reactions from partners. The intensity of obsessions leads some people with OCD to seek constant reassurance from others that their fears will not materialize, and the partner may grow weary of comforting him or her. For example, one wife repeatedly got out of bed at night to check to see if the couple's infant was breathing, in spite of the fact that the baby apparently was in good health. She was exhausted from the chronic lack of sleep, so she increasingly woke her husband and asked that he check the baby, and asked him for reassurance that the baby was going to survive the night. Her husband repeatedly tried to reassure her that her fears were unrealistic, but it was ineffective, and he became frustrated and critical of her.   In addition, the nonanxious partner might interpret irrational fears as indications that the other person is "going crazy" or is "out of control." Over time, the partner might lose respect for the person with OCD, and the partner's overt criticism of the anxious individual may increase the anxiety symptoms and obsessional thinking.

Partner-assisted and disorder-specific interventions for OCD differ from other anxiety disorders in their focus on obsessions and compulsions. Providing psychoeducation to the couple about the nature of obsessions and compulsions may alleviate a number of presenting concerns, including the nonanxious partner's interpretations that the other person doubts his or her abilities or is "losing their mind." The therapist and couple then should examine the ways in which the couple has adapted to and reinforced compulsions, in order to develop situations for exposure and response prevention. In particular, it is important for the partner not to participate in rituals or provide reassurance about the other person's fears, while encouraging the person to practice tolerating anxiety symptoms. In order to decrease conflict that may result from the anxious partner's continued requests for reassurance or participation in rituals, partners are instructed to empathize with the person's anxiety but to remind him or her gently about the treatment plan. For example, a wife might say, "I appreciate that you are scared that the stove might be on. I understand that you would like me to check to relieve your fear, but we agreed that it is best for you to learn to cope with the anxiety and confront your fear."

Although it can be tempting for a nonanxious partner to debate the logic of the obsessive thinking of an OCD individual, the couple therapist should intervene to eliminate such generally ineffective responses that actually may increase the person's anxiety. For example, when one woman's husband argued that her repeated requests to check on their sleeping baby was irrational, the woman became more concerned that her husband was blasé about dangers of sudden infant death syndrome, and she felt more responsible for monitoring the baby's well-being. The couple's therapist coached the husband in expressing empathy for his wife's distress and then reminding her of the importance of engaging in response prevention procedures.

Because general distress in a couple's relationship may increase the OCD individual's overall tension level, it can be helpful to integrate aspects of general couple therapy with partner-assisted or disorder-specific interventions. Attending to general couple issues also reduces the focus on the anxious individual as the "identified patient." Because individuals with OCD commonly evaluate themselves negatively for ritualistic behaviors that they realize are unusual (e.g., "I know it is abnormal to keep washing my hands, but I can't stop myself from doing it"), it can be helpful to their self-esteem if the therapist engages both members of the couple in resolving relationship issues for which neither person is solely responsible.

Generalized Anxiety Disorder

Individuals with GAD may appear similar to those with OCD in that they frequently worry about feared consequences and frequently seek reassurance from partners. However, GAD differs from OCD in that people worry excessively about everyday concerns in various domains of life. Whereas obsessions in OCD may appear bizarre or irrational, worries in GAD resemble mundane concerns that any person would have, although the extent of the worry in GAD exceeds the level experienced by the average person. People with GAD frequently make probabilistic predictions that the worst outcome will occur or view every problem as a catastrophe. Nevertheless, individuals with GAD may be construed (by themselves and others) as "worrywarts" or "high-stress" people, without recognition that their level of worry constitutes a psychological disorder.

Some couples seek therapy because there is pervasive tension in the household, without recognizing that one person's excessive worrying is a salient factor in creating this atmosphere. The nonanxious partner may resent being expected to remain calm and provide most of the comfort, as the anxious partner may be too focused on worries to provide support. Eventually the nonanxious partner may refuse to provide reassurance out of frustration that the other's anxiety does not decrease, or exasperation at the anxious partner's "melodrama." Indeed, many partners view the individual's worry as disproportionate, childish, and immature. Finally, individuals with GAD often experience somatic symptoms, including frequent headaches, gastrointestinal upset, muscle aches, and so forth, and their partners commonly become frustrated by the individuals' frequent complaints of not feeling good physically. Combined with the pervasive worry, somatic symptoms are likely to interfere with emotional and sexual intimacy in some couples.

Couple-based interventions can help in educating both partners about the nature of worry and in identifying couples' interaction patterns that maintain or exacerbate anxiety. Psychoeducation would highlight the interplay between thoughts and feelings in GAD. Unlike other anxiety disorders in which anxious thoughts lead to avoidance behaviors that temporarily reduce anxious feelings, worrying in GAD serves as both a trigger and an escape from anxiety. Individuals often begin worrying about one topic, become physiologically aroused, and shift their thoughts to another topic of worry as a distraction from the initial source of anxiety. Following the principles of exposure and response prevention, Brown et al. (2001) suggest a worry exposure treatment for people with GAD, in which they focus on one worry topic while they imagine the worst possible feared outcome. After spending 25 to 30 minutes on the thoughts and images of the worry, clients should habituate to the topic and experience minimal feelings of anxiety. After the exposure, clients apply cognitive restructuring to the worry by generating alternatives to the worst possible outcomes. The response prevention consists of preventing themselves from shifting to a new topic of worry or engaging in worry behaviors such as phone calls to ensure people's safety. The nonanxious partner can assist in this treatment in ways similar to interventions with other anxiety disorders, by encouraging the anxious individual to experience the anxiety until it decreases. In addition, the nonanxious partner should refrain from providing reassurance, while providing empathy for the other person's feelings rather than discounting or criticizing them. If the individual with GAD is unable to resist the urge to seek reassurance, the therapist can instruct him or her to write down the questions that normally would be directed to the partner and to ask the therapist about them at the next session. This helps to break the cycle in which the partner serves in the role of comforter. As with other anxiety disorders, it is important that the partner not alter his or her lifestyle or the couple's relationship in significant ways to alleviate the anxiety. If this has already occurred, the couple should evaluate how they have adapted their life to lessen the individual's worry and anxiety symptoms, and identify how they can make changes to promote exposure.

Other efficacious techniques for GAD include cognitive restructuring and relaxation training. In cognitive restructuring, the therapist challenges the anxious individual's cognitive errors of negative probabilistic predictions and catastrophic thinking, and then coaches the nonanxious partner in assisting the GAD individual in challenging his or her negative cognitions. One caveat to involving the partner in this type of treatment is to ensure that the partner can perform reality-testing interventions in a gentle, supportive way. Addressing somatic arousal through relaxation training doubles as a way to incorporate positive activities in the couple's relationship, as the couple may share massages, exercising, or other relaxing activities. It is important for the therapist to emphasize that relaxation strategies are not intended as a means for avoiding worry (which needs to be faced directly through exposure), but rather to reduce the somatic arousal that distracts the individual from positive life experiences. Because unpleasant somatic symptoms can interfere with a couple's intimacy, especially if the anxious individual worries about the symptoms and complains about them to the partner, it can be helpful to substitute pleasant shared relaxation experiences.

Phobias

Unlike more pervasive disorders like OCD, GAD, and panic disorder with agoraphobia, simple and social phobias (such as public speaking anxiety) might not impact a couple's relationship directly. Therapists should evaluate the extent to which any symptom–system fit has arisen concerning fears about situations or objects such as heights, insects, or public speaking. To the extent the nonanxious partner has participated in avoidance behaviors (e.g., ridding the home of any insects), the therapist should work with the couple to alter the relationship's reinforcement of avoidance. In addition, the therapist might employ a partner-assisted intervention using an exposure hierarchy to assist the individual in conquering his or her phobia. However, in other cases, a person's phobic fear is well circumscribed and does not affect the couple's relationship, nor is it reinforced by the couple's interaction patterns. In such cases, if the couple is experiencing distress in other areas of their relationship, they may benefit from couple therapy for those independent problems, with the phobic individual seeking a separate treatment for the anxiety disorder.

In contrast, some individuals' phobias may restrict the couple's life to such an extent that they need to address the problem in couple therapy. For example, couples in which one person's social phobia extends to outings with friends may have a limited social life. The partner may inadvertently reinforce avoidance by reducing social interactions with friends and acquaintances or only going to certain social settings that the anxious person considers safe. In contrast, some nonanxious partners attempt to motivate the anxious individual to attend social gatherings, either through criticism and goading or by trying to reassure the person that the other people will like him or her. In either case, the therapist can help the partner understand how these strategies tend to backfire (feedback from the anxious individual may demonstrate the negative impact). For example, criticism may lower the anxious individual's self-confidence and increase his or her fear of behaving incompetently when forced to interact with other people. Besides shifting such patterns in a disorder-specific intervention, the therapist may suggest partner-assisted exposure outings. A key aspect of partner-assisted interventions for social phobia is to phase the partner out of the exercise so that the anxious partners eventually confront his or her fears about other people's evaluations without relying on the perceived safety of the partner's presence.

Finally, couples may present with conflicts about general couple issues, only to find that the root of the problem is one person's phobia. For example, an individual might have quit a job because of a fear of taking public transportation. Whereas the couple may argue about the loss of income, the treatment might need to address the anxious individual's fears. As in any assessment for couple therapy, clinicians should examine whether an individual's psychopathology is contributing to relationship distress.

Conclusions

Regardless of the particular anxiety disorder, couple-based interventions may involve components of partner-assisted, disorder-specific, or general couple therapy approaches. Modeled after exposure and response prevention, the common denominators across disorders are the confrontation of anxiety-provoking stimuli, habituation to feelings of anxiety, and prevention of avoidance responses. Avoidance responses come in many forms, with some involving staying away from feared objects and situations (as in phobias), and others involving increases in activities (e.g., ruminative worrying in GAD and compulsive checking in OCD) that temporarily help the person stave off anxiety. Exposure and response prevention procedures reduce avoidance responses and increase the individual's ability to tolerate anxiety symptoms. Cognitive interventions involving psychoeducation for both members of the couple and cognitive restructuring for anxiety-related thought processes also are common elements of treatment. The particular symptoms of each disorder will determine the content of the exposure and response prevention, as well as the types of interventions needed to modify the way in which anxiety interacts with couple functioning. For panic disorder with agoraphobia, couples may need assistance with breaking accommodation patterns and reconnecting with the outside world. For OCD, couple-based interventions will focus on reducing partners' participation in rituals and reassurance-seeking. In GAD, frequent worrying may create a general negative atmosphere unrecognized by the couple as an anxiety disorder, and interventions focus on educating both partners about anxiety, reducing the nonanxious individual's criticism or attempts to convince the anxious person that there is no basis for worry, and coaching the nonanxious partner in encouraging "worry exposure" for the anxious individual. Phobias may restrict particular domains of the couple's lives or may have little impact on couple functioning. When a phobia is restrictive, the nonanxious partner can be involved in partner-assisted and disorder-specific interventions to support exposure and cognitive restructuring, as well as to reduce couple interactions that maintain avoidance. When a phobia has minimal impact on couple functioning, the anxious individual can be referred for individual treatment, while any couple issues that are independent of the anxiety disorder can be addressed with general couple therapy. Involvement of the nonanxious partner in specific treatments for anxiety and in treatment of other sources of overall relationship distress has great potential to facilitate improvement in anxiety disorders.

THE MANY FACES OF ANXIETY

In addition to assisting couples with Axis I anxiety disorders, clinicians often work with couples in which one or both partners experience notable subclinical anxiety that needs to be addressed in the couple's treatment. The general psychological principle of exposure for anxiety is not dependent on specific diagnostic criteria. Instead, a great deal of psychotherapy is predicated on the principle that individuals need to confront uncomfortable issues, feelings, memories, and behavioral circumstances that they have avoided. In most instances with exposure, they experience that the anticipated negative consequences do not occur or are not as aversive as anticipated.

In working with couples in which one member experiences high levels of anxiety that do not meet the full criteria for an anxiety disorder diagnosis, we explain that manifestations of anxiety result from viewing certain aspects of the world as dangerous. As a result, the couple is advised to confront situations that create anxiety so that their world does not become more constricted because of the avoidance. A major decision point for the therapist is whether to structure such interventions in a way that involves specific exposure outings on a regular basis as described previously, or whether to develop more general, informal strategies to confront anxiety-provoking situations while minimizing avoidance. For example, in the latter approach, one person might have significant anxiety about social encounters, inappropriately assuming that other individuals will focus on evaluating that person's behavior. The couple can make a joint decision that they will counteract the individual's social anxiety by incorporating various social outings into their life, both accepting invitations from others and inviting people to their home.

Not only are there individuals who demonstrate anxiety below the threshold for Axis I diagnosis, there are also individuals with Axis II diagnoses who experience significant anxiety. In particular, persons with a Cluster C diagnosis of avoidant, dependent, or obsessive–compulsive personality disorder often are fearful. Inherent in the DSM-IV diagnosis of a personality disorder is an "enduring pattern of inner experience and behavior that deviates markedly from the expectations of the individual's culture, is pervasive and inflexible, and has an onset in adolescence or early adulthood, is stable over time, and leads to distress or impairment" (American Psychiatric Association, 1994, p. 629).

Although the specific interventions must be altered to address the long-term maladaptive patterns in personality disorders, we will briefly describe treatment of persons with obsessive–compulsive personality disorders (OCPD) as an example. Individuals with OCPD are preoccupied with orderliness, perfectionism, and mental and interpersonal control. When these areas are disrupted, the individual typically experiences significant distress and anxiety. The partner with OCPD might derive a sense of control and calmness by taking charge of decision making or demanding that tasks be performed in a certain way. However, these demands may limit the person's life or create resentment in his or her partner. In therapy, the couple can be coached in altering rigid adherence to these standards, with the anticipated goal that the individual with OCPD sees that horrible consequences do not result. For example, the other partner might take responsibility for planning the details of the family vacation, with both people accepting that it might not be perfect or done in a manner that the obsessive individual would have selected. In other cases, shifting the standards for orderliness and cleanliness would provide an ongoing exposure for the compulsive individual.

CONCLUSIONS

In summary, working with couples in which one person experiences significant anxiety, whether as part of an Axis I anxiety disorder or not, involves a general set of principles. The guiding principle is that avoidance and rigid patterns of behavior develop as a way to avoid distress and anxiety. However, such strategies have the unfortunate consequence of limiting the couple's options and decreasing their overall quality of life. The most general treatment strategy for such couples is to integrate exposure to the feared situation into interventions with the couple. As the individual makes progress and becomes less avoidant, the couple therapist works with the couple to maintain the individual's progress and to take advantage of the new opportunities for relating that become available to the couple. The couple therapist helps the couple strive to understand each other's vulnerabilities, to work together to overcome these difficulties, and to cope with ongoing vulnerabilities.

REFERENCES

American Psychiatric Association (1994). *Diagnostic and statistical manual of mental disorder* (4th ed.). Washington, DC: Author.

Arnow, B. A., Taylor, C. B., Agras, W. S., & Telch, M. J. (1985). Enhancing agoraphobia treatment by changing couple communication patterns. *Behavior Therapy, 16,* 452–467.

Arrindell, W. A., Emmelkamp, P. M. G., & Sanderman, R. (1986). Marital quality and general life adjustment in relation to treatment outcome in agoraphobia. *Advances in Behavior Research and Therapy, 8,* 139–185.

Barlow, D. H. (2002). *Anxiety and its disorders: The nature and treatment of anxiety and panic* (2nd ed.). New York: Guilford Press.

Barlow, D. H., O'Brien, G. T., & Last, C. G. (1984). Couples treatment of agoraphobia. *Behavior Therapy, 15,* 41–58.

Baucom, D. H., & Epstein, N. (1990). *Cognitive behavioral marital therapy.* New York: Brunner/Mazel.

Baucom, D. H., Shoham, V., Mueser, K. T., Daiuto, A. D., & Stickle, T. R. (1998). Empirically supported couple and family interventions for marital distress and adult mental health problems. *Journal of Consulting and Clinical Psychology, 66,* 53–88.

Bernstein, D. A., & Borkovec, T. D. (1973). *Progressive relaxation training.* Champaign, IL: Research Press.

Brown, T. A., O'Leary, T. A., & Barlow, D. H. (2001). Generalized anxiety disorder. In D. H. Barlow (Ed.), *Clinical handbook of psychological disorders* (3rd ed., pp. 154–208). New York: Guilford Press.

Calvocoressi, L., Lewis, B., Harris, M., Trufan, S. J., Goodman, W. K., McDougle, C. J., & Price, L. H. (1995). Family accommodation in obsessive–compulsive disorder. *American Journal of Psychiatry, 152*(3), 441–443.

Coyne, J. C., Kessler, R. C., Tal, M., Turnbull, J., Wortman, C. B., & Greden, J. F. (1987). Living with a depressed person. *Journal of Consulting and Clinical Psychology, 55,* 347–352.

Craske, M. G., & Barlow, D. H. (2001). Panic disorder and agoraphobia. In D. H. Barlow (Ed.), *Clinical handbook of psychological disorders* (3rd ed., pp. 1–59). New York: Guilford Press.

Craske, M. G., Barlow, D. H., & Meadows (2000). *Mastery of your anxiety and panic: Therapist guide for anxiety, panic, and agoraphobia* (3rd ed.). San Antonio, TX: Graywind Psychological Corporation.

Daiuto, A. D., Baucom, D. H., Epstein, N., & Dutton, S. S. (1998). The application of behavioral couples therapy to the assessment and treatment of agoraphobia: Implications of empirical research. *Clinical Psychology Review, 18*(6), 663–687.

DeRubeis, R. J., & Crits-Cristoph, P. (1998). Empirically supported individual and group psychological treatments for adult mental disorders. *Journal of Consulting and Clinical Psychology, 66,* 37–52.

Durham, R. C., Allan, T., & Hackett, C. A. (1997). On predicting improvement and relapse in generalized anxiety disorder following psychotherapy. *British Journal of Clinical Psychology, 36*(1), 101–119.

Emmelkamp, P. M. G., de Haan, E., & Hoodguin, C. A. L. (1990). Marital adjustment and obsessive–compulsive disorder. *British Journal of Psychiatry, 156,* 55–60.

Emmelkamp, P. M. G., Van Dyck, R., Bitter, M., Heins, R., Onstein, E. J., & Eisen, B. (1992). Spouse-aided therapy with agoraphobics. *British Journal of Psychiatry, 160,* 51–56.

Epstein, N., & Baucom D. H. (2002). *Enhanced cognitive-behavioral therapy for couples: A contextual approach.* Washington, DC: American Psychological Association.

Foa, E. B., & Franklin, M. E. (2001). Obsessive–compulsive disorder. In D. H. Barlow (Ed.), *Clinical handbook of psychological disorders* (3rd ed., pp. 209–263). New York: Guilford Press.

Friedman, M. (1990). Interrelationships between biological mechanisms and pharmacotherapy of posttraumatic stress disorder. In M. E. Wolf & A. D. Mosnaim (Eds.), *Posttraumatic stress disorder: etiology, phenomenology, and treatment* (pp. 205–225). Washington, DC: American Psychiatric Press.

Fry, W. F. (1962). The marital context of an anxiety syndrome. *Family Process, 1*(2), 245–252.

Goldstein, A., & Chambless, D. (1978). A reanalysis of agoraphobia. *Behavior Therapy, 9,* 47–59.

Kessler, R. C. McGonagle, K. A., Zhao, S., Nelson,C. B., Hughes, M., Eshleman, S., Wittchen, H. U., & Kendler, K. S. (1994). Lifetime and 12-month prevalence of DSM-III-R psychiatric disorders in the United States: Results from the National Comorbidity Survey. *Archives of General Psychiarty, 51,* 8–19.

McLeod, J. (1994). Anxiety disorders and marital quality. *Journal of Abnormal Psychology, 103*(4), 767–776.

Monteiro, W., Marks, I. M., & Ramm, E. (1985). Marital adjustment and treatment outcome in agoraphobia. *British Journal of Psychiatry, 146,* 383–390.

Rankin-Esquer, L. A., Burnett, C. K., Baucom, D. H., & Epstein, N. (1997). Autonomy and relatedness in marital functioning. *Journal of Marital and Family Therapy, 23*(2), 175–190.

Regier, D. A., Narrow, W. E., & Rae, D. S. (1990). The epidemiology of anxiety disorders: The Epidemiologic Catchment Area (ECA) experience. *Journal of Psychiatric Research, 24,* 3–14.

Rohrbaugh, M., Shoham, V., Spungen, C., & Steinglass, P. (1985). Family systems therapy in practice: A systemic couples therapy for problem drinking. In B. M. Bongar & L. E. Beutler (Eds.), *Comprehensive textbook of psychotherapy: Theory and practice* (pp. 228–253). New York: Oxford University Press.

Steketee, G. (1997). Disability and family burden in obsessive–compulsive disorder. *Canadian Journal of Psychiatry, 42*(9), 919–928.

Suinn, R. M. (1990). *Anxiety management training: A behavior therapy.* New York: Plenum.

Whisman, M. A. (1999). Marital dissatisfaction and psychiatric disorders: Results from the National Comorbidity Survey. *Journal of Abnormal Psychology, 108*(4), 701–706.

CHAPTER 4

Depression

STEVEN R. H. BEACH
MAYA GUPTA

Unipolar depressive disorders are among the most prevalent of Axis I mental disorders, and, as such, are likely to be encountered by the couple therapist at some point in his or her career. These disorders represent far more than an occasional complication or variation in working with couples. Depression is a major public health problem with tremendous social, familial, and economic costs that no clinician can ignore, and the couple therapist may be in a privileged position to help ameliorate both depression and its costs. In this chapter, we hope to provide a basic understanding of depression, its interaction with couple conflict, and its treatment in couple therapy.

INTRODUCTION TO DEPRESSION

One commonly encountered form of depression, and the one about which the most has been written to date, is major depressive disorder. Its main building blocks are the cognitive, affective, and behavioral symptoms that constitute a major depressive episode: at least 2 weeks of depressed mood, a loss of interest or pleasure in activities, marked change in weight or appetite, insomnia or hypersomnia, psychomotor agitation or retardation visible to others, fatigue or loss of energy, indecisiveness, difficulty concentrating, feelings of worthlessness or guilt, or thoughts of death/suicide (American Psychiatric Association, 2000). Either depressed mood or anhedonia, along with four other symptoms, must be present to qualify for the diagnosis. Major depression is often recurrent or chronic, but may also be limited to a single episode.

Dysthymia, on the other hand, requires that symptoms persist for the greater part of at least 2 years, with any symptom-free intervals lasting no longer than 2 months. Though its symptoms are similar to those of major depressive disorder, fewer symptoms (two) are required to be present to meet DSM-IV diagnostic criteria (American Psychiatric Association, 2000); hence its primary differences from major depression are in intensity and duration.

At the least severe end of the spectrum, finally, falls dysphoria—affective distress that does not meet criteria for major depression or dysthymia but does confer an elevated risk for future clinical depression (Horwath, Johnson, Klerman, & Weissman, 1992). Recent research by Ruscio and Ruscio (2000) supports the view that depression may be distributed as a continuous, rather than as a dichotomous, variable. This concept implies that patterns observed at any given level of symptomatology may have implications for other levels of symptomatology, whether in clinical or subclinical range. For example, the discovery of an association between major depression and couple distress might suggest that an association between dysphoria and couple distress exists also. However, it is important—particularly in the context of this chapter—to note that, although such similarities have been documented, the strength of the association between a couple's relationship discord and depression may be greater when the focus is on major depression rather than on subclinical dysphoria (Whisman, 2001).

PREVALENCE ESTIMATES

Prevalence in the General Population

Data from the National Comorbidity Survey estimate the lifetime prevalence of major depression at approximately 8.3% for cases involving five to six symptoms and 7.5% for severe cases involving seven to nine symptoms (Kessler, Zhao, Blazer, & Swartz, 1997). Recent surveys estimate the lifetime prevalence of dysthymia to be 4–5% (e.g., Katon & Schulberg, 1992; Szadoczky, Rihmer, Papp, & Fueredi, 2000). Finally, although dysphoria has not been defined precisely enough to permit gathering precise prevalence data, it appears to be relatively common.

Prevalence in Specific Clinical Populations

Depression, like other mood disorders, has high rates of comorbidity with other psychiatric disorders. With regard to other Axis I disorders, this comorbidity is created, in part, as an artifact of definitions: The presence of a mood episode is a prerequisite for schizoaffective disorder, and affective distress is part of the diagnostic criteria for, or in the clinical description of, other disorders. Nonetheless, the data are noteworthy: Comorbidity between panic disorder and major depression may be 30–70%, a high figure even at the conservative end (Lesser, Rubin, Pecknold, & Rifkin, 1988), and rates of comorbidity with other anxiety disorders such as social phobia and generalized anxiety disorder (GAD) are also high. Comorbidity between depression and substance use disorders is equally well documented. Miller, Klamen, Hoffmann, and Flaherty (1996) found that 44% of alcohol/drug patients had a history of major depression. With regard to personality disorders, a meta-analysis by Corruble, Ginestet, and Guelfi (1996) found that 20–50% of inpatients with major depressive disorder, and 50–85% of outpatients, met criteria for a concurrent personality disorder; Cluster B disorders were prominent.

There is also a great deal of overlap between the mood disorders themselves. Dysthymia may often co-occur with episodes of major depressive disorder, resulting in "double depression"; affective distress is a component of the bipolar disorders (though dual diagnosis is precluded by definition); and residual depressive symptomatology is common during periods of remission from major depression. As this brief overview suggests, it may be relatively uncommon to find individuals who meet criteria for major depressive disorder without meeting criteria for any other lifetime diagnoses.

COUPLE DISCORD AND DEPRESSION

Comorbidity of Depression with Couple Distress

We begin our discussion of depression in the context of couple distress with two caveats. First, there may or may not be differences between married couples and unmarried cohabiting couples, but most data thus far have been collected on married partners. Second, research on same-sex couples has lagged far behind research on male–female couples. Accordingly, extrapolation to cohabiting or same-sex populations is somewhat risky.

However, among the heterosexual and married couples that dominate the existing distress literature, depression appears to be a relatively common phenomenon, with perhaps as many as 50% of distressed couples having one partner with substantial depressive symptomatology. When examined longitudinally, individuals in distressed marriages were at over double the risk for onset of a new episode of major depression a year later (Whisman & Bruce, 1999).

Conversely, depressed women report marital conflict at approximately the rate of 50% (Weissman, 1987), and the average depressed person scores in the distressed range of the Dyadic Adjustment Scale (Whisman, 2001). It is important to note, however, that not all depressed persons are dissatisfied with their relationships—and those who are not dissatisfied show less response to behavioral couple therapy (Jacobson, Dobson, Fruzzetti, Schmaling, & Salusky, 1991).

How strongly, then, may we claim an overall link between couple distress and depression? In a quantitative and exhaustive review of the marital literature, Whisman (2001) found that, across 26 cross-sectional studies, marital quality was negatively associated with depressive symptomatology for both women ($r = -.42$) and men ($r = -.37$), indicating a significant, albeit small gender difference. Although not directly comparable due to methodological differences, across 10 studies using diagnosed patient populations, the magnitude of this association was somewhat stronger for both women and men ($r = -.66$).

Likewise, couples' relationship distress appears to be associated with poorer outcome in response to treatment as usual. Hooley and Teasdale (1989) found that marital discord predicted 9-month relapse among formerly hospitalized depressed inpatients. Similar effects have been reported for percentage improvement in depression in response to treatment for both outpatient and inpatient settings among those persons remaining in "dysfunctional relationships" and are summarized by Whisman (2001).

Impact of Depression upon the Relationship

Depression seems particularly amenable to couple therapy because so many of the presumed mechanisms and consequences of this disorder are interpersonal. For example, Coyne (1976) gave a seminal account of depression as a process shaped largely by interpersonal factors. If, as Coyne postulated, a depressed individual's behavior (such as persistent self-derogation and attention seeking) strains even casual relationships, it is logical that an intimate relationship would evoke the same pattern in perhaps even stronger form. Indeed, depressed persons may cause their partners to feel burdened, ambivalent, and silently resentful. In addition, these feelings may often be noticeable to the partner in some form, even if the nondepressed partner attempts to conceal them. Further, even if partners were to evidence no change in behavior, the depressed person might experience them as less supportive and more critical. Zlotnick, Kohn, Keitner, and Della Grotta (2000) report that when one member of a couple has major depression or dysthymia, he or she tends to note fewer positive (and more negative) interactions with the

partner than do those with nonaffective disorders or without psychopathology. Let us now examine more closely some of the mechanisms by which depression may complicate partner interactions.

Erosion of Problem Solving and Support

Depression, problem-solving deficits, and difficulty in relationships
seem to coincide. Disagreement, ambivalence, and negative evaluation
are all common reactions of a nondepressed person to a depressed
partner when attempting to solve problems together. One can visualize
the twofold impact of such a scenario: not only does the problem remain unresolved, but also the attempt leads to negative outcomes for
the relationship. Depressed persons are often sensitive to criticism or
nonsupport from others—especially close others. Indeed, criticism
from the spouse predicts relapse in unipolar depressed patients who
return home to live with their spouse (Hooley & Gotlib, 2000). For
nondepressed persons, perceived support from a partner (which is
more important than actual support) is a buffer against stress (Lakey &
Lutz, 1996). Vaughn and Leff (1976) observed that their depressed
participants perceived nonsupport and hostility from relatives more
acutely than did nondepressed participants, and this sensitivity persist-
ed after the depressed person recovered. This result is consistent with
the difficulty depressed persons experience in disattending to negative
aspects of the environment (Gotlib & Neubauer, 2000). Additionally,
given the tendency of depressed persons to evoke negative reactions in
those with whom they interact, it is likely that some portion of the distance and negativity perceived by depressed individuals is, in fact, genuine.

The Vicious Cycle of Couple Distress and Depression

It is likely that the deterioration of the relationship through the opera-
tion of each of the above-mentioned factors serves as an additional
source of distress to the depressed partner, thereby influencing the depressive symptoms. Thus, the relationship between depression and couple distress is reciprocal: Just as a partner's depression may be the
source of interpersonal discord, couple distress may initiate, maintain,
or exacerbate depression.

   An integrative framework for understanding this process is provided by Hammen's (1991) stress generation theory. Hammen posits that
depressed individuals can, on the one hand, generate stress in their interpersonal environments in a variety of ways: They can display negative
problem solving behavior, or expect and elicit lower levels of partner

support. The increased level of stress experienced as a result of these self-created interpersonal difficulties may, in turn, intensify their depressive symptomatology. As a consequence, stress-generation theory suggests that depressed persons may be caught in a vicious cycle of creating and then reacting to interpersonal stress.

As is made clear by the stress generation formulation, when an intimate relationship is already characterized by discord, depression could easily aggravate dysfunctional interactions. Further entangling depressive symptoms and couple distress, the depressed partner may find that displays of affective distress are an effective means of delaying the non-depressed partner's criticism (Katz, Jones, & Beach, 2000). When this occurs, couple distress may provide a context that elicits and reinforces displays of depressive behavior. Clinically, therefore, stress generation theory suggests that therapists may need to be alert to a number of different processes that jointly unite depressive symptoms and couples' relationship discord.

ASSESSMENT OF DEPRESSION AND DISCORD

The assessment of suicidality, depression, and various dimensions of a couple's relationship are described at length in Beach, Sandeen, and O'Leary (1990). Below we briefly highlight key assessment considerations.

Suicidality and Other Psychopathology

For the basic safety of the depressed partner and in the overall interest of therapy, the issue of suicidality must first be addressed. As with any suicide assessment, intent, means, and plan—including reasons for dying versus reasons for living, feasibility of plan, and frequency/duration/controllability of suicidal thoughts—should be taken into account. A variety of assessment tools exist to aid in covering these dimensions, but whatever method is chosen, reassessment should continue at intervals throughout treatment so as to monitor change in suicidality over time. We also recommend a combination of clinical interviews—both unstructured and structured—and self-report measures to establish the presence of comorbid diagnoses.

Level of Discord in the Relationship

We do not expect couple interventions to be useful for all depressed persons (but see Cordova & Gee, 2001, and Coyne & Benazon, 2001, for an alternative). There is no research demonstrating the efficacy of couple therapy for depression when couples report only very low levels of conflict. Therefore, couple therapy for depression is only indicated when the couple reports significant relationship discord and the depressed person identifies this discord as salient and as a factor in the current depressive episode (Beach & O'Leary, 1992; O'Leary, Risso, & Beach, 1990). Having established that the couple is maritally distressed, the therapist should make a careful assessment of their level of functioning, including cohesion, coping, acceptance of expression, support, perceptions of dependability, and level of intimacy. Although self-report measures can often provide an overall index of relationship satisfaction, they do not always provide accurate accounts of objective information such as behavioral frequencies, because clients may underreport positive behaviors and overreport negative behaviors in their partners. Thus, both partners' reports, augmented by individual interviews with each partner and observation of couple interaction, is the best approach for comprehensive assessment.

Psychological Abuse

Psychological abuse is common in discordant couples and may also predict depression. Indeed, in many cases, psychological abuse (e.g., verbal humiliation, overcontrol, criticism by the partner) is perceived to be as harmful as the physical abuse. Linking humiliation with depression, Brown, Harris and Hepworth (1995) found that events that are generally viewed as humiliating (i.e., discovery of infidelity, husband-initiated divorce, violence by the husband) were more likely to hasten a depressive episode than were nonhumiliating events. Additionally, research by Cano and O'Leary (2000) suggests that humiliating events in marriage increase the occurrence of major depressive episodes above the effect of relationship discord alone. Accordingly, when potentially humiliating events can be identified, this factor should be an early target of therapeutic attention.

Level of Commitment

It is particularly important to ascertain whether one partner's commitment to the relationship is flagging. Low levels of commitment, whether they stem from the depressed partner's hopelessness or the nondepressed partner's frustration, predict poorer outcome and higher attrition from couple therapy (Beach & Broderick, 1983). In cases where one or both partners report disinterest in continuing the relationship, or indicate that they have no desire to invest in trying to make the relationship better, individual therapy for depression is recommended before beginning couple therapy. This reflects concern for the depressed person's well-being, because couple therapy when one or both partners have low commitment is likely to lead to demoralization for the depressed person.

At times, a couple's expressed commitment to making a relationship work actually disguises a motive (by either partner) to exit the relationship despite a willingness to participate in therapy. To forestall costly misunderstandings between partners and between clients and therapist, individual interviews conducted at the start of therapy should emphasize the importance of honesty regarding such topics. Therapists may also wish to highlight the high levels of energy and time required to participate in couple therapy, thereby drawing forth any lurking admissions of unwillingness. We currently discuss such costs and requirements of therapy using the "therapy contract" developed by Fincham, Fernandes, and Humphreys (1993). The "therapy contract" has the additional advantage of allowing various guidelines for therapy to be discussed in an open and nonjudgmental context prior to beginning couple therapy.

Affairs

Although this topic applies primarily to married couples, the issue of infidelity is of concern to the welfare of any couple in therapy. It is most likely to be discovered during individual interviews with each partner. If the unfaithful partner is willing to discontinue the affair, treatment can continue. Unwillingness to terminate the affair, on the other hand, has dire implications for therapy—in terms of both a violation of the atmosphere of openness and an obstacle to the areas in which the couple would normally seek change in treatment (such as disclosure and spending time together). Accordingly, if there is extramarital sexual activity and the partner involved is not willing to discontinue the activity, we do not recommend attempting couple therapy for depression.

TREATMENT OF DEPRESSION IN COUPLE THERAPY

Behavioral Couple Therapy

Theoretical Rationale

The theory that has guided the treatment of co-occurring couple discord and depression is a very simple one. At its base, it is a simple assertion that a couple's decreased closeness (or support) and increased conflict (or stress) tend to maintain depressive symptoms. It is also assumed that depressive symptoms tend to maintain a couple's discord, leading to a vicious cycle. By treating the relationship discord, we break the vicious cycle and allow the depressed partner to recover. Behavioral couple therapy (BCT), the best-studied couple treatment for depression, is both theory-driven and empirically grounded, as it traces its origins to behaviorism, cognitive theory, and theories of social learning and interpersonal interaction.

Techniques

BCT for depression (Beach, Sandeen, & O'Leary, 1990) is a relatively short-term treatment using skill building to change destructive behavior. A combination of social learning, behavioral exchange, and cognitive techniques are used. Immediately upon beginning therapy, severe obstacles to the relationship (e.g., an emotionally abusive environment) are addressed. In addition, adaptive interactions that may have diminished or extinguished over time are reinforced via homework (e.g., identifying and engaging in mutually pleasant activities). These changes often elicit expressions of positive feelings from both partners and improve the depressed partner's mood considerably. It is also presumed that at this stage, helping each partner view the other's change in a positive light (a cognitive intervention) should facilitate behavior that encourages the other partner to maintain those changes (a behavioral outcome). This initial boost in morale and affect provides a cooperative foundation from which the couple can better confront the second phase of therapy: restructuring of their relationship.

The second phase of treatment addresses the areas of partners' communication, problem solving, and interaction. At this stage the therapist seeks to bolster support and proactive problem-solving skills by targeting acceptance of emotional expression, actual and perceived coping assistance, perceived partner dependability, and couple intimacy. It is common in this phase to use communication training and problem-solving interventions from BCT. At this stage, there will typically be further decreases in stress within the dyad as coercive patterns of behavior are supplanted by healthier interactions. Prompting partners to provide each other with cohesion-building activities and self-esteem support remains important, but may command less in-session attention than at earlier points. This phase of therapy should leave the couple better integrated and better able to handle difficulties they may encounter in the future.

In the third and final stage of therapy, the therapist's role becomes secondary to that of the couple. Because the couple will soon end treatment, the therapist wishes to help the clients identify likely high-risk situations that may lead to either relapse of depressive symptoms or return to dissatisfaction within the relationship. The therapist prepares the couple to expect, be aware of, and be tolerant toward transitory symptoms of both depression and relationship difficulties. Appropriate ways of coping with both types of temporary setbacks are reviewed. The therapist now also helps the couple to "claim ownership" of their progress: they should leave therapy attributing their gains to their caring and love for one another. They should also have a greater sense of relationship efficacy and the conviction that they can better accommodate one partner's depression should the need arise in the future.

In recent years, BCT has undergone some changes in an effort to enhance the efficacy of therapy with couples who are less responsive to traditional approaches. Changes reflect the attempt to engage couples with lower levels of commitment, who are older, who are emotionally disengaged, or who have relatively divergent goals for the relationship. Such couples may be less likely to be able or willing to compromise, accommodate, and collaborate, all of which were required for success with traditional BCT. In addition, such couples may be less likely to respond to cohesion-building activities. One outgrowth of efforts to expand the range of BCT has been the development of integrative couple therapy (ICT) by Jacobson and Christensen (1996). In this approach, the initial focus of intervention is on helping both partners feel understood and accepted by the therapist and each other. Only after this objective is met are change-oriented interventions introduced. In this respect, ICT is somewhat like emotion-focused therapy (EFT; Greenberg & Johnson, 1988). In EFT the initial focus of therapy is on helping partners understand their problematic interactions as the outgrowth of understandable needs for safety and connection (i.e., attachment concerns), and this target precedes a focus on restructuring the relationship.

Efficacy

Three trials to date have compared BCT to individual therapy (Beach & O'Leary, 1992; Emanuels-Zuurveen & Emmelkamp, 1996; Jacobson et al., 1991). The findings suggest that couple therapy may be as effective as an individual approach in relieving a depressive episode when provided to discordant-depressed couples. In these cases, couple therapy also may have the added benefit of enhancing relationship functioning.

Interpersonal Psychotherapy–Conjoint Marital Therapy

Theoretical Rationale

Interpersonal psychotherapy for the treatment of depression (IPT; Klerman, Weissman, Rounsaville, & Chevron, 1984) is an individually based approach, developed in the 1970s, which aims to help depressed individuals understand and negotiate their interpersonal contexts, which are viewed as being associated with the onset and maintenance of their depressive symptoms. The treatment addresses four major interpersonal difficulties: grief, role disputes, role transitions, and interpersonal deficits.

More recently, IPT was modified to involve the partner of the patient in the treatment process. Whereas this approach incorporates various aspects of current couple therapies to IPT, the focus is on incorporating techniques that aim to enhance couple communication (Foley, Rounsaville, Weissman, Sholomskas, & Chevron, 1989). Accordingly, the two major goals of IPT–conjoint marital therapy (IPT-CM) are to facilitate the remission of the identified patient's depressive symptoms and to resolve a couple's disputes via role change.

Techniques

The initial phase of IPT-CM focuses on obtaining a history of the depressive symptoms from both partners, informing the couple about depression and its correlates, obtaining a history of their relationship, and identifying treatment goals. Specific techniques appropriate to this phase of therapy include establishment of the "sick role," an integral IPT concept in which the depressed patient is educated about the nature of his or her illness and its accompanying debilitation. It is equally important early on to obtain an "interpersonal inventory" in which information is gathered regarding the depressed partner's interactions with the nondepressed partner as well as with other close relations. The intermediate phase of treatment focuses on renegotiating partners' roles. The couple's level of relationship functioning is assessed in the areas of communication, intimacy, boundary management, leadership, and attainment of socially appropriate goals. When members of a couple differ in their expectations of what one another's roles should be, the therapist intervenes by clarifying these differences and exploring alternative options. At this stage, therapist-facilitated exploration of the partners' and couple's patterns of behavior in other relationships (using the "interpersonal inventory" from the first phase) may be useful in illuminating unrealistic expectations and assumptions that govern the depressed person's interactions. The therapist also aids the couple in making a transition to new roles and new expectations, providing support as old roles may be abandoned with regret and new roles approached with hesitancy. In particular, the therapist may explore with the couple why they are not changing. An initial approach in this regard is to ask the couple to imagine in detail how things would be different and what new behaviors would take the place of old symptomatic behaviors. Any concerns or fears related to change could be explored. The IPT therapist also refuses to accept partners' global negative labeling of themselves or their relationship, tries to provide more constructive rules to guide discussions, and projects confidence that interpersonal problems can be solved. Accordingly, there are a number of potential points of conceptual overlap with approaches used in BCT. The termination phase also resembles BCT insofar as it involves reviewing the couple's progress, identifying potential obstacles, and evaluating solutions. As in earlier phases of IPT-CM, possible feelings of loss—here with respect to the discontinuation of regular sessions—may be addressed during the termination phase.

A feature that may distinguish IPT-CM from other couple approaches in both theory and technique is its relatively greater focus on the individual problems of the identified patient. The IPT-CM therapist is careful to distinguish between individual problems of each partner and conjoint problems of their relationship. Accordingly, the therapist shifts between focusing on the individual problems of each partner and the couple's issues.

Efficacy

IPT has been well validated as an individual psychotherapy. IPT-CM is less established, but one study has laid a good foundation. Foley et al. (1989) randomly assigned 18 depressed outpatients to either individual IPT or IPT-CM. Compared to individual therapy, IPT-based couple therapy proved as effective in reducing depressive symptomatology and somewhat more effective in enhancing the couple's relationship.

ADJUNCTIVE THERAPIES

Behavioral Couple Therapy Plus Individual Cognitive Therapy

Jacobson and colleagues' (1991) study, described earlier, included a combined component of behavioral couple therapy and individual cognitive therapy, and compared the efficacy of the combined approach with each of the component treatments. The combined group was similar or slightly worse in treating depression in the nondistressed couples;

in terms of relationship satisfaction, the combined treatment did not work as well as BCT with the dissatisfied couples. In reviewing this work, Whisman and Uebelacker (1999) suggest that clinicians need not give up on combined treatments, emphasizing that when attempting to integrate different therapies, it is crucial to strive for a harmonious blend of the elements of the different therapies rather than simply adding disparate elements together. This idea is given additional force by Teichman, Bar-El, Shor, Sirota, and Elizur (1995), who appeared successful in combining elements of cognitive therapy and couple therapy. Likewise, insight-oriented couple therapy (Snyder & Wills, 1989), emotion focused couple therapy (Greenberg & Johnson, 1988), and integrative couple therapy (Jacobson & Christensen, 1996) offer interesting and apparently successful models for integrating a focus on individual vulnerabilities but with a focus on a couple's interactions. Thus, there is some basis for optimism that an integrative intervention targeting both individual vulnerabilities and partners' interactions could work.

Behavioral Couple Therapy Plus Pharmacotherapy

Attrition rates for outpatient clinical trials of psychotropic medications are 30–40% (Thase & Kupfer, 1997), and family conflicts are associated with poorer outcome to antidepressant trials (e.g., Rounsaville, Sholomskas, & Prusoff, 1980). It is possible that stress-generation processes within the family form an impediment to successful medication management. If so, couple and parenting interventions might be seen as an avenue for increasing the effectiveness of antidepressant medication while decreasing stress within the family. Alternatively, antidepressant medications might provide a method for dealing with individual vulnerability to depression, whereas family intervention furnishes a method for dealing with the stress-generation processes that are common in depression. If so, one might hypothesize that relapse and recurrence rates might be reduced when efficacious family interventions are combined with antidepressant medication. Because no adequate trial of this hypothesis has been reported in the literature, this is an important area for future investigation.

SPECIFIC CIRCUMSTANCES IN WHICH TO CONSIDER TREATMENT MODIFICATIONS

Suicidality

Clearly, the most pressing of complications in working with depressed clients is the issue of suicide. For a significant portion of depressed individuals, the ultimate outcome is suicide, with some estimates suggesting that the lifetime risk of suicide is as high as 15% (Hirschfeld & Goodwin, 1988). Due to the danger an actively suicidal patient faces, and because behavioral couple therapy does not appear to work as well as cognitive therapy for acutely suicidal patients, we do not recommend attempting couple therapy until the patient's safety has been ensured. Once beyond this practical concern, however, there is no evidence to contraindicate couple therapy for even fairly severe cases of depression (Beach, 1996).

Comorbidity

Given the high associations between depressive and other disorders documented earlier in this chapter, the couple therapist may expect to tailor treatment somewhat to specific circumstances indicated by people with dual (or multiple) diagnoses. For example, a depressed person with social phobia may be understandably recalcitrant when asked to undertake an evening out at a party or nightclub as an activity with his or her partner. Alternatively, withdrawal symptoms or drug-related behaviors in a depressed person who uses substances may interfere with activity planning or even with couple rapport. However, in outcome studies of couple therapy for depression, the presence of comorbid conditions had no greater impact on the efficacy of couple therapy than on individual therapy (Beach, 1996). However, for both couple therapy and individual therapy, comorbid conditions were associated with somewhat lower levels of recovery.

Concurrence of other disorders, such as psychosis or bipolar symptomatology, may require referrals for medication. Because behavioral couple therapy has many didactic elements, we do not recommend beginning couple therapy until the active symptoms of psychosis or mania have been controlled. At the same time, even when psychopharmacological treatment is clearly required, the presence of the partner and the focus on listening skills and problem solving may facilitate medication compliance. Therefore, there is no necessary conflict between referral for medication and the use of behavioral couple therapy.

When personality diagnoses are present, treatment can often continue as usual, with the possible exception of slowing the course of therapy, increasing attention to maintenance of the dual alliance, or adding elements that may address concerns central to the personality disorder. However, severe personality complications or even specific disorders—such as the borderline or histrionic disorders—may make it extremely difficult for the therapist to devote an equal amount of attention to each partner without being accused of favoritism or conspiratorial behavior by the partner with the personality disorder. Unfortunately, Cluster B diagnoses are common in depressed patients (Corruble et al., 1996), creating challenges for optimally tailoring treatment. It appears, nonetheless, that one may still be successful by incorporating individual sessions as needed, adopting an accepting and nonjudgmental stance toward both partners, and facilitating more benign attributions for partner behavior before attempting to produce change in therapy.

Male versus Female Depressed Partner

Models of depression in couples—both formal models and unofficial representations in clinicians' minds—have tended to operate from the presupposition that it is the female partner who is depressed. The rate of depression in women is twice that of men (Weissman, 1987). However, there are only modest gender differences in the magnitude of the cross-sectional relationship between marital discord and depression (Whisman, 2001). Still, women are more likely to take on the role of maintaining the relationship and, therefore, might have a sense of increased responsibility both for their relationships and for the status of their relationships (Lerner, 1987). This sense of responsibility, coupled with women's preferential use of emotion-focused coping, might lead women to blame themselves for relationship problems, consequently placing them at greater risk of depression (Nolen-Hoeksema, 1987). As a result, one might hypothesize a relatively stronger longitudinal effect of couple discord on depressive symptomatology for women than for men (Fincham et al., 1997), and a stronger cross-sectional relationship between depressive symptoms and couple discord for women than for men (Whisman, 2001). For female clients whose depression stems largely from their relationship difficulties, couple therapy may therefore seem more appropriate as a treatment for their symptoms.

By contrast, the male gender role is more consistent with activity and displays of anger and retaliation (Kuebli & Fivush, 1992). Thus, men might be less likely to take responsibility for the couple's relationship discord and more likely to minimize the seriousness of partner concerns. Likewise, men's greater tendency to withdraw from discussions of problems, a tendency that may be intensified by feelings of depression, also is consistent with a relatively stronger effect of depression on later relationship satisfaction for men than for women. It is thus possible that treating men's relationship dissatisfaction alone may fail to address preexisting (and causal) depression.

Although these gender differences in the importance of certain intraindividual variables, such as coping (for women) and withdrawal (for men), underscore the potential complexity of attempting to intervene with depressed and discordant couples, there is no evidence that couple therapy has different effects for depressed men than for depressed women. Thus, although therapists need to be alert to the possibility that somewhat different forms of couple intervention may be indicated when the depressed partner is male rather than female, there is little empirical guidance available at this time. Anecdotally, it has been noted that wives of depressed men often may be relatively unaccepting of their husband's depression, perhaps because depression is incompatible with the traditional male gender role. This suggests the potential importance of an early educational component focusing on reducing blame of the depressed partner for being depressed, and the possibility that this may be a more important component of treatment when the male partner is the depressed member of the dyad.

Both Partners Depressed

When both partners are depressed, the clinical picture can change, and there may be additional points of clinical intervention. No studies have specifically examined couples in which both partners were depressed, but some such couples have been included as part of the outcome research in this area. Indeed, it seems likely that couple therapists will encounter couples in which both members meet criteria for depression (or have a lifetime diagnosis). Without empirical support, it is difficult to advise modifications to the course of couple therapy in this scenario. However, it may be speculated that if both partners suffer from the same disorder, they may be better able to understand one another, avoiding the potential obstacle of one partner's depressive behavior worsening the dissatisfaction of a nondepressed partner. Likewise, it may be easier for the therapist to elicit more benign attributions for the partner's behavior, thereby setting the stage for change.

ADDITIONAL RESOURCES FOR CLIENTS

Couples may understandably wish to educate themselves about depression in their time between sessions. This initiative, besides sparing valuable session time for goal-directed therapeutic work, may have the added benefit of providing (1) an activity partners can do together, and (2) a means of fostering the understanding and empathy that so often appears to be lacking in a nondepressed partner's attitudes toward a depressed partner.

A fairly comprehensive summary of facts and topics related to depression, useful as a first reading list for couples discovering they are facing a depressive disorder, is located at *www.surgeongeneral.gov/library/mentalhealth/chapter4/sec3.html*. Because this is a U.S. government website, it is likely to be well-maintained and relatively permanent. Clients may also be directed to the updated lists of depression links on the Internet (*www.psychcentral.com/resources/Depression*).

For more targeted information, PlanetTherapy.com maintains a lay section devoted specifically to couples and depression (*www.planettherapy.com/circle/couples/depression.html*). Also, *www.intimacyanddepresion.com* is an outreach site sponsored in part by the National Depressive and Manic Depressive Organization. The National Foundation for Depressive Illness maintains a list of support groups for depression (800-248-4344). Alternatively, for those who may wish to discuss their experiences with a depressed partner in a forum with others in such a role, the newsgroup *www.soc.support.depression.family*—part of the popular Usenet system—may be a valuable resource.

ADDITIONAL RESOURCES FOR THERAPISTS

Couple therapists who desire to learn more about depression are encouraged to consult the Internet as well. The nonprofit National Depressive and Manic–Depressive Organization (*www.ndmda.org* or 800-826-3632), also mentioned above, works with health care professionals as well as with the public. For updated references on depression research, *www.WebMD.com* and the online *Physicians' Desk Reference* located at *www.pdr.net* usually list the most recent articles and often make full text available.

For training in the specific therapeutic approaches presented in this chapter, several excellent references exist in print. Therapists interested in the details of BCT treatment for depression are directed to *Depression in Marriage* by Beach et al. (1990). Those interested in IPT-CM should consult the IPT manual, *Interpersonal Psychotherapy of Depression* by Klerman et al. (1984). Of course, no text or Internet source can substitute for case-by-case consultation, and some form of supervised experience is likely to be useful in learning to untangle the complex web of depression in intimate relationships.

CASE ILLUSTRATION

Jim and Teresa presented for couple therapy with both reporting significant relationship distress. Teresa had a history of depression and currently met criteria for major depression. Her most recent episode began shortly after the couple relocated and it became clear that Jim was planning an academic career. Teresa believed her current depressive episode began after the relationship problems began. Their relationship, which was quite positive, had been deteriorating for the past year and this was a concern to both of them. Both felt frustrated and at an impasse. Despite Jim's reluctance to seek couple therapy, they recently decided that something had to be done.

As the following case illustrates, even when couples are no longer overtly displaying their feelings of caring and there is significant relationship conflict, there is often a deep reservoir of positive connection in the couple that can be tapped by the alert therapist early in treatment. Doing so is critically important to the success of couple therapy for depression because it is an antidote for the global pessimism about the relationship that may otherwise cause therapeutic efforts, particularly those focused on resolving problems and disagreements, to bog down.

Getting Couple Therapy for Depression Started

THERAPIST: I would like to start off by summarizing what I know about the two of you from your questionnaires and giving you a chance to correct or add to the things I have summarized from them. Then I would to get a better sense from the two of you how you met and your relationship developed. Finally, I would like to talk about some possible initial constructive steps the two of you may be able to take in getting started. How does that sound?

JIM: That sounds fine. (*Teresa nods.*)

THERAPIST: OK. The two major issues that were highlighted in the questionnaires were conflict around finances and conflict around career decisions. You, Jim, are pretty happy with what you are doing career-wise. You recognize that staying with your current career choice, an academic career, would involve moving around the country and in the long run might involve making less money than some other options, but these are both consequences that seem OK to you. But you, Teresa, would much prefer settling down in one place, and the possibility of greater long-term income also is important. Moving around has negative implications for your personal career options and you feel isolated. The two of you also raise problems related to differences in personality, and different backgrounds. You, Jim, describe yourself as more gregarious and outgoing whereas you, Teresa, describe yourself as more at ease with a few stable friends and more comfortable with a stable, constant lifestyle. You also said that you, Teresa, have been moody and brooding about your being upset with the way things are going, and may have started to withdraw. On the other hand, Jim, you may have come to dominate the discussion of these issues. So, neither of you feel that your discussions have gone very well. So, those are some of the issues that struck me. How am I doing so far?

TERESA: Very good.

JIM: Right.

THERAPIST: OK, well, instead of me continuing further, what I would like to do now is to invite the two of you to tell me more about the problems that are bringing you in, maybe even things you haven't told each other before. And I will leave it up to you as to who starts—but I do want to make sure you both have a chance to add things.

TERESA: You can start.

JIM: Well, everything you said is true except for one thing about my current income; it is actually higher now than if I went into business for myself. Of course, in the long run I agree that I would make more money in business for myself. But it's not so much the money as the style of life that. . . .

THERAPIST: The hours?

JIM: No, the hours are infinitely better they way I do it now, except this month is bad. Really there are many, many advantages to the job I have now, except that we have to live here.

THERAPIST: Where are you from originally?

JIM: I'm from Pittsburgh and we met in St. Louis. We talked about living in California or Texas, or maybe Washington, DC.

THERAPIST: And is it fair to say that you (*looking at Teresa*) would like to go back to Texas?

TERESA: Very much.

JIM: Well, we could go live in Texas, but I would have to give up my career entirely and I find that completely unpalatable.

THERAPIST: Teresa, could you tell me a little more about your views on this? You have heard what Jim has been saying and I assume this is not new ground for you, or is it?

TERESA: No, we have these conversations all the time. This particular issue didn't come to a head until this past year. I had always assumed that Jim would go into business for himself and that we would move, maybe back to Pittsburgh, and that's where we would establish roots and become part of a community and our boys would go to school. This business of his wanting an academic career, to me, sort of came out of left field.

JIM: Though that's not exactly true because you knew I was thinking about a fellowship, you just didn't believe I was really going to do it.

TERESA: Right.

JIM: (*to therapist*) We talked about this and I mentioned getting a fellowship where I could make more money and stay in Pittsburgh, and she said, "No. If you are going to do a fellowship you should do the best one you can. We will move anywhere and I'll take a job and we'll do anything we need to do to get you the fellowship."

TERESA: That's true. But I guess I didn't think the idea of going into academics would really win in the end. And then, we had a very traumatic move here. Looking at a lifetime of moves was something else that was entirely unpalatable to me. So, this is now looking at "the rest of our lives" and I am not happy with what I am seeing. Let's say that I do get back into the job market. It's not unlikely that we would then move to another part of the country, and that is all very unpleasant for me.

THERAPIST: So, would it be fair to say that the issue of careers and moving is the main issue right now for the two of you?

TERESA: Yes, and what we are doing right now is just sweeping it under the carpet. We aren't doing anything about it; we are just living day to day.

JIM: That's right.

TERESA: (*to Jim*) We don't talk about it because you don't like unpleasantness, so we try not to confront unpleasant issues.

JIM: (*to therapist*) We talked about it for 6 hours on the way to Pittsburgh, but it gets Teresa upset. So I don't like to pursue it too much. (*He goes on to describe a number of nuances about their situation and gives both his own view of the problem and Teresa's view of the problem. During this time Teresa is silent, and a little withdrawn.*)

THERAPIST: (*turning to Teresa*) Well, Teresa, let me ask you a couple of tough questions. Sorry they are tough, but first, how do you feel about Jim saying so much about all this and actually speaking for you at times? And second, do you think he is accurately understanding your view, or is he missing some things?

TERESA: Well, Jim speaks for me all the time. Jim is always speaking for me, so I am used to that.

THERAPIST: How do you feel about that?

At this point in the session, the therapist shifted the discussion to process and affect. By moving away from the impasse itself and toward the issue of process and associated feelings, the therapist both laid the groundwork for communication training later in therapy and demonstrated for the couple that there were new possibilities to be explored. At the same time, this served as an early direct attempt to change habitual patterns, and so required some persistence by the therapist. When successful, as in this case, a shift to process and affect has the beneficial effect of opening the couple to a shift toward a positive focus as well; that is, it suggests the possibility that things can change and the therapist can help the couple effect this change.

Later in the session, the therapist moved to initiate a positive focus. In most cases, this is done by reviewing courtship history and using that focus to draw out things about the partner that were attractive and led to the relationship deepening. Because a number of positive elements, and positive beliefs about the partner, seemed buried just below the surface, and because it appeared these positive views were being missed by both partners, in this case the therapist moved in a more direct manner to elicit a positive focus.

THERAPIST: Let me stop you there and switch gears. What I would like you to do now is to describe the best aspects of each other. Just for a few minutes, and I would like to start with you, Jim. What are Teresa's best aspects; what are her best qualities, the ones that you have admired most or that you still admire the most? Just focus on those things with no "buts" like "yes, but." Just say what you admire most.

JIM: Well, I have always been physically attracted to Teresa. I know she doesn't believe it anymore, but it's true. And she's interesting and different. We also share some joint interests like cooking and traveling, which are fun.

THERAPIST: What makes her interesting and different?

JIM: She has something I never had before . . . she has helped me be a better person, a better father, helped me be more mature about my studies. She also loves our boys and I love them too. I really love her family. I enjoy visiting with them. And she does take good care of me, and I guess I like that. Maybe I was looking for someone to take care of me. And she is intelligent and we can have intelligent discussions.

THERAPIST: (to Teresa) What are your views about Jim, about his best attributes, things that you like about him?

TERESA: One of the things that attracted me to Jim is that he is genuinely a good person. I see that every day. It is not just a façade. He is genuinely a good person and he is charismatic and he attracts people. He is also very good verbally. I like to listen to him talk. As much as I complain about it, I do enjoy listening to him. I think he is very intelligent and I enjoy listening to his discussions of various things. He also makes a good gin and tonic . . . and he takes care of me too. He's a romantic and that was the other thing that I liked about him. He swept me off my feet when we met.

THERAPIST: What were the circumstances? How did you first meet?

At this point the therapist returned to the more usual pattern of exploring the courtship and relationship history with the couple. However, the tone of the session was noticeably changed. The therapist had found a broad vein of positive affect that could be used to shift the momentum in therapy toward building cohesion, approach, and support. At the end of the session the therapist gave an assignment to the couple for the intervening week before their next session.

"OK, now I would like to tell you a little more about what you can expect from this experience and what you can do this week. Perhaps each of you could write down things you could do that you think would have a positive impact on the other. These would be little things that would show the caring the two of you clearly have for each other. You might also try one or two of the things out, also see if you notice the things your partner does. If you bring lists next time I will ask about them first thing at the beginning of the session. [For a more complete discussion of the "caring items" intervention, see Beach et al., 1990.]"

Jim and Teresa went on to rebuild a positive focus in the relationship. In their fourth session they began to focus on their communication and developed ways that helped Teresa feel that her concerns were being heard and dealt with. As they worked through a process of problem solving, they reported growing closer and continuing to engage in caring activities. By the end of therapy Teresa was no longer depressed, her Beck Depression Inventory (BDI) score having fallen from 35 to 2. Both reported that their relationship was strong and they were optimistic about their future. At 1-year follow-up, Teresa continued to be nondepressed and both continued to report high levels of relationship satisfaction.

CONCLUDING COMMENTS

Working with clients who are depressed and relationally discordant is clearly a more complex problem that working with uncomplicated couple discord. However, it is clear that we have several effective ways to intervene in the intimate relationships of depressed patients. Although the current level of success should not be oversold (Coyne & Benazon, 2001), it is clear that a solid conceptual foundation supports the use of couple therapy for depressed patients. A large and robust literature indicates that couples' relationships are often problematic for depressed persons, and difficulties in their relationships are likely to continue for many depressed patients even after successful individual or pharmacological treatment. At the same time, there is good evidence that these problematic relationships can be repaired and it seems appropriate to recommend an efficacious, targeted intervention to bring about that repair. Accordingly, couple therapists should not shy away from offering couple therapy in the context of depression.

REFERENCES

American Psychiatric Association. (2000). *Diagnostic and statistical manual of mental disorders* (4th ed., text rev.). Washington, DC: Author.

Beach, S. R. H. (1996). Marital therapy in the treatment of depression. In C. Mundt, M. J. Goldstein, K. Hahlweg, & P. Fiedler (Eds.), *Interpersonal factors in the origin and course of affective disorders* (pp. 341–361). London: Gaskell.

Beach, S. R. H., & Broderick, J. E. (1983). Commitment: A variable in women's response to marital therapy. *American Journal of Family Therapy, 11,* 16–24.

Beach, S. R. H., & O'Leary, K. D. (1992). Treating depression in the context of marital discord: Outcome and predictors of response for marital therapy versus cognitive therapy. *Behavior Therapy, 23,* 507–528.

Beach, S. R. H., Sandeen, E. E., & O'Leary, K. D. (1990). *Depression in marriage.* New York: Guilford Press.

Brown, G. W., Harris, T. O., & Hepworth, C. (1995). Loss, humiliation and entrapment among women developing depression: A patient and non-patient comparison. *Psychological Medicine, 25,* 7–21.

Cano, A., & O'Leary, K. D. (2000). Extramartal affairs precipitate major depressive episodes and symptoms of non-specific depression and anxiety. *Journal of Consulting and Clinical Psychology, 68,* 774–781.

Cordova, J. V., & Gee, C. B. (2001). Couples therapy for depression: Using healthy relationships to treat depression. In S. R. H. Beach (Ed.), *Marital and family processes in depression* (pp. 185–203). Washington, DC: American Psychological Association.

Corruble, E., Ginestet, D., & Guelfi, J. D. (1996). Comorbidity of personality disorders and unipolar major depression: A review. *Journal of Affective Disorders, 37,* 157–170.

Coyne, J. C. (1976). Toward an interactional description of depression. *Psychiatry, 39,* 28–40.

Coyne, J. C., & Benazon, N. R. (2001). Coming to terms with the nature of depression in marital research and treatment. In S. R. H. Beach (Ed.), *Marital and family processes in depression* (pp. 25–43). Washington, DC: American Psychological Association.

Emanuels-Zuurveen, L., & Emmelkamp, P. M. (1996). Individual behavioral–cognitive therapy vs. marital therapy for depression in maritally distressed couples. *British Journal of Psychiatry, 169,* 181–188.

Fincham, F. D., Beach, S. R. H., Harold, G. T., & Osborne, L. N. (1997). Marital satisfaction and depression: Different causal relationships for men and women? *Psychological Science, 8,* 351–356.

Fincham, F. D., Fernandes, L. O. L., & Humphreys, K. (1993). *Communicating in relationships.* Champaign, IL: Academic Press.

Foley, S. H., Rounsaville, B. J., Weissman, M. M., Sholomaskas, D., & Chevron, E. (1989). Individual versus conjoint interpersonal psychotherapy for depressed patients with marital disputes. *International Journal of Family Psychiatry, 10,* 29–42.

Gotlib, I. H., & Neubauer, D. L. (2000). Information-processing approaches to the study of cognitive biases in depression. In S. L. Johnson, A. M. Hayes, T. M. Field, N. Schneiderman, & P. M. McCabe (Eds.), *Stress, coping, and depression* (pp. 117–143). Mahwah, NJ: Erlbaum.

Greenberg, L. S., & Johnson, S. M. (1988). *Emotionally focused therapy for couples.* New York: Guilford Press.

Hammen, C. (1991). *Depression runs in families: The social context of risk and resilience in children of depressed mothers.* New York: Springer-Verlag.

Hirschfeld, R. M. A., & Goodwin, F. K. (1988). Mood disorders. In J. A. Talbott, R. E. Hales, & S. C. Yudofsky (Eds.), *Textbook of psychiatry* (pp. 403–441). Washington, DC: American Psychiatric Press.

Hooley, J. M., & Gotlib, I. H. (2000). A diathesis-stress conceptualization of expressed emotion and clinical outcome. *Applied and Preventive Psychology, 9,* 135–151.

Hooley, J. M., & Teasdale, J. D. (1989). Predictors of relapse in unipolar depressives: Expressed emotion, marital distress, and perceived criticism. *Journal of Abnormal Psychology, 98,* 229–235.

Horwath, E., Johnson, J., Klerman, G. L., & Weissman, M. M. (1992). Depressive symptoms as relative and attributable risk factors for first-onset major depression. *Archives of General Psychiatry, 49,* 817–823.

Jacobson, N. S., & Christensen, A. (1996). *Integrative couple therapy: Promoting acceptance and change.* New York: Norton.

Jacobson, N. S., Dobson, K., Fruzzetti, A. E., Schmaling, K. B., & Salusky, S. (1991). Marital therapy as a treatment for depression. *Journal of Consulting and Clinical Psychology, 59,* 547–557.

Katon, W. J., & Schulberg, H. (1992). Epidemiology of depression in primary care. *General Hospital Psychiatry, 14,* 237–247.

Katz, J., Jones, D. J., & Beach, S. R. H. (2000). Distress and aggression during dating conflict: A test of coercion hypothesis. *Personal Relationships, 7,* 391–402.

Kessler, R. C., Zhao, S., Blazer, D. G., & Swartz, M. (1997). Prevalence, correlates, and course of minor depression and major depression in the national comorbidity survey. *Journal of Affective Disorders, 45,* 19–30.

Klerman, G. L., Weissman, M. M., Rounsavile, B. J., & Chevron, E. (1984). *Interpersonal psychotherapy of depression.* New York: Basic Books.

Kuebli, J., & Fivush, R. (1992). Gender differences in parent–child conversations about past emotions. *Sex Roles, 27,* 683–698.

Lakey, B., & Lutz, C. J. (1996). Social support and preventive and therapeutic interventions. In G. R. Pierce, B. R. Sarason, & I. G. Sarason (Eds.), *Handbook of social support and the family* (pp. 435–465). New York: Plenum Press.

Lerner, H. G. (1987). Female depression: Self-sacrifice and self betrayal in relationships. In R. Formanek & A. Gurian (Eds.), *Women and depression: A lifespan perspective* (pp. 200–221). New York: Springer.

Lesser, I. M, Rubin, R. T, Pecknold, J. C., & Rifkin, A. (1988). Secondary depression in panic disorder and agoraphobia: I. Frequency, severity, and response to treatment. *Archives of General Psychiatry, 45,* 437–443.

Miller, N. S., Klamen, D., Hoffmann, N. G., & Flaherty, J. A. (1996). Prevalence of depression and alcohol and other drug dependence in addictions treatment populations. *Journal of Psychoactive Drugs, 28,* 111–124.

Nolen-Hoeksema, S. (1987). Sex differences in unipolar depression: Evidence and theory. *Psychological Bulletin, 101,* 259–282.

O'Leary, K. D., Risso, L. P., & Beach, S. R. H. (1990). Attributions about the marital discord/depression link and therapy outcome. *Behavior Therapy, 21,* 413–422.

Rounsaville, B. J., Sholomskas, D., & Prusoff, B. A. (1980). Chronic mood disorders in depressed outpatients: Diagnosis and response to pharmacotherapy. *Journal of Affective Disorders, 2,* 73–88.

Ruscio, J., & Ruscio, A. M. (2000). Informing the continuity controversy: A taxometric analysis of depression. *Journal of Abnormal Psychology, 109,* 473–487.

Snyder, D. K., & Wills, R. M. (1989). Behavioral versus insight-oriented marital therapy: Effects on individual and interspousal functioning. *Journal of Consulting and Clinical Psychology, 57,* 39–46.

Szadoczky, E., Rihmer, Z., Papp, Z., & Fueredi, J. (2000). Epidemiology of dysthymic disorder. *Psychiatria Hungarica, 15,* 66–75.

Teichman, Y., Bar-El, Z., Shor, H., Sirota, P., & Elizur, A. (1995). A comparison of two modalities of cognitive therapy (individual and marital) in treating depression. *Psychiatry, 58,* 136–148.

Thase, M. E., & Kupfer, D. J. (1997). Recent developments in the pharmacotherapy of mood disorders. *Journal of Consulting and Clinical Psychology, 64,* 646–659.

Vaughn, C. E., & Leff, J. P. (1976). The influence of family and social factors on the course of psychiatric illness: A comparison of schizophrenic and depressed neurotic patients. *British Journal of Psychiatry, 129,* 125–137.

Weissman, M. M. (1987). Advances in psychiatric epidemiology: Rates and risks for major depression. *American Journal of Public Health, 77,* 445–451.

Whisman, M. A. (2001). The association between depression and marital dissatisfaction. In S. R. H. Beach (Ed.), *Marital and family processes in depression: A scientific foundation for clinical practice* (pp. 3–24). Washington, DC: American Psychological Association.

Whisman, M. A., & Bruce, M. L. (1999). Marital dissatisfaction and incidence of major depressive episode in a community sample. *Journal of Abnormal Psychology, 108,* 674–678.

Whisman, M. A., & Uebelacker, L. A. (1999). Integrating couple therapy with individual therapies and antidepressant medications in the treatment of depression. *Clinical Psychology: Science and Practice, 6,* 415–429.

Zlotnick, C., Kohn, R., Keitner, G., & Della Grotta, S. (2000). The relationship between quality of interpersonal relationships and major depressive disorder: Findings from the National Comorbidity Survey. *Journal of Affective Disorders, 59,* 205–215.

CHAPTER 5

Bipolar Disorder

DAVID J. MIKLOWITZ
CHAD D. MORRIS

Bipolar disorder is characterized by wide swings of mood from severe depressions to highly activated "manic" periods. The symptoms associated with bipolar disorder have wide-ranging effects on the life of the affected individual. But like other biologically based illnesses, the symptoms are seldom confronted in isolation. Those individuals closest to the person with bipolar illness—notably partners—must also struggle with the realities of this serious and persistent illness and its effects on couple, social, and occupational functioning.

There has been relatively little attention paid to couples facing the challenges presented by bipolar disorder. This chapter explains the rationale and key techniques of a specific approach to couple therapy: family-focused psychoeducational treatment (FFT; Miklowitz & Goldstein, 1997). FFT is delivered in conjunction with pharmacotherapy and is designed for patients who have had a recent episode of bipolar, manic, mixed, or depressed disorder and recover from this episode in a couple or family-of-origin context.

FFT assists partners in building a knowledge base about bipolar disorder and developing communication and problem-solving skills to cope with the challenges posed by the illness. It consists of up to 21 sessions delivered in three relatively discrete modules: psychoeducation, communication enhancement training, and problem-solving skills training. The psychoeducational approach that FFT employs is based in a long research and clinical tradition in schizophrenia (for a review, see Goldstein & Miklowitz, 1995).

PREVALENCE AND COMORBIDITY
OF BIPOLAR DISORDER

Bipolar disorder affects about 1.2% of the population over 18 (Kessler et al., 1994; Regier et al., 1993). Its typical onset is between the ages of 15 and 19 (Goodwin & Jamison, 1990). Men and women appear to have equal rates of bipolar I disorder, which involves cycling between extremes of depression, mania, or mixed disorder (depression and mania simultaneously; American Psychiatric Association, 1994; Goodwin & Jamison, 1990). In contrast, women appear to have higher rates of bipolar II disorder, involving cycling from severe depression to milder, less debilitating periods of activation called hypomania (American Psychiatric Association, 1994; Liebenluft, 1996). Despite the lesser severity of the illness, patients with bipolar II disorder often have unremitting periods of depression that negatively affect couple functioning.

Bipolar disorder is highly recurrent. Over periods of 2 years, relapse rates average about 60%, and over 5 years, about 75% (e.g., Gelenberg et al., 1989; Gitlin, Swendsen, Heller, & Hammen, 1995). The disorder is also associated with significant marital, interpersonal, and occupational impairment (Coryell et al., 1993; Goldberg, Harrow, & Grossman, 1995). Given the degree of individual and interpersonal turmoil that manic and depressive symptoms can cause, it is not surprising that it is a major contributor to the worldwide disease burden of mental illness. It is second only to cardiovascular conditions in causing lost years of healthy life worldwide (Murray & Lopez, 1996).

BIPOLAR DISORDER AND COUPLE FUNCTIONING

Bipolar Disorder and Marital Distress

Clinicians who work with couples struggling with bipolar disorder readily provide examples of the chaotic nature of these relationships. Brodie and Leff (1971) reported that 57% of bipolar marriages ended in divorce, versus only 8% of the marriages of persons with major depressive disorder. Of course, this rate of 57% is not substantially higher than the 50% population rate of divorce. In a 3-year follow-up, Carlson, Kotin, Davenport, and Adland (1974) reported that 19 of 47 bipolar marriages ended in divorce. When divorce did not occur, the caregiving spouse often reported remaining in the marriage only out of a sense of duty. Targum, Dibble, Davenport, and Gershon (1981) found that 53% of the well spouses of bipolar partners claimed they would not have originally married had they known more about the bipolar disorder prior to becoming engaged, in contrast with 5% of the patient partners. In a 5-year follow-up of patients initially assessed during a period of illness, Coryell et al. (1993) found that among patients who had been married, those with bipolar disorder were more likely (45%) to become separated or divorced than patients with unipolar depression (26%) or matched healthy comparison subjects (18%).

Not all studies find that bipolar disorder negatively affects relationships. For example, Ruestow, Dunner, Bleecker, and Fieve (1978) reported that bipolar marriages are better adjusted than marriages containing a depressed member. Frank et al. (1981) found that bipolar marriages do not differ from normal marriages when the patient is asymptomatic. Differences among studies may be in part a function of whether marital adjustment is studied during manic–depressive states or during the patient's remitted periods. Couples will almost certainly appear more dysfunctional during and after a major episode than during a period of stability.

Mechanisms by Which Bipolar Disorder Can Affect Couple Functioning

Because its onset is typically in mid- to late adolescence, bipolar disorder can disrupt the successful resolution of developmental tasks related to establishing and maintaining long-term relationships and developing skills related to emotional self-regulation. As a result, persons with the disorder often fall behind, sometimes irreparably, in interpersonal functioning. Further, prior to the first manic episode, many individuals experience depression, anxiety, attention-deficit/hyperactivity disorder, or other disruptive behavior disorders, all of which can negatively impact interpersonal relationships (Geller & Luby, 1997; Lish, Dime-Meenan, Whybrow, Price, & Hirschfeld, 1994; Strober, 1992). Delays in social–emotional development, in turn, can negatively affect the stability of subsequent marriages or long-term relationships.

Couples often feel the repercussions of depressive or manic episodes long after the acute symptoms have remitted. The impulsive acts accompanying mania often lead to legal, financial, and occupational problems that create an undercurrent of tension and magnify normal daily stressors. Partners are often uncertain of the future and fearful of the impact of the next episode on couple or family life.

Manic states, even those which have largely resolved and would be considered within the "subsyndromal" range, are often characterized by significant irritability in the patient, who may be easily provoked by minor slights (see the case study). In contrast, depressive states often generate sympathy from a caregiving partner at first, but then lead to feelings of frustration and rejection (Coyne, Downey, & Boergers, 1992). A partner may have little knowledge of the syndrome and assert that the individual with bipolar disorder is purposefully creating conflict or chaos in the relationship.

Expressed Emotion Research

The association between patients' symptomatic behaviors and couple or family functioning has been studied most consistently with the expressed emotion (EE) construct. Levels of EE criticism, hostility, or emotional overinvolvement are usually observed in a caregiving parent or spouse in the context of a structured interview, in which he or she talks about a concurrently ill relative. EE is a well-established predictor of relapse among families containing a member with schizophrenia, major depressive disorder, or bipolar disorder (Butzlaff & Hooley, 1998; Miklowitz, Goldstein, Nuechterlein, Snyder, & Mintz, 1988). The mechanisms by which EE affects the course of psychiatric disorders are unclear, but hypotheses about individual vulnerability and family stress interactions have been articulated (Hooley & Gotlib, 2000).

The interactions of high-EE couples and families can be distinguished from the interactions of low-EE couples and families by the frequency and duration of verbal conflicts ("point/counterpoint" battles). Simoneau, Miklowitz, and Saleem (1998) found that families and couples who were rated high-EE when the patient was in an acute bipolar episode showed an increased rate of "reciprocal dependencies" during problem-solving tasks conducted during the postepisode recovery period: When one family member criticized the other, the other family member reciprocated the criticism, which led to a further criticism from the first member, and so forth. Low-EE couples or families were more able to discourage conflict from escalating. Possibly, members of these couples have learned to set limits with each other or call for a time-out. Collectively, these findings suggest a target for psychoeducational treatment: interrupting destructive patterns of verbal communication and teaching effective conflict resolution skills during the emotionally charged postepisode period.

Wendel, Miklowitz, Richards, and George (2000) clarified the cognitive-attributional processes that may be occurring among relatives rated high versus low-EE. When interacting with the bipolar patient, high-EE parental and spousal relatives make more "controllability attributions" about the patient's negative behaviors than low-EE parental or spousal relatives (e.g., "You try to do so many things at once that you can never stop and focus on one thing"). Hooley and Gotlib (2000) explain that high-EE relatives are more likely than low-EE relatives to view the patient's behavior—including illness-related behaviors or symptoms—as intentional and under his or her personal control. In contrast, low-EE relatives are more prone to attributing negative patient behaviors to uncontrollable factors such as a biologically based illness. This research suggests a target for couple therapy: educating couples about which aspects of the ill partner's behavior are truly controllable by him or her, versus which behaviors are best attributed to an unresolved illness.

CLINICAL IMPLICATIONS FOR WORKING WITH COUPLES CONTAINING A BIPOLAR PARTNER

Theoretical Rationale for FFT

Couple dysfunction usually reflects a crisis introduced by the cycling of a partner's bipolar disorder. The FFT clinician does not view marriages or relationships as "dysfunctional." Rather, healthy relationships are often damaged by the partners' mutual and often discrepant attempts to cope with symptoms that are foreign to them. The bipolar individual whose symptoms have not yet remitted often provokes his or her partner by behaving aggressively toward him or her. In turn, the partner may resort to blame and anger toward the patient when his or her attempts to solve symptom-related problems repeatedly prove ineffective.

The primary assumptions of the FFT model are that couples benefit from (1) empathic understanding by a concerned professional; (2) knowledge and acceptance of the syndrome of bipolar disorder (including how to recognize and intervene when "prodromal symptoms" of relapse appear); and (3) learning skills for resolving conflicts that often arise in reaction to expressions of the disorder. Accomplishing these goals can help keep the couple environment "low key" and hospitable to sustained remissions of the illness.

Part of the repair of family or couple relationships involves clarifying that at least some of the patient's behavior is biologically based and is not intended to hurt the caregiving partner. At the same time, the bipolar partner is not taken off the hook: he or she is encouraged to take steps to control the disorder through learning as much as possible about it, communicating regularly with a physician, remaining adherent to medications, maintaining a balanced lifestyle, and implementing stress management strategies. The latter strategies can involve couple communication skills and taking a structured approach to problem solving.

The Six Objectives of FFT

FFT has six interrelated goals that apply to most couples. First, the couple is encouraged to make sense of the most recent episode of the bipolar illness, including what symptoms were present, what psychosocial stressors served as eliciting stimuli, and how biological factors (including nonadherence to medications) contributed to the episode's onset. Second, the clinician encourages the patient and his or her partner to recognize that the patient is vulnerable to future episodes. Third, the clinician makes clear that long-term drug treatment will be a necessary component of the management of the disorder.

Most patients are not surprised to learn that the FFT clinician recommends medication. However, accepting that the disorder is recurrent and requires continuous drug treatment is a "hard pill to swallow." Some patients strongly object to this idea, and press the notion that the illness was a once-only occurrence. The FFT clinician offers a realistic view of drug treatment: Medications will not prevent relapses altogether, but they will lead to longer periods of wellness and lessen the severity of episodes that do occur. At the same time, the clinician acknowledges the emotional conflicts inherent in accepting a long-term drug regimen.

The fourth objective is to help participants to distinguish the patient's personality from his or her disorder. Patients often complain that their partner or parents have confused the two: "Everything I do is now attributed to my disorder" is a common statement by patients. FFT helps the couple to make "person versus disorder" distinctions (e.g., what is "manipulativeness" vs. "a sudden increase in mood lability"?). It also addresses the issues about identity and fear of the future that often underlie questions about such distinctions.

The fifth issue, regarding coping with psychosocial stressors, must be individualized to the patient. Some bipolar patients are strongly affected by even minor events that affect sleep/wake rhythms, such as a flight to a different time zone (Malkoff-Schwartz et al., 1998). Others experience manic symptoms after events that promote goal directedness, such as getting a new job (Johnson et al., 2000). Part of the educational work involves helping the couple to identify what stressors have affected the patient in the past, and which are likely to cause him or her trouble in the future.

Finally, the overarching goal of FFT is to restore functional couple and family relationships after the episode. Achieving this goal involves didactic training in coping strategies (e.g., how to identify early warning signs) and in communication and problem-solving skills. It may also involve coaching the couple on parenting styles, including how best to explain the disorder to children (see the case study).

Treatment Context: Structure, Duration, and Participants

FFT usually involves 12 weekly sessions, followed by 6 biweekly sessions, and then 3 monthly sessions (21 sessions over 9 months). First, educational information (7 or more sessions) is provided about the symptoms, prodromal signs, course, etiology, and treatment of the disorder, with a focus on the patient's and partner's own experiences. Second, couples are given standard communication tools (e.g., active listening, making requests for changes in a partner's behavior) to help resolve conflicts during the postepisode period (7–10 sessions). Third, couples are taught problem-solving skills for negotiating specific conflicts, usually those that are the direct or indirect result of the disorder (4–5 sessions). The degree to which each of these modules dominates the treatment is a function of the couple's preexisting knowledge or skill, usually as revealed during pretreatment assessments (see below).

Typically, patients who are referred for couple therapy are also seeing a psychiatrist for drug treatment (see "Additional Treatment Considerations," below). If the patient is not already in drug treatment, he or she is referred to a medical practitioner, usually one who has expertise in the mood disorders.

Participants in FFT treatment can include the patient's marital or romantic partner, siblings, or parents. Occasionally, we have conducted treatments in which the patient's partner and parents were both involved. With time, these arrangements usually evolve into couple therapy, depending on which relatives are the most active in the patient's care. Offspring of the patient can be included if (in the patient's or partner's estimation) their involvement would be beneficial to them.

Pretreatment Assessment Procedures

FFT, like other approaches to couple treatment of bipolar disorder (e.g., Clarkin, Carpenter, Hull, Wilner, & Glick, 1998), begins with a series of assessments of individual and couple or family functioning. Assessments are typically positioned during the immediate postacute illness period, when the patient has residual symptoms and has begun the often lengthy process of symptomatic recovery (extended symptom remission) and functional recovery (reestablishing prior levels of functioning; Keck et al., 1998). The assessment sessions, including a standard diagnostic interview (e.g., the Structured Diagnostic Interview for DSM-IV; First, Spitzer, Gibbon, & Williams, 1995), provide a regularity of contact with clinicians from the outset.

In conducting individual diagnostic assessments, the clinician should be attuned not only to verifying the diagnosis of bipolar disorder but also to documenting comorbid disorders or other historical factors that may impact the couple's ability to benefit from treatment. For example, if the bipolar partner also has attention deficit hyperactivity disorder, he or she will have a more difficult time focusing on the education or communication skill assignments. If he or she has a history of alcohol or drug abuse, the course of the therapy may be marked by frequent lapses into mood episodes interwoven with substance use, suicidal preoccupations, and medication nonadherence.

Pretreatment assessments of couple functioning are focused on three primary questions:

1. How much do the partners understand about bipolar disorder?
2. How well do they communicate and solve problems?
3. To what degree is the couple environment facilitative of versus destructive toward the patient's process of recovery?

Assessments often include a Camberwell Family Interview for assessing EE in the caregiver (Vaughn & Leff, 1976) or the briefer 5-minute speech sample assessment (Magana et al., 1986).

Equally or even more informative are observations of the couple's interaction patterns, as reflected in couple discussions of relationship problems that have arisen during the immediate postillness phase. These observations, which can be made with formalized assessment and coding procedures (see, e.g., Simoneau et al., 1998) or through informal observation by the clinician, can elucidate the extent to which interactions are heated versus low key and whether conflicts resolve amicably or escalate into unproductive, escalating verbal exchanges. Interactional assessments can also elucidate differences between the patient and caregiving partner in attributional patterns: Are negative events attributed to internal, stable, or controllable factors of the patient, or to external or less controllable factors, including the illness?

Typically, the patient's level of residual symptoms of depression or mania has effects on these variables. For example, couples that have tremendous difficulty solving problems when the patient is depressed may regain preexisting skills once the patient has fully stabilized. Couples who have heated interchanges when the patient is hypomanic may become more conciliatory when the patient is in remission.

Early Phases of Psychoeducation

As in any couple treatment, the clinician develops an alliance with both members of the couple from the outset. This alliance building can be as simple as joking with the partners, asking them questions about their lives apart from the illness, and self-disclosing as appropriate. The bipolar partner will greatly value any attempts by the clinician to express interest in him or her as a person beyond the clinical disorder.

FFT begins with a discussion with the couple of goals and expectations (Miklowitz & Goldstein, 1997). The clinician explains the tasks of therapy as follows:

"When one person in a couple begins to recover from an episode of mania or depression, there is a 'getting reacquainted' period in which you have to get to know each other all over again, and try to make sense as a couple of what just happened. This is a tough time for any couple, and part of our purpose here is to make this period of getting reacquainted less disturbing to the two of you."

The patient and caregiving partner are then encouraged to describe the most recent episode of mania or depression. How did the caregiving person know that his or her bipolar partner was becoming ill? How did the bipolar partner recognize that something was wrong? Were any environmental stressors operating prior to the episode? Were there problems of substance or alcohol abuse, or nonadherence with medication regimens?

Gradually, the couple defines a *prodromal* phase of the patient's episodes, which usually consists of their observations about changes in mood (sudden irritability, reactivity, gloominess, or giddiness), sleep, levels of sociability, thought patterns (racing vs. slowed down), and sexual drive or activity. This discussion leads into the *relapse drill*, in which participants define a series of steps to take if the patient starts to become ill again: how to arrange an emergency medical appointment to get the patient's medication changed; how to manage certain controllable forms of stress (e.g., excessive work demands); arranging for extra childcare should the patient have difficulty with parenting; and using effective communication to help derail a worsening episode (see the case study).

Later Phases of Psychoeducation

As the education progresses, the clinician turns to issues concerning the etiology and treatment of the disorder. This includes coverage of the vulnerability mechanisms underlying illness cycles (e.g., reviewing the patient's family history of mood disorder); identifying relevant psychosocial stressors (e.g., frequent travel involving changes in time zones); defining the patient's risk factors for increased cycling (e.g., sudden disruptions of sleep/wake rhythms, alcohol or drug abuse, couple conflicts); and protective factors (e.g., compliance with medication regimens, keeping track of moods on a mood chart, staying on consistent sleep/wake routines, using couple communication and problem-solving strategies).

FFT assumes that members of a couple will have significant emotional reactions to the information they have been provided, including resistances to the illness notion and painful apprehensions about what the illness means for their lives. Sometimes, these reactions result in missed sessions, coming late, or constant rescheduling. In other cases, the clinician will simply perceive that the couple is not relating well to the sessions or their structure, that they don't perceive the relevance of the sessions to their lives, or that other issues are more pressing. Dealing with these reactions is as much a part of FFT as is the provision of didactic material. FFT is delivered with a "psychotherapeutic attitude," such that clinicians are continually sensitive to the affective issues that are aroused by the information they provide. The clinician must address the patient's or partner's disbelief in the diagnosis, their mistrust of the therapist, or other impediments to skill acquisition.

One way to address resistances is to *anticipate* them before they occur, and *reframe* them as healthy and expectable. For example, the clinician can say,

> "As we go through this educational material, you may have a lot of questions about how the bipolar diagnosis applies to you. After a couple has experienced a manic episode, it's completely understandable to be confused and to think that what happened didn't really happen, that it was just a fluke and won't happen again. It's healthy to have these questions and confusions. If these questions come up for you here, let's talk about them."

This intervention makes it safe for members of the couple to express their disagreements about the reality of the diagnosis or their different predictions about the future.

Communication Enhancement Training (CET)

CET is introduced and initiated toward the end of the psychoeducation module (typically session 7 or 8), by which point the patient has usually achieved a degree of clinical stability. Nonetheless, patients who are not fully stable may still benefit from exercises that promote mutuality within the relationship and foster a sense of collaboration. By this point in treatment, the clinician has gained a good sense of the couple's communication patterns, and has some ideas as to where to intervene.

The clinician introduces CET as follows:

"Now that you know some things about bipolar disorder, we think you'll appreciate the second major component of our treatment together, which is called communication enhancement training. We want to help you communicate in the most clear and least stressful way possible, so that everyone's voice is heard and problems get solved. We'll do a series of exercises called 'role playing.' This means we'll be asking you to turn your chairs to each other and practice new ways of talking among yourselves." (Miklowitz & Goldstein, 1997, pp. 191–193)

The clinician then systematically acquaints the couple with four basic communication skills: *expressing positive feelings* (compliments, positive acknowledgement of a partner's behavior); *active listening* (paraphrasing, keeping good eye contact, nodding, asking clarifying questions); making *positive requests for changes in a partner's behavior* (diplomatically asking the partner to do something differently); and *expressing negative feelings* (constructive criticisms paired with an encouragement to problem solve). As is true for couples coping with other kinds of relationship distress, communication skills are best learned in a role-playing/behavioral rehearsal format, in which the clinician models a specific skill and then encourages the partners to rehearse the skill with each other.

Some couples benefit from going slowly through each skill and practicing until each comes naturally. For other couples—particularly those for whom verbal conflicts have escalated and the patient's disorder is not yet stable—the clinician may choose to focus CET on altering a specific communication pattern. Consider, for example, a couple containing a partner with ongoing mixed (irritable, depressed, goal-directed, racing) symptoms. The hypomanic or mixed patient presents difficulties in the skill rehearsal format: he or she may be easily provoked by the caregiving partner, magnify the significance of various complaints, or go off on many tangents. In turn, the caregiving partner may be intimidated by the patient's aggressiveness, and respond with equal rancor. The patient may then bemoan the lack of support from his or her partner, who then withdraws.

It is always possible that such a patient has an ineffective medication regimen, and that an increase in mood stabilizer dosage or the addition of a second mood stabilizing or antipsychotic agent will alter this communication pattern. Regular communication with the treating psychiatrist is essential to assure consideration of these treatment options. But even in this case, the clinician should forge ahead with the skill training agenda. The structure and focus of these exercises may help the patient achieve greater mood stability, at least in the presence of his or her partner. The key is to move slowly. For example, the clinician may simply ask the partners to paraphrase each other before making their next counterargument, or to phrase criticisms of each other in a more constructive manner (e.g., "I'd be of more help to you if you could talk to me in a softer tone of voice and wait for me to finish my thought").

During these exercises, the clinician points out that the patient's unresolved symptoms are probably reflected in his or her excessive reactivity to the caregiver. The clinician also predicts that the couple's interchanges will become less toxic and more rewarding once the bipolar partner more fully stabilizes. Stating, "It's very understandable for couples to have this level of conflict after an episode" is usually experienced by both partners as supportive. Patients are often calmed by "normalizing" of the couple's conflicts. Beneath his or her aggressiveness, forcefulness, and bravado is often the patient's fear that the caregiving partner will choose to leave.

As for couples coping with other kinds of distress, practicing the communication skills between sessions is central to making them "stick." The clinician assigns homework after each communication enhancement session, usually involving setting a time to have a weekly couple "appointment" to practice the skills and record each partner's efforts on a homework sheet (see Miklowitz & Goldstein, 1997, for examples of these sheets).

FFT can include an exploration of the couple's resistances to skill training on an insight-oriented level. For example, in response to the couple that expresses reluctance to role-play or repeatedly forgets to do homework, the clinician may say, "Perhaps using these skills feels awkward and uncomfortable because you're both angry about things that happened when [the patient] was not doing so well. Would it be helpful for us to talk about some of those things first before we proceed?" Candid discussions about underlying issues related to conflicts over intimacy or trust often "unlock" the partners' resistances to learning new skills and to applying them outside of the sessions.

Problem-Solving Skills Training

The final phase of FFT is usually undertaken by session 15, or even earlier if the clinician deems it appropriate. Problem solving involves encouraging the couple to identify concrete conflict topics and then to submit each topic to a set of steps: agreeing on the definition of a problem; brainstorming several possible solutions; evaluating the advantages and disadvantages of each proposed solution; agreeing on one solution or a set of solutions; developing an implementation plan (Who will do what? What resources are needed?); and reviewing the status of the original problem (Falloon, Boyd, & McGill, 1984; Liberman, Wallace, Falloon, & Vaughan, 1981). During the phases following a hospitalized manic or mixed episode, typical couple problems include the patient's medication use (e.g., inconsistent medication habits), his or her problems related to resuming work and social roles, combating unresolved symptom states (e.g., irritability, lethargy), and specific relationship or living situation conflicts.

For example, Lew, age 29, had been hospitalized for a manic episode and then cycled into a depressive period. As his depression began to remit, his wife Marianna began to voice complaints about the lack of physical contact between the two of them. Lew acknowledged that he still felt attracted to her and also wanted physical contact, but that his depression and low self-concept made it difficult for him to be comfortable being physically or emotionally close to anybody.

The clinician began by normalizing Lew's withdrawal and reluctance as common behaviors among patients or caregiving partners in the aftermath of a bipolar episode. He spent the first portion of a problem-solving session encouraging the couple to simply define this problem. Marianna made clear that she was not necessarily talking about sex, but rather, hugging, cuddling, and touching each other. Lew expressed the view that it might be helpful for Marianna to be more direct about when she wanted or needed physical contact. They generated a variety of solutions, which included (1) Lew agreeing to express physical affection spontaneously, at least when he felt comfortable with it; (2) Marianna being direct about asking for contact, and, if necessary, for Lew to explain why it was uncomfortable for him at that particular moment; and (3) for the couple to schedule an evening or afternoon together, away from the kids, in which physical contact might occur more spontaneously. The couple chose to implement the first and last options after Marianna expressed discomfort with asking Lew for physical affection (from Miklowitz & Goldstein, 1997). Problem solving usually works best when the partners generate and choose their own solutions, while the clinician keeps a low profile.

Because problem solving is usually begun once FFT sessions have been titrated to biweekly or monthly, it is usually essential that the couple do some of the work between sessions. A problem-solving worksheet (Falloon et al., 1984; Miklowitz & Goldstein, 1997) helps generalize the skills to the home setting.

Termination

In the final sessions, the clinician reviews with the couple the six goals of FFT (see above) and helps the partners determine the extent to which each has been addressed. If the couple still has ongoing conflicts or the patient is still not clinically stable, "booster" sessions can be scheduled in the months that follow. Referrals to support groups (see below), additional couple therapy, or individual therapy for one or both partners (see the case study) are often made. The patient's continued participation in pharmacotherapy sessions is strongly encouraged and verified with the physician.

EMPIRICAL FINDINGS REGARDING TREATMENT EFFICACY

Two experimental studies have examined the efficacy of FFT. In the first, the Colorado Treatment Outcome Project (CTOP; Miklowitz, Simoneau, et al., 2000), 101 patients were randomly assigned to 21 sessions of FFT with standard medications, or to a comparison condition involving crisis management with medication maintenance. Patients began the study in an acute, usually hospitalized bipolar I manic, mixed, or depressed episode, and were discharged to homes containing spouses, parents, or other relatives. Patients in crisis management received two sessions of family education and crisis intervention sessions on an as-needed basis for 9 months. At minimum, a clinician telephoned patients in the crisis management group every month. All treatments in both conditions were done in the couple's or the family's home.

Rates of relapse by 1 year were lower in the FFT/medication condition (29%) than in the crisis management/medication condition (53%). Patients receiving FFT also had less severe depressive symptoms by 9 months, a group difference which remained over a 24-month follow-up (Miklowitz, Richards, et al., 2001). The differences between the FFT and crisis management groups did not vary by whether the family unit was spousal or parental.

Simoneau, Miklowitz, Richards, Saleem, and George (1999) examined 44 patients and families from the CTOP who completed pretreatment and posttreatment assessments of interactional behavior. Patients and relatives in FFT showed increases from pretreatment to posttreatment in the frequency of positive interactional behaviors (particularly nonverbal acknowledgements), but patients and relatives in crisis management did not. Notably, increases in levels of positive nonverbal behavior among patients were correlated with the degree of symptom improvement over the first study year. FFT did not lead to greater reductions in negative family interactional behaviors (e.g., frequency of criticisms, negative looks, disagreements, or negative solutions to problems) than those observed in crisis management.

The CTOP study could be criticized on the grounds that the FFT and crisis management comparison groups were not matched on the number of therapy sessions. A randomized trial of FFT conducted in an outpatient clinic at the University of California, Los Angeles (UCLA; Rea et al., in press) compared 21 sessions of FFT (with maintenance medication) to a comparably paced individual therapy (education, case management, and problem solving) with maintenance medication. The majority of these patients lived with their parents rather than spouses.

Results of the UCLA study indicated that rates of relapse and rehospitalization were lower among FFT-treated patients than among patients treated with individual therapy, although only during the second year of the study. Patients in FFT were also less likely to be hospitalized when they did relapse than those in individual therapy. Thus, participants in FFT may have learned to recognize emerging symptoms early and obtain emergency medical treatment.

The results of both studies are consistent in suggesting that FFT is an efficacious adjunct to pharmacotherapy for couples and families containing a member with bipolar disorder. Interestingly, both studies suggested that FFT has delayed effects. Possibly, the education and skills training central to the FFT approach must be "absorbed" before their clinical effects relative to comparison interventions can be observed.

ADDITIONAL TREATMENT CONSIDERATIONS

Adjunct Treatments

Pharmacotherapy is the first-line treatment for bipolar disorder. Thus, patients see a psychiatrist for medication management while in FFT. Nowadays, typical drug treatment regimens include lithium carbonate or the anticonvulsants (usually divalproex sodium [Depakote], carbamazepine, or lamotrigine [Lamictal]), alone or in various combinations. Adjunctive agents can include antidepressants, atypical antipsychotics, anxiolytic medications, or thyroid supplements.

A good relationship between the FFT clinician and the treating psychiatrist is essential. Regular dialogue between them should occur regarding the patient's style of approaching treatment, consistency with recommended drug regimens, and clinical status. In addition to assuring continuity of care and appropriate management of emergencies, ongoing collaboration between the FFT clinician and physician can help unlock the patient's resistances to medications or, for that matter, to couple therapy.

Special Populations

Certain populations of bipolar patients may be less likely to benefit from FFT. Patients who refuse to comply with their medication regimens at the outset are unlikely to be stable enough to engage in or contribute productively to the educational or skill training tasks. In contrast, other patients enter FFT fully compliant with medications but uncertain as to whether they have bipolar disorder, often due to misunderstandings about what the diagnosis means. These patients may benefit a great deal from educational sessions to help them come to terms with the illness. In either case, the clinician must make clear at the outset that FFT is not a substitute for medication. Rather, a primary goal is to help both members of the couple accept the need for medication in the disorder's maintenance.

Patients with active substance abuse or alcohol dependence disorders are not good candidates for FFT. First, mood stabilizing medications are not as efficacious with patients who have comorbid substance disorders. Substance abuse has been consistently associated with shorter intervals prior to mood disorder relapses (e.g., Tohen, Waternaux, & Tsuang, 1990). Second, if the patient is actively using alcohol or other substances, it may be impossible to determine whether the real diagnosis is bipolar disorder versus a substance-induced mood disorder. Educating the couple about bipolar disorder will be unproductive if the diagnosis is wrong. Third, alcohol- or substance-dependent patients usually deny the reality of the disorder and the necessity of drug or psychosocial treatments. Nonetheless, patients who are remitted from earlier bouts with drug or alcohol problems may benefit from FFT, especially if they are simultaneously engaged in an outpatient chemical dependency program.

FFT within the Managed Care Setting

In the managed care era there are systemic fiscal incentives to use brief or time-limited psychotherapy modalities. Although not created in response to managed care, the objectives of FFT and its time line are consistent with the realities imposed by utilization management reviews. In many cases, managed care organizations authorize an initial number of sessions (e.g., 4–8) and then provide reauthorizations based on documented need until a maximum mental health policy benefit is met. FFT modules have "detachability"; that is, individual modules within FFT can be self-standing and fit within a set number of authorized visits. Based on initial functional assessments of the couple (e.g., reasons for seeking services at this time), treatment plans can prioritize the FFT modules or abbreviate them (e.g., provide communication training only, or brief education followed by more extensive problem solving).

Utilization management usually requires documentation of a clear, specific, and time-limited focus. Ongoing evaluation of goal attainment is a core feature of FFT and consistent with the behavioral tracking mechanisms emphasized in the managed care world. Reauthorization offers clinicians an opportunity to determine if a module has been successfully integrated or must be revisited before moving on to the couple's next level of skill development.

FFT clinicians often form long-term relationships with couples and offer maintenance sessions when requested (the "general practitioner" model). For example, a couple may seek out the clinician when the bipolar partner has relapsed or is in the process of relapsing. The clinician then assists the partners to expand their knowledge of the factors affecting the current mood cycling, to revise their relapse prevention plans, and solidify their repertoire of coping strategies. Using FFT in such a manner can increase short-term care utilization but decrease costly emergency and inpatient service use (Rea et al., in press). By these means, FFT has the potential to address the realities of the mental health system in the context of an evidence-based treatment modality.

Additional Resources for the Individual, Couple, or Clinician

A number of national organizations serve as resources for clinicians and couples in treatment. These organizations provide up-to-date information about the disorder, and in some cases provide local support groups. These include the National Institute of Mental Health (website: *www.nimh.nih.gov*), the Child and Adolescent Bipolar Foundation (*www.bpkids.org*), the Depression and Related Affective Disorders Association (*www.drada.org*), the National Alliance for the Mentally Ill (*www.nami.org*), the Depression and Bipolar Support Alliance (*www.ndmda.org*), the National Foundation for Depressive Illness, Inc. (*www.depression.org*), the National Alliance for Research on Schizophrenia and Depression (*www.narsad.org*), and the National Mental Health Association (*www.nmha.org*).

CASE ILLUSTRATION

Melanie, a 44-year old woman with bipolar II disorder, lived with her husband of 15 years, Ben, age 46, and their three children. Melanie worked part time at a clothing store and Ben managed an apartment building. Her most recent depression had a "mixed" quality to it—there were elements of hypomania (agitation, irritability, and anxiety) co-occurring with depression (e.g., feelings of worthlessness). The physician managing her drug regimen felt that Melanie and Ben had significant relationship problems that were contributing to her mood cycling, and referred her for FFT. She took the mood stabilizer Trileptal (oxcarbazepine), and a selective serotonin reuptake inhibitor, Paxil.

Initial observations of the couple's communication patterns during a pretreatment assessment revealed that Melanie tended to "overpower" Ben, often talking over him loudly and aggressively, even when she was agreeing with him. His response style was to withdraw, which made her feel that he was uninterested in her. According to the couple, their style was more mutual when Melanie was in a remission from her disorder, but neither of them could clearly pinpoint when that had last occurred.

During the initial phases of FFT psychoeducation, the clinician asked Melanie and Ben to describe their experiences of Melanie's most recent illness. Melanie focused on her feelings of depression, suicidal preoccupations, anxiety, and agitation, but also described her episode as "a sort of spiritual awakening . . . letting go of my attachments to people, places, and things." Ben had a rudimentary understanding of bipolar disorder but had difficulty distinguishing what were and were not her symptoms. He described her, when hypomanic, as "overwhelming, intrusive . . . she comes up with these ideas that she insists are brilliant—like converting our storage shed into a spare bedroom—and when I don't latch onto them right away, she gets incredibly irritated and self-destructive." He explained that she had angrily run out of the house the last time this had occurred, cursing him, and exclaiming that he showed no interest in the things that made her life enjoyable.

It became clear to the FFT clinician that Ben thought much of Melanie's behavior was purposeful and that she was bent on "getting revenge" for his lack of emotional availability. The clinician offered him an alternative explanation: that Melanie's hypomanic or depressive states reflected an inborn predisposition interacting with specific environmental stressors. Ben showed interest in these notions but had difficulty applying them to his individual situation: "If this is really her biology, why can she keep it together with other people but not with me?" Melanie explained that she did indeed have a difficult time not tearing into other people, particularly her employer. She added that her greater expressiveness with Ben reflected the fact that she felt safer with him.

An early task in the psychoeducation involved getting Melanie to keep track of her own mood states through a mood chart (Sachs, 1996; see the down-loadable version at *www.manicdepressive.org*). This exercise required that Melanie rate her daily moods on a 7-point scale from –3 (depressed) to + 3 (manic), and to record her sleep/wake patterns, use of medications, alcohol use, and psychosocial stressors (including marital arguments). After a month of keeping the chart, both partners made an observation they hadn't made before: Melanie's moderate use of alcohol in social situations presaged several days of irritable, depressed mood. Melanie did not agree to stop using alcohol, but decided to limit her consumption to one beer early in the evening, and to evaluate its effects on her mood as reflected on her chart.

Later in psychoeducation, Melanie and Ben developed a relapse prevention plan. The nature of this plan was less focused on depressive episodes than on dealing as a couple with her brief hypomanic periods. The couple identified rules for dealing with Melanie's hypomanic escalation when it was starting to occur. These rules included allowing Ben to "escape" to another part of the house when conflicts escalated, both partners attempting to use self-quieting techniques to keep arguments from spiraling (self-talk, pausing, reframing the situation to themselves), and Melanie or Ben calling her physician to have her medications reevaluated if her moods were getting out of control.

As the couple began communication enhancement training, the partners identified two goals: to develop better skills for addressing couple conflicts, especially those that occurred when Melanie was cycling, and to practice explaining Melanie's disorder to their children. Communication training involved role-playing of specific skills and homework assignments between sessions. The couple benefited most from exercises directed at active listening and diplomatic limit-setting.

Melanie showed a great deal of sensitivity to the issues that her children would find salient about her disorder. She role-played explaining the disorder to them as if they were present: "I have a chemical imbalance that makes my moods go up and down, probably something I inherited. . . . When I get real irritable or down it's not your fault, but you may need to leave me alone for awhile or try not to provoke me." She decided they were too young to understand that they might be at high risk for developing the disorder, but did decide to encourage them to avoid alcohol and drugs that, in her experience, "consistently put me over the edge."

In the final stages of FFT, Melanie and Ben used problem solving to focus on an issue that had been in the background throughout the treatment: Ben's lack of direction in his career. He acknowledged that helping Melanie deal with her disorder had enabled him to avoid dealing with problems of his own. In problem solving, the clinician encouraged Ben to break this issue down into a number of smaller, component problems: the fact that he needed to develop a résumé, that he resented working in the mornings, and that he was confused as to how and where to look for a job. These problems became more clearly defined as the couple attempted to solve them one by one. The outcome was that Ben agreed to search for part-time work in computer programming, with a focus on locating work with flexible hours.

At the conclusion of FFT, Melanie's illness was relatively stable. She was still prone to exhaustion, depression, and irritability when she worked too hard, which still led to couple conflict. The couple, however, had an easier time identifying when Melanie's mood was escalating and to avoid the verbal brawls that had formerly accompanied these episodes. They felt that their communication had become more collaborative and mutual. As stated by Melanie, "We can now talk about both of our problems, not just mine."

For his part, Ben became more willing to acknowledge the role of Melanie's inborn disorder in determining her behavior, and less likely to view her outbursts as due to meanness or insensitivity. He acknowledged for the first time that he had his own problems with depression, and that "some of this is about me and where I wanted to be at this point in my life." He had not found a suitable job but had been actively looking. The clinician referred Ben to an individual therapist and encouraged Melanie to continue her medical treatment sessions. He also referred her to a support group for persons with bipolar disorder.

CONCLUSIONS

Couples coping with bipolar disorder face significant stress in the aftermath of episodes. Ordinary couple conflicts become magnified by the patient's unresolved symptoms and the caregiving partner's attributions about the causes of these behaviors. A program of family-focused psychoeducation accompanied by drug treatment may contribute to longer periods of wellness in the patient and significantly lower levels of couple distress.

Much remains to be learned about family interventions with this population. The patients and family constellations that are most likely to benefit, and the optimal duration and intensity of therapy, need to be clarified. Little work has been done to identify the mechanisms by which treatment achieves its effects, which may include improving communication and problem solving, enhancing the couple's ability to recognize emergent symptoms of relapse, or enhancing the patient's adherence to drug regimens. Finally, the cost-effectiveness of treatment may be maximized by providing FFT in a multifamily group format in which several couples meet and simultaneously receive education and skills training. Multifamily groups have been found to be highly effective for patients with schizophrenia (McFarlane et al., 1995). These questions are best addressed in the context of controlled community effectiveness studies.

ACKNOWLEDGMENTS

Preparation of this chapter was supported in part by National Institute of Mental Health Grant Nos. MH55101 and MH62555, and by a Distinguished Investigator Award to David J. Miklowitz from the National Alliance for Research on Schizophrenia and Depression.

REFERENCES

American Psychiatric Association. (1994). *Diagnostic and statistical manual of mental disorders* (4th ed.). Washington, DC: Author.

Brodie, H. K. H., & Leff, M. J. (1971). Bipolar depression: A comparative study of patient characteristics. *American Journal of Psychiatry, 127,* 1086–1090.

Butzlaff, R. L., & Hooley, J. M. (1998). Expressed emotion and psychiatric relapse: A meta-analysis. *Archives of General Psychiatry, 55,* 547–552.

Carlson, G. A., Kotin, J., Davenport, Y. B., & Adland, M. (1974). Follow-up of 53 bipolar manic–depressive patients. *British Journal of Psychiatry, 124,* 134–139.

Clarkin, J. F., Carpenter, D., Hull, J., Wilner, P., & Glick, I. (1998). Effects of psychoeducational intervention for married patients with bipolar disorder and their spouses. *Psychiatric Services, 49,* 531–533.

Coryell, W., Scheftner, W., Keller, M., Endicott, J., Maser, J., & Klerman, G. L. (1993). The enduring psychosocial consequences of mania and depression. *American Journal of Psychiatry, 150,* 720–727.

Coyne, J. C., Downey, G., & Boergers, J. (1992). Depression in families: A systems perspective. In D. Cicchetti & S. L. Toth (Eds.), *Developmental perspectives on depression* (pp. 211–249). Rochester, NY: University of Rochester Press.

Falloon, I. R. H., Boyd, J. L., & McGill, C. W. (1984). *Family care of schizophrenia: A problem-solving approach to the treatment of mental illness.* New York: Guilford Press.

First, M. B., Spitzer, R. L., Gibbon, M., & Williams, J. B. W. (1995). *Structured clinical interview for DSM-IV axis I disorders.* New York: Biometrics Research Department, New York State Psychiatric Institute.

Frank, E., Targum, S. D., Gershon, E. S., Anderson, C., Stewart, B. D., Davenport, Y., Ketchum, K. L., & Kupfer, D. J. (1981). A comparison of nonpatient and bipolar patient–well spouse couples. *American Journal of Psychiatry, 138,* 764–767.

Gelenberg, A. J., Kane, J. N., Keller, M. B., Lavori, P., Rosenbaum, J. F., Cole, K., & Lavelle, J. (1989). Comparison of standard and low serum levels of lithium for maintenance treatment of bipolar disorders. *New England Journal of Medicine, 321,* 1489–1493.

Geller, B., & Luby, J. (1997). Child and adolescent bipolar disorder: A review of the past 10 years. *Journal of the American Academy of Child and Adolescent Psychiatry, 36,* 1168–1176.

Gitlin, M. J., Swendsen, J., Heller, T. L., & Hammen, C. (1995). Relapse and impairment in bipolar disorder. *American Journal of Psychiatry, 152*(11), 1635–1640.

Goldberg, J. F., Harrow, M., & Grossman, L. S. (1995). Course and outcome in bipolar affective disorder: A longitudinal follow-up study. *American Journal of Psychiatry, 152,* 379–385.

Goldstein, M. J., & Miklowitz, D. J. (1995). The effectiveness of psychoeducational family therapy in the treatment of schizophrenic disorders. *Journal of Marital and Family Therapy, 21,* 361–376.

Goodwin, F. K., & Jamison, K. R. (1990). *Manic–depressive illness.* New York: Oxford University Press.

Hooley, J. M. & Gotlib, I. H. (2000). A diathesis-stress conceptualization of expressed emotion and clinical outcome. *Applied and Preventive Psychology, 9,* 131–151.

Johnson, S. L., Sandrow, D., Meyer, B., Winters, R., Miller, I., Solomon, D., & Keitner, G. (2000). Increases in manic symptoms following life events involving goal-attainment. *Journal of Abnormal Psychology, 109,* 721–727.

Keck, P. E. J., McElroy, S. L., Strakowski, S. M., West, S. A., Sax, K. W., Hawkins, J. M., Bourne, M. L., & Haggard, P. (1998). Twelve-month outcome of patients with bipolar disorder following hospitalization for a manic or mixed episode. *American Journal of Psychiatry, 155,* 646–652.

Kessler, R. C., McGonagle, K. A., Zhao, S., Nelson, C. B., Hughes, M., Eshelman, S., Wittchen, H. U., & Kendler, K. S. (1994). Lifetime and 12-month prevalence of DSM-III-R psychiatric disorders in the United States: Results from the National Comorbidity Survey. *Archives of General Psychiatry, 51,* 8–19.

Liberman, R. P., Wallace, C. J., Falloon, I. R. H., & Vaughn, C. E. (1981). Interpersonal problem-solving therapy for schizophrenics and their families. *Comprehensive Psychiatry, 22,* 627–629.

Liebenluft, E. (1996). Women with bipolar illness: Clinical and research issues. *American Journal of Psychiatry, 153,* 163–173.

Lish, J. D., Dime-Meenan, S., Whybrow, P. C., Price, R. A., & Hirschfeld, R. M. (1994). The National Depressive and Manic–Depressive Association (NDMDA) survey of bipolar members. *Journal of Affective Disorders, 31,* 281–294.

Magana, A. B., Goldstein, M. J., Karno, M., Miklowitz, D. J., Jenkins, J., & Falloon, I. R. H. (1986). A brief method for assessing expressed emotion in relatives of psychiatric patients. *Psychiatry Research, 17,* 203–212.

Malkoff-Schwartz, S., Frank, E., Anderson, B., Sherrill, J. T., Siegel, L., Patterson, D., & Kupfer, D. J. (1998). Stressful life events and social rhythm disruption in the onset of manic and depressive bipolar episodes: A preliminary investigation. *Archives of General Psychiatry, 55,* 702–707.

McFarlane, W. R., Lukens, E. P., Link, B., Dushay, R., Deakins, S. A., Newmark, M., Dunne, E. J., Horen, B., & Toran, J. (1995). Multiple-family groups and psychoeducation in the treatment of schizophrenia. *Archives of General Psychiatry, 52,* 679–687.

Miklowitz, D. J., & Goldstein, M. J. (1997). *Bipolar disorder: A family-focused treatment approach.* New York: Guilford Press.

Miklowitz, D. J., Goldstein, M. J., Nuechterlein, K. H., Snyder, K. S., & Mintz, J. (1988). Family factors and the course of bipolar affective disorder. *Archives of General Psychiatry, 45,* 225–231.

Miklowitz, D. J., Richards, J. A., George, E. L., Simoneau, T. L., Powell, K., & Suddath, R. (2001, July). *Treating bipolar patients with medication and family psychoeducation: Results of a randomized clinical trial.* Paper presented at World Congress of Behavioral and Cognitive Therapies, Vancouver, BC.

Miklowitz, D. J., Simoneau, T. L., George, E. A., Richards, J. A., Kalbag, A., Sachs-Ericsson, N., & Suddath, R. (2000). Family-focused treatment of bipolar disorder: One-year effects of a psychoeducational program in conjunction with pharmacotherapy. *Biological Psychiatry, 48,* 582–592.

Murray, C. J. L., & Lopez, A. D. (1996). *The global burden of disease: A comprehensive assessment of mortality and disability from diseases, injuries, and risk factors in 1990 and projected to 2020.* Cambridge, MA: Harvard University Press.

Rea, M. M., Tompson, M., Miklowitz, D. J., Goldstein, M. J., Hwang, S., & Mintz, J. (in press). Family-focused treatment vs. individual treatment for bipolar disorder: Results of a randomized clinical trial. *Journal of Consulting and Clinical Psychology.*

Regier, D. A., Narrow, W. E., Rae, D. S., Manderscheid, R. W., Locke, B. Z., & Goodwin, F. K. (1993). The de facto mental and addictive disorders service system: Epidemiologic catchment area prospective 1-year prevalence rates of disorders and services. *Archives of General Psychiatry, 50,* 85–94.

Ruestow, P., Dunner, D. L., Bleecker, B., & Fieve, R. R. (1978). Marital adjustment in primary affective disorder. *Comprehensive Psychiatry, 19,* 565–571.

Sachs, G. S. (1996). Bipolar mood disorder: Practical strategies for acute and maintenance phase treatment. *Journal of Clinical Psychopharmacology, 16* (Suppl. 1), 33–47.

Simoneau, T. L., Miklowitz, D. J., Richards, J. A., Saleem, R., & George, E. L. (1999). Bipolar disorder and family communication: Effects of a psychoeducational treatment program. *Journal of Abnormal Psychology, 108,* 588–597.

Simoneau, T. L., Miklowitz, D. J., & Saleem, R. (1998). Expressed emotion and interactional patterns in the families of bipolar patients. *Journal of Abnormal Psychology, 107,* 497–507.

Strober, M. (1992). Relevance of early age-of-onset in genetic studies of bipolar affective disorder. *Journal of the American Academy of Child and Adolescent Psychiatry, 31,* 606–610.

Targum, S. D., Dibble, E. D., Davenport, Y. B., & Gershon, E. S. (1981). The family attitudes questionnaire: Patients and spouses' views of bipolar illness. *Archives of General Psychiatry, 38,* 562–568.

Tohen, M., Waternaux, C. M., & Tsuang, M. T. (1990). Outcome in mania: A 4-year prospective follow-up of 75 patients utilizing survival analysis. *Archives of General Psychiatry, 47,* 1106–1111.

Vaughn, C. E., & Leff, J. P. (1976). The influence of family and social factors on the course of psychiatric illness: A comparison of schizophrenia and depressed neurotic patients. *British Journal of Psychiatry, 129,* 125–137.

Wendel, J. S., Miklowitz, D. J., Richards, J. A., & George, E. L. (2000). Expressed emotion and attributions in the relatives of bipolar patients: An analysis of problem-solving interactions. *Journal of Abnormal Psychology, 109,* 792–796.

CHAPTER 6

Schizophrenia-Spectrum Disorders

KIM T. MUESER
MARY F. BRUNETTE

Schizophrenia is a severe psychiatric disorder that has a broad impact on all aspects of personal and social functioning. Because of the disabling nature of schizophrenia, it can have a major effect on the ability to establish and maintain close relationships, and is a major consideration in conducting couple therapy. In this chapter we provide an introduction to schizophrenia and related disorders, and consider the implications of these for conducting couple therapy when one or both partners has the disorder. We discuss the broad treatment needs of individuals with schizophrenia, and address principles for assessing these needs in the context of work with couples. We present an approach to treating couples in which one partner has schizophrenia—behavioral family therapy—and we review the research supporting this model. We conclude by considering the adjunctive treatment needs of people with schizophrenia-spectrum disorders and resources for clients, their partners, and clinicians working with such couples.

CONCEPTUALIZATION

Description of the Disorder

Schizophrenia is a major mental illness that can affect all aspects of functioning. The psychopathology of schizophrenia is characterized by three clusters of symptoms: positive symptoms, negative symptoms, and cognitive impairment. *Positive symptoms* (or psychotic symptoms) refer to hallucinations (i.e., false perceptions, such as hearing voices when no one is around); delusions (i.e., false beliefs, such as believing that others are persecuting you or that your partner has been unfaithful when this is not true); and bizarre behavior (e.g., collecting odd scraps of paper). *Negative symptoms* are symptoms characterized by deficits in emotional experience, behavioral expressiveness, and energy level. Common negative symptoms include anhedonia (diminished experience of pleasure); asociality (reduced social drive); anergia (decreased ability to initiate and follow through with plans); alogia (poverty of speech or content of speech); and blunted affect (diminished emotional expressiveness). *Cognitive impairments* span the range of different cognitive functions including speed of information processing, attention and concentration, memory, abstract reasoning, and planning ability.

The diagnostic criteria for schizophrenia emphasize the presence of positive and negative symptoms (American Psychiatric Association, 1994), although there is growing evidence that cognitive impairment is extremely common (Green & Nuechterlein, 1999). Typically, the positive symptoms of schizophrenia are episodic, with severity fluctuating over time, although these symptoms are persistent in 25–40% of clients. Negative symptoms, in contrast, tend to be more stable and more pervasive, and few clients experience full remission of these symptoms between episodes of psychosis. The cognitive symptoms in schizophrenia tend to persist throughout the course of the illness, although their severity also increases during exacerbation of positive symptoms.

In addition to the characteristic symptoms of schizophrenia, diagnostic criteria also require impairment in psychosocial functioning in major role functioning (e.g., as worker, student, parent, or partner), maintaining good interpersonal relationships, caring for oneself, and enjoying leisure activities. In addition to the characteristic symptoms and impairments, the diagnosis of schizophrenia requires a 6-month period of impaired functioning. Therefore, at least some chronicity is incorporated into the definition of the disorder. Because some impairment in functioning is required for the diagnosis of schizophrenia, it is tautological to say that the disorder affects functioning. However, it should also be noted that for many clients, problems in social functioning long precede the onset of their illness, which then exacerbates a preexisting impairment.

Schizophrenia is closely related to three other disorders: schizoaffective disorder, schizopheniform disorder, and schizotypal personality disorder. Based on studies of mental illness in families and response to treatment, these disorders are grouped together as *schizophrenia-spectrum disorders,* and are treated following the same principles. Individuals who meet the symptom and impaired functioning criteria for the disorder, but whose impairment is of less than 6 months' duration (or who experience a full remission of symptoms with episodes lasting less than 6 months) meet diagnostic criteria for *schizopheniform disorder.* Individuals who meet criteria for schizophrenia during periods when their mood is normal, but who also have significant episodes of depression or mania, meet diagnostic criteria for *schizoaffective disorder. Schizotypal personality disorder* resembles schizophrenia in many ways, although the severity of symptoms tends to be lower, and its course is less episodic and marked by less flagrant positive symptoms.

Because schizophrenia affects so many different areas of functioning, it is not surprising that there are many other comorbid disorders and associated problems with the illness. Substance abuse and dependence are very common in clients with schizophrenia, with lifetime rates approximately 50% and recent rates of abuse or dependence at 25–35%, in considerable excess of the rate of lifetime substance use disorder of approximately 16% in the general population (Regier et al., 1990). Depression is very common in schizophrenia, with most clients experiencing at least some symptoms of depression over the course of their illness, and a lifetime suicide rate of approximately 10% (Roy, 1986). Problems with anxiety are high, including increased rates of trauma and posttraumatic stress disorder (Mueser, Rosenberg, Goodman, & Trumbetta, 2002), obsessive–compulsive disorder (Tibbo, Kroetsch, Chue, & Warneke, 2000), social anxiety (Penn, Hope, Spaulding, & Kucera, 1994), and panic disorder (Argyle, 1990). These associated symptoms of schizophrenia can be as debilitating or more so than the characteristic symptoms of schizophrenia, and can have a major impact on quality of life and social relationships.

PREVALENCE, COURSE, AND IMPACT OF DISORDER ON THE RELATIONSHIP

The prevalence of schizophrenia is approximately 1% in the general population. Onset of the illness typically occurs between the ages of 16 and 30, with onset after the age of 35 being relatively rare. In general, women have a later age at onset of schizophrenia, and they tend to have a more benign course of illness, including fewer hospitalizations and better social functioning (Haas & Garratt, 1998). Although the course of illness is episodic, it varies substantially from one person to the next. Over a lifetime, symptoms tend to gradually diminish with significant numbers of clients achieving sustained remissions of their symptoms (Harding & Keller, 1998).

There are many ways in which the symptoms and associated problems of schizophrenia can interfere with the quality of close relationships and marriage. Perhaps most fundamentally, impairments in role functioning and self-care skills commonly result in a shifting of major responsibilities to the healthy or less impaired partner. This shift can be burdensome to the partner and a source of tension in the relationship. Specific symptoms and impairments can create additional problems in relationships. Positive symptoms, such as firmly held delusions, can have a major impact on maintaining a close relationship, and can interfere with sharing a common outlook on the world with another person. The effects of negative symptoms on social relationships are more insidious and can be more devastating. Lack of engagement in and enjoyment of shared activities including sexual relations, due to schizophrenia, can threaten the formation or maintenance of solid emotional bonds. Diminished responsiveness to the partner, either behavioral or emotional, can render a person with schizophrenia unrewarding to interact with, and lead to avoidance and termination of a close relationship. A particularly thorny problem associated with negative symptoms is that relatives of clients often do not recognize these symptoms as part of the illness, and instead perceive them as under clients' voluntary control, resulting in blame and criticism (Weisman, Nuechterlein, Goldstein, & Snyder, 1998).

Cognitive impairment can interfere with solving problems together, and the ability to accurately perceive and process relevant social information, including the partner's emotions, beliefs, and concerns. Cognitive impairment can also contribute to poor social skills, making it more difficult to establish and maintain close relationships. Problems with insight, including the recognition that one has a psychiatric illness, can create further difficulties in a close relationship with someone with schizophrenia.

With respect to common associated problems, substance abuse can have a wide range of negative effects in close relationships with persons with schizophrenia. Relatives are often critical about clients' abuse of alcohol and drugs, and substance abuse can contribute to symptom relapses and rehospitalizations, increased violence toward partners, diminished judgment, legal and financial problems, and unstable housing and homelessness (RachBeisel, Scott, & Dixon, 1999). Depression can have a negative effect on the partner by inducing similar dysphoria, whereas suicide attempts may be traumatic for the healthy partner, leading to hypervigilance and anxiety about subsequent attempts.

Most of the research on close relationships in persons with schizophrenia pertains to marriage. Schizophrenia has a well-established impact on the likelihood of marriage, marital adjustment and satisfaction, and the longevity of the relationship. Less than 25% of men with schizophrenia marry, whereas 50–70% of women marry (Loranger, 1984). Aside from marriage, women with schizophrenia are also more likely than men to have been involved in heterosexual relationships, either before or after onset of the illness (Goldstein, Tsuang, & Farone, 1989). The difference in marriage rates appears to be partly due to the later age of onset of schizophrenia for women, and different sex roles in the mate selection process whereby men take a more active role in courtship then women. In line with this, the wives of men with schizophrenia report that they were more active in pursuing their husbands than women married to men who do not have schizophrenia (Planansky & Johnson, 1967).

Research suggests that maintaining a close relationship with someone with schizophrenia can be difficult. Marital distress is common (Hafner, 1986) and divorce rates are high. More symptomatic clients are more likely to separate (Clausen, 1986). Although the development of a mental illness can be a major stress on a couple, some couples report that a psychotic episode in one partner can have a positive effect on the relationship by drawing the couple together.

Marital outcomes in women and men with schizophrenia appear to be different. On average, married men with schizophrenia tend to fare better than married women (Jablensky & Cole, 1997). This difference in outcome could be due to the fact that better premorbid adjustment is related to marriage more strongly in men than women with schizophrenia, or the tendency for wives of men with schizophrenia to be more sympathetic to their husbands about their illness than the husbands of women with schizophrenia.

Relationships with children are important to clients with schizophrenia. In their interactions with children, women with schizophrenia tend to express more tension and inappropriate behaviors as well as less attention, interaction, and reciprocity when compared to matched controls (Persson-Blennow, Naslund, McNeil, & Kaij, 1986). Parenting skills vary depending on premorbid functioning and symptom severity, with parenting functioning requiring several months to recover following a relapse (Rodnick & Goldstein, 1974). Many women with schizophrenia were poorly parented themselves and experienced abuse or neglect (Brunette & Drake, 1997). These childhood experiences may contribute to lack of knowledge about effective parenting. Because of the problems experienced by persons with schizophrenia, many give up or lose custody of their children (Miller & Finnerty, 1996), especially if they require psychiatric hospitalization early in their children's life. Multiple factors, including illness severity and timing, the parent's knowledge and skills related to parenting, and the presence of supports and services affect a client's ability to maintain custody.

Qualitative aspects of a close relationship can influence the onset and course of schizophrenia. Marital distress, conflict, and turmoil frequently precede the onset of psychosis and subsequent relapses and rehospitalizations. Abundant research shows that negative affect in a close family member (i.e., expressed emotion), especially a spouse or parent, can precipitate symptom relapses in people with schizophrenia (Butzlaff & Hooley, 1998).

Mechanisms by Which Schizophrenia Affects Relationships

By its very nature and the criteria used to diagnose it, schizophrenia can have a profound effect on close relationships. These relationships can, in turn, influence the course of the illness. Understanding how relationships affect schizophrenia, for better or worse, can enable clinicians and partners to take steps to stabilize the disorder and minimize symptom relapses.

A useful model for conceptualizing the interactions between the biological factors, the environment (including close relationships), and the course of schizophrenia is the *stress–vulnerability model* (Zubin & Spring, 1977). According to this model, the course and severity of schizophrenia are determined by the dynamic interplay between biological vulnerability, environmental stress, and coping skills. Biological vulnerability is assumed to be determined early in life by a combination of genetic and perinatal factors. This biological vulnerability is critical to the development of schizophrenia and without it the illness will not develop. When an individual has a biological vulnerability to schizophrenia, that vulnerability can be triggered by environmental stress, leading to the emergence of symptoms and characteristic impairments. Common examples of stress include major life events (moving away from home, starting a job, death of a loved one), tense and critical relationships with significant others, and lack of meaningful structure. After the onset of schizophrenia, exposure to stress can precipitate symptom exacerbations and further impair psychosocial functioning. Last, the more effective coping skills the client has, the less susceptible he or she will be to stress-induced relapses, as successful coping can either eliminate the sources of stress or minimize its negative effects.

The stress–vulnerability model has important implications for conducting couple therapy when one individual has the disorder. According to the stress–vulnerability model, outcomes can be improved through modifying biological factors (increasing medication adherence, decreasing substance abuse); the environment (decreasing tension in relationships, increasing social support); or the client (increasing coping skills and social skills). In order to address successfully the range of factors that can influence schizophrenia, clients and partners need to be engaged in a cooperative venture designed to teach them the requisite information and skills needed to manage the illness, to minimize its disruptive effects on their relationship, and to work toward achieving shared and individual goals.

Interventions designed to teach couples information and skills for managing schizophrenia must also take into account the symptoms and liabilities of the illness. This work aims to avoid precipitating relapses by helping the couple to maintain low levels of interpersonal stress while improving skills for resolving interpersonal conflict. Because of cognitive impairments, clients with schizophrenia may have difficulty grasping abstract concepts sometimes used in traditional couple therapy, requiring a greater emphasis on more concrete and behavioral skills. In addition, problems in social perception in persons with schizophrenia, including impaired emotion recognition, insensitivity to hints, and trouble understanding a partner's point of view, emphasize the importance of working on basic communication skills. Keeping the stress–vulnerability model and the characteristic symptoms of schizophrenia in mind, couple work focuses on teaching partners how to manage the illness and to develop better communication and problem-solving skills, with a deemphasis on fostering insight into relationship dynamics.

CLINICAL IMPLICATIONS FOR COUPLE THERAPY

Assessment

Because schizophrenia affects so many different areas of functioning, couple work requires careful attention to both the management of the illness and associated comorbidities, as well as relevant dimensions of the relationship. Therefore, assessment in couple therapy is necessarily broad based, because suboptimal treatment of the disorder will have a profound impact on the functioning of the client and their relationship. With respect to assessing the disorder, the evaluation must cover the core psychopathology of the illness (positive symptoms, negative symptoms, cognitive impairment), role functioning (e.g., as parent or student), social relationships, and self-care skills.

The ability to effectively manage the psychiatric illness and to work collaboratively with professionals is an important goal in couples work for schizophrenia, because some form of ongoing monitoring and treatment is usually required. To evaluate needs related to participation in treatment, each partner's understanding of schizophrenia and the principles of its treatment should be assessed. Participation in recommended treatments, especially adherence to prescribed medications, is another important topic for assessment. Just as the characteristic symptoms and impairments of schizophrenia should be assessed, so too should associated problem areas. Depression, substance abuse and dependence, past and current exposure to trauma (and aggression toward the partner), and posttraumatic stress disorder should be routinely assessed in clients with schizophrenia who are participating in couple therapy.

In terms of the couple's relationship, the usual dimensions of relationship satisfaction should be assessed, including satisfaction with shared leisure activities, distribution of household responsibilities, intimacy and sexual relations, child rearing, and relationships with in-laws. Because of the negative symptoms and social impairment characteristic of schizophrenia, role strain is common due to the tendency for the less ill partner to "pick up the slack," doing more household and parental tasks, working more, and initiating more communication and shared activities in the couple. Therefore, evaluating the extent of role strain and desired changes is crucial in couple work. Family planning needs also require special attention, because use of birth control is often sporadic, unplanned pregnancies are common, and as a result more stress is added to the relationship.

Although the partners of people with schizophrenia often take on a disproportionate share of responsibility in the relationship, it should also be noted that many such individuals have their own psychiatric problems (Shanks & Atkins, 1985), and that the psychological and psychiatric needs of these partners also require careful assessment. Especially common among partners of persons with schizophrenia are problems with substance abuse, depression or bipolar disorder, schizophrenia, and antisocial personality disorder. Just as schizophrenia can have a major impact on the relationship, so can another disorder in the other partner. If such a disorder is detected, appropriate steps should be taken to evaluate whether the individual is receiving appropriate treatment for that disorder. Furthermore, teaching the couple how to manage the partner's disorder needs to be incorporated into treatment.

Assessment methods rely primarily on interviews, conducted both conjointly and individually. Advantages of conducting individual interviews with each partner are that (1) some people feel more free to discuss certain concerns when alone with a therapist (e.g., domestic violence, substance abuse, blame, psychotic symptoms); (2) individual meetings serve to solidify the working relationship between each partner and the therapist; and (3) independent perspectives on the same issues can be assessed, thereby enabling the therapist to see where partners agree or disagree with one another. Individual interviews should be supplemented by a review of any available records and discussions with other persons involved in the treatment of the partner with schizophrenia. Specific forms and instruments for assessing couples in which one partner has schizophrenia or another major illness can be found in Mueser and Glynn (1999).

Treatment

The most important treatment implication for working with couples in which one partner has schizophrenia is the necessity for the dyad to be able to manage the disorder in collaboration with professionals. Because many difficulties in the relationship may stem from poorly managed symptoms, characteristic impairments, and misunderstandings about the illness that may lead to blame, most couple work in schizophrenia must first attend to developing an understanding of the illness and the skills needed to manage it. Only after such skills have been developed can effective work be done to address any remaining relationship problems. As previously described, the stress–vulnerability model provides a general heuristic in guiding couple work in schizophrenia, with the goals of reducing biological vulnerability and stress, and increasing coping skills and social support.

The most well-established intervention for families in which one member has schizophrenia, including couples, is behavioral family therapy (BFT) for psychiatric disorders (Mueser & Glynn, 1999). BFT is a variant of behavioral couple therapy, developed in the 1970s (Jacobson & Margolin, 1979). The goals of BFT are to teach the couple basic information about the nature and management of schizophrenia, to improve skills for communicating with each other, and to teach strategies for effective problem solving. The intervention typically takes between 9 months and 2 years (although ongoing maintenance sessions may be required for some couples), with sessions occurring on a declining contact basis (e.g., 13 weekly sessions, 13 biweekly sessions, followed by monthly sessions). Sessions can be conducted either at home or the clinic, with session duration approximately 1 hour. Although the focus of couple work is naturally on the couple, if other family members are closely involved, such as parents, in-laws, siblings, or adolescent or adult children, those individuals may be involved in some of the sessions.

BFT is divided into six components that are covered in sequence, with review and retraining conducted as necessary: engagement, assessment, psychoeducation, communication skills training, problem-solving training, and special problems. Educational handouts, worksheets, and homework assignments are routinely used to teach the information and skills. The elements of each component of the model are briefly described below.

Engagement

Successful engagement is critical to providing intervention, and care must be taken to present couple work as an integral part of treatment. Engagement is usually accomplished by first presenting a treatment overview to the client, followed by presenting it to the partner, and then arranging an orientation meeting to review the BFT program and set positive expectations for change. When engaging the client, the goals of BFT should be explained as teaching them information about how to manage schizophrenia, reducing stress, and increasing family support for pursuing individual and shared goals. It is important to emphasize that the focus of couple work is not just on the management of the client's disorder, but also on improving the overall quality of the relationship. Engagement of the partner follows a similar process, emphasizing the goals of avoiding relapses and rehospitalizations, improving the skills and functioning of the partner with schizophrenia, and helping the partner achieve personal and shared goals.

One common problem in working with couples in which one member has schizophrenia is that the healthy partner may experience significant bouts of demoralization and despair due to having witnessed and sought treatment for symptom relapses, mood problems, or problems meeting role expectations in their partner with schizophrenia. Instilling hope in the healthy partner that positive change and more effective management of the illness are possible, becomes a critical task in the engagement process. For example, the wife of a patient with schizophrenia was both anxious about and dubious of the potential benefits of couple work. Exploration of her concerns revealed that her husband had made numerous unannounced suicide attempts that left her feeling worried and helpless. The therapist was able to validate the wife's concerns, and explain that an important goal of couple work would be to develop effective strategies for responding to symptom relapses at the earliest possible time to avoid crises such as suicide attempts. This assurance was helpful in engaging the wife in couple therapy.

Assessment

After orienting the couple to the goals and expectations of BFT, individual meetings are set up with each partner. During these individual meetings, the therapist learns each person's perspective, including knowledge of schizophrenia and the principles of its treatment, perceived problem areas, and desired goals for treatment. At the completion of each individual assessment, each person is requested to identify between one and three personal goals to work toward over the next 6 months. Reassessments are conducted at least every 6 months, either on a joint or individual basis. Assessment information based on the interviews is supplemented by behavioral observations of communication and problem-solving skills in session.

Although couples benefit from working on mutual goals, setting individual goals for each person is also crucial for a healthy relationship. Furthermore, each person can obtain support and help from the other in working toward these goals. Examples of goals for individuals include completing high school or college, joining an exercise class, taking dance lessons, quitting smoking, getting a job or promotion, developing a new hobby, and saving for a new car.

Psychoeducation

Psychoeducational sessions are taught in a lively, interactive style, supplemented by handouts summarizing critical information. Three to six sessions are usually devoted to educating the couple about schizophrenia and its treatment, with major topics including diagnosis, symptoms, and course of schizophrenia; medications; the stress–vulnerability model; the role of the family; and drug and alcohol abuse. The client is identified as the "expert" concerning the illness and is relied on to share his or her expertise by helping describe symptoms and experiences related to the illness. Frequent questions are asked to evaluate the couple's understanding of the information and to help them see how it relates to their own situation. A premium is placed in psychoeducational sessions on establishing a calm, mutually respectful atmosphere in which information can be discussed and different perspectives aired without creating tension or conflict.

A unique issue that sometimes arises when conducting psychoeducation is that the client may not acknowledge having the illness, even after being informed of his or her diagnosis and after reviewing the symptoms. It is helpful for the therapist to conceptualize such denial of illness as an ego-preserving strategy whereby the client maintains self-esteem by not accepting the fact that he or she has a serious, socially stigmatizing disease. In the face of denial, the therapist should avoid trying to persuade the client that he or she has schizophrenia, which is usually unsuccessful, but instead should seek to find a term that the client feels more comfortable with, such as "nervous condition," "mental illness," or "stress problem." If the healthy partner attempts to convince the client of the diagnosis, the therapist should intervene by pointing out that what is important is that the client has agreed to couple work aimed at achieving shared goals. When the client does not accept the diagnosis, the therapist should nevertheless provide the same basic educational information about schizophrenia to the couple, while substituting the new term. Most clients who deny having schizophrenia are willing to acknowledge having some other difficulty that has interfered with their functioning and may have resulted in hospitalizations. By seeking common ground in psychoeducation and avoiding unnecessary conflict, the therapist models for the healthy partner how to communicate collaboratively with the client, while identifying and working toward agreed-upon goals.

Communication Skills Training

Some couples benefit from supplementary skills training in communication, whereas others do not need this. Indicators of the need for communication training include pejorative put-downs, frequent arguments, hostility, excessive criticism, and raised voices or frequent negative voice tone. When communication skills training is warranted, between four and eight sessions are usually spent teaching skills. Specific skills taught include active listening, expressing positive feelings, making positive requests, expressing negative feelings, compromising, negotiation, and requesting a time-out. These skills are taught following the steps of social skills training including modeling, role playing, positive and corrective feedback, and homework assignments to practice the skill on their own.

Communication skills training with couples in which one person has schizophrenia may require more time and patience than with other couples. The process of learning new skills is an arduous one for many clients, further slowed when cognitive impairment is prominent. Skills training may be needed over multiple sessions; even after training in problem-solving skills has begun, refresher sessions may need to be devoted to communication skills. The therapist can explain to couples that information-processing problems are common in schizophrenia, that communication must be direct, behaviorally specific, and include feeling statements (when appropriate) to be effective.

Problem-Solving Training

Training in problem-solving skills involves teaching the couple to solve problems or work toward goals following a six-step process: (1) define the problem; (2) identify possible solutions; (3) evaluate solutions; (4) select the best solution; (5) plan on how to implement the solution; and (6) follow up with implementation of the plan and conduct additional problem solving as necessary.

For each problem or goal, a "chair" is selected who guides the couple through the steps of problem solving, with either the chair or partner keeping a written record of each step. At the beginning of problem-solving training, the clinician models the skills for the couple, taking the role of chair, with subsequent problem-solving efforts chaired by the couple. Over time, increasingly more difficult problems are addressed. For most couples, the majority of sessions in BFT are devoted to training in problem solving, with 5 to 20 sessions spent developing this skill.

For most couples, teaching problem solving assumes that each partner is able to contribute equally to the process, and that each person is capable of "chairing" a problem-solving meeting. Although this is often the case when one partner has schizophrenia, when the disorder is severe it may compromise one partner's ability to take the lead in problem solving. In such cases, the therapist may work toward developing the skill of chairing problem-solving meetings in the healthy partner, while involving the person with schizophrenia in the steps of problem solving itself. Similarly, memory deficits in people with schizophrenia may interfere with conducting problem solving outside of sessions, and the healthy partner may need to be relied on more to initiate such meetings.

Special Problems

This final component of BFT involves teaching additional skills or using supplementary strategies to help the couple deal with problems not adequately addressed in the preceding components. Examples of special problems include contingency contracting, cognitive restructuring to deal with persistent depression or anxiety, graduated exposure therapy for anxiety problems, teaching parenting skills, and developing strategies to manage cravings for alcohol or drugs.

The evidence supporting BFT for schizophrenia is based mainly on controlled studies of families including clients living with or in ongoing contact with parents, spouses, siblings, or children. No studies have examined the impact of BFT on couples alone, although most have included couples as one of the family constellations involved in treatment. Treatment duration of BFT ranges between 6 and 24 months, with follow-up periods (posttreatment initiation) ranging from 6 months to 5 years. The most common outcome measured has been relapse and rehospitalization.

Comprehensive reviews of family intervention for schizophrenia have been published elsewhere (Pitschel-Walz, Leucht, Bäuml, Kissling, & Engel, 2001). Briefly, eight randomized controlled studies have been published examining the effects of outpatient BFT for schizophrenia. Among these studies, five included couples and compared BFT with standard care, with long-term (18 months or longer) outcomes across the studies favoring the BFT group in relapses, rehospitalizations, increased knowledge about mental illness, improved social functioning of the client, and decreased distress among relatives. In summary, the research provides support for the effects of BFT in families, including couples, in which one member has schizophrenia.

ADDITIONAL TREATMENT CONSIDERATIONS

Adjunctive Treatment

Couple work for schizophrenia needs to take place in the context of comprehensive treatment that attends to a wide range of clients' needs, including medical, psychopharmacological, and psychosocial concerns. Comprehensive case management is required to assess basic needs and to coordinate care. Because medical problems are frequently neglected in clients with schizophrenia, routine exams are needed to monitor physical health, including screening for infectious diseases. Pharmacological treatment with antipsychotic medications is the mainstay of treatment, with the vast majority of clients experiencing at least some benefit.

With respect to psychosocial treatment, several interventions in addition to family work have been shown to improve outcomes in controlled research trials (Mueser, Bond, & Drake, 2001). *Assertive community treatment* (ACT) is a case management model characterized by an intensive team approach to managing severe mental illness, in which caseloads are shared across clinicians, most services are provided in the community (e.g., clients' homes), and services are given directly by the team rather than being brokered to other providers. ACT has been found to reduce rehospitalizations and symptom severity, and to improve housing stability in multiple studies. *Supported employment* is an approach to vocational rehabilitation that focuses on rapid search for competitive work in integrated community settings, provision of follow-along supports, and integration with other treatments, and deemphasizes length of prevocational assessment and skills training. Abundant research shows that supported employment is more effective than other approaches to vocational rehabilitation.

Social skills training involves teaching new interpersonal skills, based on the principles of social learning theory, for improving social relationships and getting basic needs met. Multiple studies have shown that skills training is effective, especially when provided over long periods of time (e.g., more than 6 months). *Integrated treatment* of dual disorders (mental illness and substance use disorders) involves the use of assertive outreach to engage clients in treatment, motivational strategies, nonconfrontational approaches, and group, individual, and family approaches, and has been found to reduce substance abuse in clients with schizophrenia. *Cognitive-behavioral therapy* for psychosis, in which clients are helped to evaluate the evidence supporting delusional beliefs, has also been shown to reduce severity of psychosis, and in some studies to lower risk of relapses and rehospitalizations. There are many other potentially helpful adjunctive therapies for persons with schizophrenia, but which currently lack a strong empirical basis.

Clients who show needs in the areas addressed by these interventions may benefit from referral to additional services. At this time, there is little evidence to guide clinicians in determining when clients should be referred to a service. Although clients may be able to benefit from participating in several different interventions, it is prudent not to initiate too many new services at the same time, because clients may find this stressful.

Additional Resources for Couples

Couples may benefit from joining the National Alliance for the Mentally Ill (NAMI), an organization with regional chapters throughout the United States that provides education and advocacy services for persons with mental illness and their families. Local affiliates of NAMI usually conduct monthly meetings that provide education and support. Referrals for treatment and other resources are also available.

The self-help movement for severe mental illness has grown in recent years, with psychosocial clubhouses and "consumer"-run drop-in centers becoming increasingly available. Clients may find it useful to explore these programs because they offer hope, support from peers, and transitional employment opportunities across a range of jobs that help to develop work experience (Macias, Kinney, & Rodican, 1995). An important message of hope in self-help programs is that of *recovery* from mental illness, which is conceptualized as the process of clients taking control of their own lives and pursuing their own goals and interests, even in the face of a major mental illness.

Numerous books are available aimed at helping families of persons with schizophrenia learn and cope more effectively with the illness

(Keefe & Harvey, 1994; Mueser & Gingerich, 1994; Torrey, 1995; Woolis, 1992). Although no books are currently available that focus solely on the needs of couples, useful information is provided about the illness, medication, other treatments, and coping with symptoms and common problems. Family members can also find it useful to learn more about the experience of schizophrenia and to read other families' accounts of the relative's illness (Daveson, 1991; Kytle, 1987; Schiller & Bennett, 1994; Swados, 1991; Vine, 1982).

Resources for Couple Therapists

Therapists working with persons with schizophrenia and their partners need to become as familiar as possible with this complex illness and the broad range of effective treatments. Therapists should be familiar with the books listed in the previous section for families so that they can make specific recommendations. In addition to two books that serve as treatment manuals for BFT (Falloon, Boyd, & McGill, 1984; Mueser & Glynn, 1999), therapists may benefit from consulting several others books about the effects of mental illness on the family (Hatfield & Lefley, 1987, 1993; Lefley, 1996; Lefley & Johnson, 1990), and working with such families (Anderson, Reiss, & Hogarty, 1986; Barrowclough & Tarrier, 1992; Kuipers, Leff, & Lam, 1992; Marsh, 1998). Two professional journals are also devoted to schizophrenia, *Schizophrenia Bulletin* and *Schizophrenia Research*. Finally, numerous educational films and websites are available that provide useful information and resources about schizophrenia.

In addition to learning more about schizophrenia, the most valuable resource to the therapist is other people in the lives of the couple. Schizophrenia affects many areas, and effective treatment requires careful coordination between both professionals and significant others. Reaching out to and involving other caring individuals in treatment is critical to effective management and improvement of the illness. In addition to informal contacts with these individuals, it may be critical to involve such persons in some couple sessions so they can become more knowledgeable about the illness and play a constructive role in the client's rehabilitation. Examples of potentially important people include extended family members, friends, clergy, and other professionals such as other therapists and physicians.

CASE ILLUSTRATION

Nora was a 28-year-old married woman with schizophrenia who lived with her husband, James, and two children ages 18 months and 5 years old. Nora and James were referred for couple therapy shortly after Nora had been treated for a relapse of her psychosis that required a psychiatric hospitalization for 2 weeks.

Nora had been hospitalized first at age 24 and had experienced three hospitalizations prior to her most recent one. Each rehospitalization was associated with the development of paranoid delusions and auditory hallucinations, including command hallucinations to kill herself. Nora's symptoms were relatively well managed by antipsychotic medications, with only transient paranoid symptoms occasionally present. Her negative symptoms were less successfully treated and included blunted affect, apathy, and anhedonia. These symptoms had a profound impact on her functioning in the family, including her ability to care for her two children and her relationship with James. Although Nora showed some concreteness in thinking, her cognitive impairment was not prominent. She was intermittently compliant with prescribed medications. Nora drank alcohol with James, but not on a daily basis.

James was 32 years old and had alcohol dependence. He drank alcohol on a daily basis, intermittently used drugs (mainly marijuana, with some cocaine abuse), and described a pattern of erratic work due to his alcohol problem. James was aware of his alcoholism and expressed motivation to work on it. He had several periods of abstinence in the past several years, including one period of 8 months approximately 4 years before.

The couple experienced significant strain in their relationship. Nora's negative symptoms interfered with her ability to function as a mother, and made her an unrewarding companion for her husband. James's alcohol dependence resulted in inconsistent employment and contributed to the couple's financial strain. In addition, James's drinking frequently precipitated fights, which occasionally escalated into physical confrontations involving pushing and occasional blows. Child and protective services had been repeatedly called because of neighbors' concerns over the neglect of the children, although no legal action had ever been taken. The couple maintained close contacts with Nora's family including her mother, sister, and brother. These relatives were involved in helping Nora care for the children, stepping in during crises to take over her responsibilities.

After individual contacts with James, Nora, and Nora's relatives, the purposes of the family program (behavioral family therapy) were explained and everyone expressed interest in participating. Individual assessments with each person were scheduled to evaluate his or her understanding of schizophrenia, motivation for treatment, and to identify treatment goals. Because Nora's relatives were peripherally involved, the therapist elected to involve them in the educational sessions and some of the problem-solving sessions, while conducting most of the work with the couple.

The educational sessions went smoothly. The family discussion about the nature of schizophrenia and its characteristic symptoms was the first time any members had talked together about Nora's psychiatric illness. Although she expressed doubt that she had schizophrenia, she acknowledged having a "nervous condition" and was willing to serve as the "expert" in explaining the nature of the symptoms she experienced. Family members were interested to learn that medication is effective in reducing symptoms and preventing relapse, and James was corrected in his misconception that antipsychotic medications are addictive. Family members found the stress–vulnerability model especially useful, and Nora's sister noted that some of the relapses had occurred after stressful life events, including the death of their mother. Family members also found the information about the effects of alcohol on decreasing the benefits of antipsychotic medication useful. James commented that he sometimes noticed that Nora's symptoms seemed worse the day after they had been drinking together.

Four weeks were devoted to training the couple in communication skills. One major source of problems was that Nora had prominent blunted affect, including flattened facial expressiveness and lack of vocal inflection. James perceived Nora's lack of expressiveness as reflecting her disinterest. The therapist explained that blunted affect is a symptom of schizophrenia that often disguises an individual's true feelings, and that individuals with schizophrenia who display blunted affect can nevertheless experience the full range of human emotions (Berenbaum & Oltmanns, 1992). In order to help Nora compensate for her blunted affect in her interactions with James, communication skills training focused on helping her make clear the verbal feeling statements, both positive and negative, to better convey her moods.

The expression of negative feelings was especially difficult for James. He had been physically abused as a child and grew up in a home in which the open expression of negative feelings was punished. Instead of expressing negative feelings directly, he escaped by "drinking his feelings away." The therapist worked with the couple to provide them with better skills for expressing negative feelings, and encouraged James to check in with Nora after expressing a negative feeling to her to determine whether he had made his point without offending her. Because James had difficulty identifying and articulating his feelings, the therapist encouraged him to start a feeling log, and to include in this log situations in which he felt an urge to drink.

The couple had poor skills for resolving problems. As they became more able to express feelings directly, open conflicts decreased, but frustration was still evident in their inability to formulate and follow through on plans. Training in problem solving, which initially included the other family members, provided a much needed structure. After several weeks of training and graded homework assignments to practice the skill, the couple began to have meetings on their own to work on problems and goals together. Initially, challenging problems were avoided, with a focus on goals such as doing a leisure activity together or agreeing on a bedtime for their older daughter. Over time, as their skills developed, they began to address more difficult problems including distribution of the housework, childcare responsibilities, learning parenting skills to deal with common problems (e.g., bedtime), and getting help from Nora's relatives in baby-sitting.

Eventually, the couple raised the problem of their poor financial situation, which led to discussion of James' alcohol dependence. James had been recording his feelings in his log and had begun to track his daily drinking. He recognized that he had a problem and expressed motivation to become abstinent. In problem solving, different solutions were identified to the problem of alcoholism, and he chose to try and cut down his alcohol use gradually. James was unsuccessful at meeting his goals of reduced drinking, and after several weeks alternative solutions were reconsidered. James chose to participate in an inpatient detoxification program. He followed up on his plan and began regular attendance at Alcoholics Anonymous. In one session, the therapist and Nora helped James develop a relapse prevention plan for his alcoholism.

Treatment was provided over an 18-month period, including 32 sessions, with monthly booster sessions continued for an additional 6 months. Substantial gains were made in many areas that were maintained at a 2-year follow-up. Nora had no rehospitalizations, and on two occasions partial relapses were detected and responded to quickly, averting full-blown relapses. James's efforts to achieve abstinence were largely successful, and he obtained work several weeks after completing the detoxification program. He had one relapse of 4 days of drinking after 6 months of sobriety, and then regained abstinence in part through the support of his AA sponsor. He continued to be abstinent at follow-up, and had moved on to a higher paying job. The couple reported better confidence in their ability to care for their children, which was corroborated by the other relatives and the lack of any further involvement with child protective services. The couple also reported significantly greater satisfaction with their relationship, including more closeness and a better understanding of each other.

CONCLUSIONS

Because schizophrenia is defined in part based on social dysfunction, relationship problems are pervasive in this population. Couple therapy in which one individual has schizophrenia requires a comprehensive approach that includes teaching the couple information and skills for more effectively managing the illness, for resolving conflict, and for making progress toward individual and shared goals. Behavioral family therapy is a model for conducting couple work in which one person has schizophrenia that has been shown to improve the outcome of the illness. Through collaborative couple work and comprehensive treatment that includes medication and access to other evidence-based rehabilitation methods (e.g., supported employment, social skills training, integrated dual diagnosis treatment, cognitive therapy for psychosis), the long-term functioning of persons with schizophrenia can be optimized, paving the way to personal recovery from the illness and clients reclaiming control over their lives.

REFERENCES

American Psychiatric Association. (1994). *Diagnostic and statistical manual of mental disorders* (4th ed.). Washington, DC: Author.

Anderson, C. M., Reiss, D. J., & Hogarty, G. E. (1986). *Schizophrenia and the family*. New York: Guilford Press.

Argyle, N. (1990). Panic attacks in chronic schizophrenia. *British Journal of Psychiatry, 157*, 430–433.

Barrowclough, C., & Tarrier, N. (1992). *Families of schizophrenic patients: Cognitive behavioural intervention*. London: Chapman & Hall.

Berenbaum, H., & Oltmanns, T. F. (1992). Emotional experience and expression in schizophrenia and depression. *Journal of Abnormal Psychology, 101*, 37–44.

Brunette, M. F., & Drake, R. E. (1997). Gender differences in patients with schizophrenia and substance abuse. *Comprehensive Psychiatry, 38*, 109–116.

Butzlaff, R. L., & Hooley, J. M. (1998). Expressed emotion and psychiatric relapse. *Archives of General Psychiatry, 55*, 547–552.

Clausen, J. A. (1986). A 15- to 20-year follow-up of married adult psychiatric patients. In L. Erlenmeyer-Kimling & N. E. Miller (Eds.), *Life-span research on the prediction of psychopathology* (pp. 175–194). Hillsdale, NJ: Erlbaum.

Daveson, A. (1991). *Tell me I'm here: One family's experience of schizophrenia*. New York: Penguin Books.

Falloon, I. R. H., Boyd, J. L., & McGill, C. W. (1984). *Family care of schizophrenia: A problem-solving approach to the treatment of mental illness*. New York: Guilford Press.

Goldstein, M. J., Tsuang, M. T., & Farone, S. V. (1989). Gender and schizophrenia: Implications for understanding the heterogeneity of the illness. *Psychiatry Research, 28,* 243–253.

Green, M. F., & Nuechterlein, K. H. (1999). Should schizophrenia be treated as a neurocognitive disorder? *Schizophrenia Bulletin, 25*(2), 309–318.

Haas, G. L., & Garratt, L. S. (1998). Gender differences in social functioning. In K. T. Mueser & N. Tarrier (Eds.), *Handbook of social functioning in schizophrenia* (pp. 149–180). Boston: Allyn & Bacon.

Hafner, R. J. (1986). *Marriage and mental illness: A sex roles perspective.* New York: Guilford Press.

Harding, C. M., & Keller, A. B. (1998). Long-term outcome of social functioning. In K. T. Mueser & N. Tarrier (Eds.), *Handbook of social functioning in schizophrenia* (pp. 134–148). Boston: Allyn & Bacon.

Hatfield, A. B., & Lefley, H. P. (1987). *Families of the mentally ill: Coping and adaptation.* New York: Guilford Press.

Hatfield, A. B., & Lefley, H. P. (1993). *Surviving mental illness: Stress, coping, and adaptation.* New York: Guilford Press.

Jablensky, A., & Cole, S. W. (1997). Is the earlier age at onset of schizophrenia in males a confounded finding?: Results from a cross-cultural investigation. *British Journal of Psychiatry, 170,* 234–240.

Jacobson, N. S., & Margolin, G. (1979). *Marital therapy: Strategies based on social learning and behavior exchange principles.* New York: Brunner/Mazel.

Keefe, R. S. E., & Harvey, P. D. (1994). *Understanding schizophrenia: A guide to the new research on causes and treatment.* New York: Free Press.

Kuipers, L., Leff, J., & Lam, D. (1992). *Family work for schizophrenia: A practical guide.* London: Gaskell.

Kytle, E. (1987). *The voices of Robby Wilde.* Washington, DC: Seven Locks Press.

Lefley, H. P. (1996). *Family caregiving in mental illness.* Thousand Oaks, CA: Sage.

Lefley, H. P., & Johnson, D. L. (1990). *Families as allies in treatment of the mentally ill: New directions for mental health professionals.* Washington, DC: American Psychiatric Press.

Loranger, A. W. (1984). Sex differences at age of onset of schizophrenia. *Archives of General Psychiatry, 41,* 157–161.

Macias, C., Kinney, R., & Rodican, C. (1995). Transitional employment: An evaluative description of Fountain House practice. *Journal of Vocational Rehabilitation, 5,* 151–158.

Marsh, D. T. (1998). *Serious mental illness and the family: The practitioner's guide.* New York: Wiley.

Miller, L. J., & Finnerty, M. (1996). Sexuality, pregnancy, and childrearing among women with schizophrenia-spectrum disorders. *Psychiatric Services, 4*(5), 502–506.

Mueser, K. T., Bond, G. R., & Drake, R. E. (2001). Community-based treatment of schizophrenia and other severe mental disorders: Treatment outcomes. *Medscape Mental Health* [online journal], *6, www.psychiatry.medscape.com.*

Mueser, K. T., & Gingerich, S. L. (1994). *Coping with schizophrenia: A guide for families.* Oakland, CA: New Harbinger.

Mueser, K. T., & Glynn, S. M. (1999). *Behavioral family therapy for psychiatric disorders* (2nd ed.). Oakland, CA: New Harbinger.

158   TREATMENTS FOR EMOTIONAL AND BEHAVIORAL DISORDERS

Mueser, K. T., Rosenberg, S. D., Goodman, L. A., & Trumbetta, S. L. (2002). Trauma, PTSD, and the course of severe mental Illness: An interactive model. *Schizophrenia Research, 53*, 123–143.

Penn, D. L., Hope, D. A., Spaulding, W., & Kucera, J. (1994). Social anxiety in schizophrenia. *Schizophrenia Research, 11*, 277–284.

Persson-Blennow, I., Naslund, B., McNeil, T. F., & Kaij, L. (1986). Offspring of women with nonorganic psychosis: Mother–infant interaction at one year of age. *Acta Psychiatrica Scandinavica, 73*, 207–213.

Pitschel-Walz, G., Leucht, S., Bäuml, J., Kissling, W., & Engel, R. R. (2001). The effect of family interventions on relapse and rehospitalization in schizophrenia—A meta-analysis. *Schizophrenia Bulletin, 27*, 73–92.

Planansky, K., & Johnson, R. (1967). Mate selection in schizophrenia. *Acta Psychiatrica Scandinavica, 43*, 397–409.

RachBeisel, J., Scott, J., & Dixon, L. (1999). Co-occurring severe mental illness and substance use disorders: A review of recent research. *Psychiatric Services, 50*, 1427–1434.

Regier, D. A., Farmer, M. E., Rae, D. S., Locke, B. Z., Keith, S. J., Judd, L. L., & Goodwin, F. K. (1990). Comorbidity of mental disorders with alcohol and other drug abuse: Results from the Epidemiologic Catchment Area (ECA) study. *Journal of the American Medical Association, 264*, 2511–2518.

Rodnick, E. H., & Goldstein, M. J. (1974). Premorbid adjustment and the recovery of mothering function in acute schizophrenic women. *Journal of Abnormal Psychology, 83*(6), 623–628.

Roy, A. (Ed.). (1986). *Suicide in schizophrenia.* Baltimore: Williams & Wilkins.

Schiller, L., & Bennett, A. (1994). *The quiet room: A journey out of the torment of madness.* New York: Warner.

Shanks, J., & Atkins, P. (1985). Psychiatric patients who marry each other. *Psychological Medicine, 15*, 377–382.

Swados, E. (1991). *The four of us: A family memoir.* New York: Farrar, Straus & Giroux.

Tibbo, P., Kroetsch, M., Chue, P., & Warneke, L. (2000). Obsessive–compulsive disorder in schizophrenia. *Journal of Psychiatric Research, 34*, 139–146.

Torrey, E. F. (1995). *Surviving schizophrenia: A manual for families, consumers and providers* (Third Edition). New York: HarperPerennial.

Vine, P. (1982). *Families in pain: Children, siblings, spouses, and parents of the mentally ill speak out.* New York: Pantheon.

Weisman, A. Y., Nuechterlein, K. H., Goldstein, M. J., & Snyder, K. S. (1998). Expressed emotion, attitudes, and schizophrenic symptom dimensions. *Journal of Abnormal Psychology, 107*, 355–359.

Woolis, R. (1992). *When someone you love has a mental illness.* New York: Jeremy P. Tarcher/Perigee.

Zubin, J., & Spring, B. (1977). Vulnerability: A new view of schizophrenia. *Journal of Abnormal Psychology, 86*, 103–126.

CHAPTER 7

Alcohol and Other Substance Abuse

WILLIAM FALS-STEWART
GARY R. BIRCHLER
TIMOTHY J. O'FARRELL

Although alcoholism and drug abuse have been historically viewed as individual problems best treated on an individual basis (e.g., Jellinek, 1960), a large and growing body of literature suggests the family often plays a crucial role in the lives of alcoholics and drug abusers (Stanton & Heath, 1997). An increasing number of investigators and treatment providers have explored the interrelation of family factors and substance abuse, with the clinical applications of couple and family therapy to treatment of alcoholism and drug abuse increasing considerably over the last three decades. In fact, the Joint Commission on Accreditation of Health Care Organizations (JCAHO) standard for accrediting substance abuse treatment programs in the United States now requires that an adult family member who lives with an identified substance-abusing patient be included at least in the initial assessment (Brown, O'Farrell, Maisto, Boies, & Suchinski, 1997).

Enthusiasm for understanding the role family members may play in the development, maintenance, and treatment of alcoholism and drug abuse has not been limited to the research community. The sheer volume of texts in the lay press that have appeared on the topics of codependency, adult children of alcoholics, addictive personality, enabling, and so forth, is staggering. For example, an Internet search of a large online book retailer revealed that over 250 books were currently available for purchase on the topic of codependency alone. Moreover, self-help support groups for family members of alcoholics and drugs abusers (e.g., Al-Anon) are available in virtually every community.

Because relationship problems and substance use disorders so frequently co-occur, it would be very difficult to find clinicians who specialize in the treatment of adult substance use disorders or relationship problems who have not had to address concurrently both sets of issues for many clients seeking help. The purpose of the present chapter is to provide an overview of a behaviorally oriented couple-based treatment for substance use that would be useful to both specialists in either the treatment of alcoholism and drug abuse or the treatment of marital/relationship distress. Our goal is to provide an integrated conceptualization of substance use problems and dyadic relationships grounded in the empirical literature that has evolved over the last 30 years and thus is an alternative to the psychology of family and addiction that dominated the popular press for much of the late 20th century.

ALCOHOLISM AND DRUG ABUSE: A RELATIONSHIP-BASED CONCEPTUALIZATION

Before examining the interrelation of substance abuse and relationship functioning, it is important to provide contemporary diagnostic definitions of alcoholism and drug addiction.

Defining Alcohol and Drug Use Disorders

There are actually several different definitional frameworks for these disorders that have appeared in the literature. The most widely used is the psychiatric diagnostic approach, exemplified in the fourth edition of the *Diagnostic and Statistical Manual of Mental Disorders* (DSM-IV; American Psychiatric Association, 1994) and the 10th edition of the *International Classification of Diseases* (ICD-10; World Health Organization, 1992). Using the DSM-IV system as an example, the diagnosis of alcohol or psychoactive substance use disorders includes two general subcategories: abuse and dependence. *Substance dependence* is marked by a cluster of cognitive, behavioral, and physiological symptoms indicating that the individual continues to use a given psychoactive substance despite significant substance-related problems. To meet diagnostic criteria for dependence on a psychoactive substance, an individual must display at least three of the following seven symptoms: (1) physical tolerance; (2) withdrawal; (3) unsuccessful attempts to stop or control substance use;

(4) use of larger amounts of the substance than intended; (5) loss or reduction in important recreational, social, or occupational activities; (6) continued use of the substance despite knowledge of physical or psychological problems that are likely to have been caused or exacerbated by the substance; and (7) excessive time spent using the substance or recovering from its effects.

In contrast, the essential feature of *substance abuse* is a maladaptive pattern of problem use leading to significant adverse consequences. This includes one or more of the following: (1) failure to fulfill major social obligations in the context of work, school, or home; (2) recurrent substance use in situations that create the potential for harm (e.g., drinking and driving); (3) recurrent substance-related legal problems; and (4) continued substance use despite having persistent social or interpersonal problems caused or exacerbated by the effects of the substance.

Although the ICD-10 and DSM-IV definitions of alcohol and drug use disorders were claimed to be largely atheoretical by their developers, some have argued that the classifications arise from a medical model orientation (e.g., Pattison, Sobell, & Sobell, 1977). In turn, behavioral scientists have proposed an alternative approach to the disease concept of alcoholism and drug abuse that underlies the DSM classifications (e.g., Adesso, 1995; Nathan, 1981). In this framework, alcohol and drug use disorders are not defined as a unitary disease, nor is it implicitly assumed that the observed substance use symptoms are the manifestation of a disease state. Symptoms are viewed as acquired habits that emerge from a combination of social, pharmacological, and behavioral factors. Emphasis is placed on environmental, affective, and cognitive antecedents and reinforcing consequences of substance use. The outgrowth of this functional conceptualization of substance use is that drinking and drug use are ruled by motivation and learning principles, as are other human behaviors (Wulfert, Greenway, & Dougher, 1996).

Prevalence of Alcohol and Drug Use Disorders and Comorbidity with Relationship Problems

Epidemiological surveys of alcohol and drug use disorders indicate they are among the most common psychiatric disorders in the general population. The most recent national survey on the prevalence of alcohol and drug use disorders is the National Longitudinal Alcohol Epidemiologic Survey (NLAES; Grant et al., 1994), in which 42,862 noninstitutionalized respondents living in the contiguous United States, aged 18 years and older, were interviewed regarding their use of alcohol and other substances, using DSM-IV classification criteria. According to the

NLAES, the past year combined prevalence of alcohol abuse and dependence was 7.4%, representing more than 13 million Americans; the lifetime rate was 18.2%, or nearly 34 million Americans.

Prevalence rates of DSM-IV drug use disorders were much lower than those reported for alcohol use disorders. Rates for past year abuse and dependence for most drugs were less than 1%, with the exception of cannabis abuse and dependence combined (1.2%). The prevalence of past year abuse or dependence on any drug was 1.5%. Overall, the lifetime rate of any drug abuse or dependence was 6.1%.

There are several lines of converging evidence that indicate substance abuse and relationship distress covary. Although individuals diagnosed with alcohol abuse or dependence are just as likely to marry as the rest of the population, they are more likely to divorce or separate (Nace, 1982). Moreover, men and women with drinking problems are more likely to divorce than individuals with any other type of psychological disorder (Reich & Thompson, 1985). Several studies have found that levels of relationship distress among alcoholic and drug-abusing dyads are high (e.g., Fals-Stewart, Birchler, & O'Farrell, 1999; O'Farrell & Birchler, 1987). Relationship problems are predictive of a poor prognosis in alcohol and drug abuse treatment programs (Fals-Stewart & Birchler, 1994; Vanicelli, Gingerich, & Ryback, 1983). Finally, poor response to substance abuse treatment is predictive of ongoing marital difficulty (e.g., Billings & Moos, 1983; Finney, Moose, Cronkite, & Gamble, 1983).

In clinical samples, we also see indications that a high comorbidity exists between relationship distress and substance use disorders. In our studies, among adult substance-abusing clients entering treatment, roughly one third are married or cohabiting in stable relationships with romantic partners, with most of these couples reporting moderate to severe relationship distress (e.g., Fals-Stewart, Birchler, & O'Farrell, 1999). Moreover, in a study of 56 men seeking marital therapy, Halford and Osgarby (1993) found that more than one third met the criterion for alcoholism on a standard alcoholism screening interview, one fifth reported drinking at unsafe levels (i.e., 20 alcoholic drinks per week), and more than four-fifths reported frequent marital disagreements about alcohol use.

The Interrelation between Substance Use and Relationship Distress

The causal connections between substance use and relationship discord are complex and appear to interact reciprocally. For example, chronic drinking outside the home is correlated with reduced relationship satisfaction for spouses (e.g., Dunn, Jacob, Hummon, & Seilhamer, 1987). At the same time, however, stressful marital interactions are related to increased problematic substance use and are related to relapse among alcoholics and drug abusers after treatment (e.g., Fals-Stewart & Birchler, 1994; Maisto, O'Farrell, McKay, Connors, & Pelcovitz, 1988). Thus, the relation between substance use and relationship problems is not unidirectional, with one consistently causing the other, but rather each can serve as a precursor to the other.

Viewed from a family perspective, there are several antecedent conditions and reinforcing consequences of substance use. Poor communication and problem solving, arguing, financial stressors, and nagging are common antecedents to substance use. Consequences of substance use can be positive or negative. For instance, certain behaviors by a non-substance-abusing partner, such as avoiding conflict with the substance-abusing partner when he or she is intoxicated, are positive consequences of substance abuse and can thus inadvertently reinforce continued substance-using behavior. Partners who avoid the substance abuser or make disapproving verbal comments about his or her alcohol or drug use are among the most common negative consequences of substance abuse (e.g., Becker & Miller, 1976). Other negative effects of substance use on the family, such as psychological distress of the spouse and social, behavioral, academic, and emotional problems among children, increase stress in the family system and may therefore lead to or exacerbate substance use (Moos, Finney, & Cronkite, 1990).

CLINICAL IMPLICATIONS FOR COUPLE THERAPY

Our behaviorally oriented approach to couple therapy, which we refer to as behavioral couple therapy (BCT), with substance-abusing clients and their romantic partners does not have a unique set of assumptions about how people change but rather encompasses current notions about how people change in terms of the widely known stages-of-change model (Prochaska & DiClemente, 1983). In this model, individuals progress through different stages of change: (1) precontemplation, in which the individual is not concerned about changing his or her behavior; (2) contemplation, in which the individual becomes concerned about and begins to consider changing the behavior; (3) action, in which the individual changes the behavior and stabilizes this change for an initial period; (4) maintenance, in which the behavior change remains stable; and (5) relapse, in which the individual returns to the problem behavior. The family model we espouse in this chapter emphasizes the role of the spouse in influencing a person's progression through these stages. For example, a spouse's concern about their partner's alcohol or drug problem may move the individual from the precontemplation into the contemplation stage of change. In turn, this stages-of-change model helps guide the assessment and treatment of substance-abusing clients with couple-based therapy, whether the married or cohabiting substance-abusing individual is initially seeking substance abuse treatment or relationship therapy.

Assessment

The multifaceted aspects of both substance using behavior and relationship adjustment are targets of assessment procedures with alcoholic and drug-abusing couples. We advocate a multimethod assessment approach with these couples, typically including semistructured conjoint and individual interviews, paper-and-pencil questionnaires, and observed samples of couple problem-solving communication. Although beyond the scope of the present chapter, Fals-Stewart, Birchler, and Ellis (1999) provide a detailed description of assessment procedures often recommended with couples in which partners abuse alcohol or drugs.

The assessment phase includes both an evaluation of substance use severity and dyadic adjustment. The assessment of substance use involves inquiries about recent types, quantities, and frequencies of substances used, whether the extent of physical dependence on alcohol or other drugs requires detoxification, what led to help seeking at this time, the outcomes of prior efforts to seek help, and the goals of the substance abuser and the family member (e.g., reduction of substance use, temporary or permanent abstinence). Along with alcohol and drug use severity, it is strongly recommended that assessment include an evaluation of problem areas likely to be influenced by substance use, including (1) medical problems; (2) legal entanglements; (3) financial difficulties; (4) psychological distress; and (5) social/family problems (McLellan et al., 1985).

Concurrently, various aspects of partners' dyadic adjustment are also assessed. Birchler and Fals-Stewart (2000) have developed a conceptual framework called the "7 Cs," which describes seven critical elements of a long-term intimate relationship that need to be evaluated as part of any comprehensive couple assessment: (1) character features (e.g., personality traits); (2) cultural and ethnic factors (i.e., cultural, racial, ethnic, religious, family-of-origin, and socioeconomic variables); (3) contract (i.e., explicit and implicit expectations about partners' roles and what they expect to derive from the relationship); (4) commitment (i.e., to be involved, remain loyal, and to maintain the stability and quality of the relationship over time); (5) caring (i.e., partners' abilities to express relational behaviors that promote emotional and physical intimacy); (6) communication (i.e., open and honest sharing of information between partners); and (7) conflict resolution (e.g., skills in the areas of problem solving, decision making, and anger management). This would include a multimethod evaluation of partners' general relationship satisfaction and stability of the relationship (i.e., current or planned separations as well as any past separations) along with an assessment of each partner's psychological and personality functioning. Furthermore, several studies now suggest that spousal violence is alarmingly high among both alcohol- and drug-abusing couples (e.g., O'Farrell & Murphy, 1995); thus, evaluation of family violence and fears of recurrence must be assessed.

In our first meeting with clients, we typically inform them that the first two to three sessions are used to gather assessment information and that neither they nor the therapist are committing to engaging in treatment. After the assessment phase is complete, the partners and the therapist mutually determine whether the data gathered as part of the assessment suggest that treatment would be helpful, with the information garnered from the assessment used to develop and implement couple-specific treatment plans. Because there are clear therapeutic benefits to participating in the assessment (i.e., increased knowledge about substance use, rapport building, facilitating the contemplation of change) the discrimination between assessment and treatment is, in reality, a false dichotomy. But making this distinction serves an important purpose; for many clients, participating in an "initial assessment" is less threatening than delving directly into treatment.

After assessment information has been gathered, the clients and therapists meet for a feedback session, which we refer to as a "roundtable discussion," in which the therapist provides an overview of the findings from the evaluation, including impressions of the nature and severity of both the substance abuse and relationship problems. Partners are asked to be active participants in this discussion, sharing their impressions and providing any critical information they deem to be missing, inaccurate, or incomplete. The goals of this feedback session are to (1) provide the partners with objective, nonjudgmental information about the couple's relationship functioning and the negative consequences of the substance misuse, and (2) increase motivation for treatment.

Treatment

Nearly 30 years ago, the National Institute on Alcohol Abuse and Alcoholism (NIAAA) described couple and family therapy for alcohol dependent clients as "one of the most outstanding current advances in the area of psychotherapy of alcoholism" and called for controlled clinical trials to evaluate the effectiveness of this class of interventions (Keller, 1974, p. 161). Of the many forms of family-based therapies, one that held particular promise was BCT, also referred to as behavioral marital therapy (BMT), which has been shown to produce superior dyadic functioning among distressed couples compared to no treatment or nonspecific control conditions (Hahlweg & Markman, 1988), and to be equally or more effective than other therapies in terms of reducing relationship distress (Gurman, Kniskern, & Pinsof, 1986). Since the time NIAAA called for empirical examinations of family-based treatments for alcoholism, BCT has been evaluated rigorously in several controlled clinical trials. Results from these studies, which are summarized later in the chapter, provide very strong empirical support for the effectiveness of BCT with substance-abusing clients and their intimate partners.

Typical Treatment Goals

The two primary goals of BCT are to (1) eliminate abusive drinking and drug use and support the substance abuser's efforts to change, and (2) alter dyadic and family interaction patterns to promote a family environment that is more conducive to sobriety. Viewed from a relationship context, a high priority is to change substance-related interaction patterns between partners, such as nagging about past drinking and drug use and ignoring or otherwise minimizing positive aspects of current sober behavior. The stance we recommend treatment providers assume is to encourage abstinent alcohol- and drug-abusing clients and their partners to engage in behavior more pleasing to each other. Continued discussions about and focus on past or "possible" future drinking or drug use increases the likelihood of relapses (Maisto et al., 1988).

Therapists also help partners begin the process of repairing the extensive relationship damage that is often incurred over many years of conflict resulting from drinking and drug use. This is typically the most difficult aspect of treatment and involves not only allowing the non-substance-abusing partner to discuss the emotional pain they incurred during the course of their partner's drinking, but also eventually working toward a certain degree of forgiveness (while not committing to the unrealistic goal of forgetting the past). In turn, the substance-abusing partner must be able to tolerate the negative affect of these exchanges. It is the role of the therapist to help the non-substance-abusing partner modulate his or her negative affect, which can be very strong, so that these interactions are not overwhelming or otherwise destructive, while also assisting the substance-abusing partner to process the affect and express his or her feelings within the context of a constructive dialogue. Moreover, therapists help partners find solutions to relationship difficulties that may not be directly related to substance abuse. As therapy progresses, partners learn to confront and resolve relationship conflicts while avoiding relapse.

BCT works directly to increase relationship factors conducive to abstinence. A behavioral approach assumes that family members can reward abstinence—and that alcohol- and drug-abusing clients from happier, more cohesive relationships with better communication have a lower risk of relapse. The substance-abusing client and the partner are seen together in BCT, typically for 15–20 outpatient couple sessions over 5–6 months. Generally couples are married or cohabiting for at least a year, without current psychosis, and one member of the couple has a current problem with alcoholism, drug abuse, or both. The couple starts BCT soon after the substance user seeks help.

BCT Treatment Methods

BCT sees the substance-abusing client with the partner to build support for sobriety. The therapist arranges a daily sobriety contract in which the client states his or her intent not to drink or use drugs that day (in the tradition of one day at a time), and the partner expresses support for the client's efforts to stay abstinent. For alcoholic clients who are medically cleared and willing, daily Antabuse ingestion witnessed and verbally reinforced by the partner also is part of the sobriety contract. The partner records the performance of the daily contract on a calendar provided by the therapist. Both members of the couple agree not to discuss past drinking or fears about future drinking at home to prevent substance-related conflicts that can trigger relapse, but rather to reserve these discussions for the therapy sessions. At the start of each BCT couple session, the therapist reviews the sobriety contract calendar to see how well each member of the couple has done their part. If the sobriety contract includes 12-step meetings or urine drug screens, these are also marked on the calendar and reviewed. The calendar provides an ongoing record of progress that is rewarded verbally at each session. The couple performs the behaviors of their sobriety contract in each session to highlight its importance and to let the therapist observe how the couple does the contract, providing corrective feedback as needed.

Using a series of behavioral assignments, BCT increases positive feelings, shared activities, and constructive communication because these relationship factors are conducive to sobriety. *Catch Your Partner Doing Something Nice* has each partner notice and acknowledge one pleasing behavior performed by the other person each day. In the *Car-*

ing Day assignment, each person plans ahead to surprise their partner with a day when they do some special things to show their caring. Planning and doing *Shared Rewarding Activities* is important because many substance abusers' families have stopped shared activities that are associated with positive recovery outcomes (Moos et al., 1990). Each activity must involve both partners, either by themselves or with their children or other adults, and each activity can be carried out at home or away from home. Teaching *Communication Skills* can help partners deal with stressors in their relationship and in their lives, and this may reduce the risk of relapse.

Relapse prevention is the final activity of BCT. At the end of weekly BCT sessions, each couple completes a *Continuing Recovery Plan* that is reviewed at quarterly follow-up visits for an additional 2 years.

Typical Structure of Therapy Sessions

BCT sessions tend to be moderately to highly structured, with the therapist setting the agenda for the sessions from the outset of each meeting. A typical BCT session begins with an inquiry about any drinking or use of drugs that has occurred since the last session. Compliance with any sobriety contract that has been negotiated is also reviewed and any difficulties with compliance are discussed and addressed. The session then moves to a detailed review of homework assigned during the previous session and the partners' success in completing the assignment. The therapist then identifies any relationship or other types of problems that may have arisen during the last week that can be addressed in session, with the goal of resolving the problems and designing a plan for resolution. Therapists then introduce new material, such as instruction in and rehearsal of skills to be practiced at home during the week. Toward the end of the session, partners are given specific homework assignments to complete during the subsequent week.

During initial sessions, BCT therapists focus on decreasing negative feelings and interactions about past and possible future drinking or drug use and increasing positive behavioral exchanges between partners. Later sessions move to engaging partners in communication skills training, problem-solving strategies, and negotiating behavior change agreements.

Research on BCT with Alcoholism

A series of studies has compared drinking and relationship outcomes for alcoholic clients treated with BCT or individual alcoholism counseling. Outcomes have been measured at 6-month follow-up in earlier studies and at 18–24 months after treatment in more recent studies. The studies show a fairly consistent pattern of more abstinence and fewer alcohol-related problems, happier relationships, and lower risk of marital separation for alcoholic clients who receive BCT than for clients who receive only individual treatment (Azrin, Sisson, Meyers, & Godley, 1982; Bowers & Al-Rehda, 1990; Hedberg & Campbell, 1974; McCrady, Stout, Noel, Abrams, & Nelson, 1991; O'Farrell, Cutter, Choquette, Floyd, & Bayog, 1992). Domestic violence, with more than 60% prevalence among alcoholic couples before entering BCT, decreased significantly in the 2 years after BCT and was nearly eliminated with abstinence (e.g., O'Farrell & Murphy, 1995). Cost outcomes in small scale studies show that reduced hospital and jail days after BCT save more than five times the cost of delivering BCT for alcoholic clients and their partners (O'Farrell et al., 1996). Finally, for male alcoholic clients, BCT improves the psychosocial adjustment of couples' children more than does individual-based treatment (Kelley, Fals-Stewart, Clarke, Cooke, & Winters, 2000), even though children are not directly treated in either intervention. Thus, there may be a "trickle down" effect of the communication skills training used as part of BCT, with improved methods of interacting permeating the whole family system.

Research on BCT with Drug Abuse

The first randomized study of BCT with drug-abusing clients compared BCT plus individual treatment to an equally intensive individual-based treatment (Fals-Stewart, Birchler, & O'Farrell, 1996). Clinical outcomes in the year after treatment favored the group that received BCT on both drug use and relationship outcomes. Compared to those who participated in individual-based treatment, BCT participants had significantly fewer cases that relapsed, fewer days of drug use, fewer drug-related arrests and hospitalizations, and longer time to relapse. Couples in BCT also had more positive relationship adjustment on multiple measures and fewer days separated due to relationship discord than couples whose partners received individual-based treatment only.

Cost–benefit outcomes analyses of participants in this study also favor BCT over individual treatment (Fals-Stewart, O'Farrell & Birchler, 1997). Social costs in the year before treatment for drug abuse-related health care, criminal justice system use for drug-related crimes, and income from illegal sources and public assistance averaged about $11,000 per case for clients in both treatment groups. In the year after treatment, for the group that received BCT, social costs decreased significantly to about $4,900 per case, with an average cost savings of about $6,600 per client.

Results of cost-effectiveness analyses also favored the BCT group. BCT produced greater clinical improvements (e.g., fewer days of substance use) per dollar spent to deliver BCT than did individual treatment. Therefore, this study showed that in treating drug abuse, BCT as part of individual-based treatment is significantly more cost-effective and cost-beneficial than individual treatment alone.

Domestic violence outcomes in this same study also favored BCT (O'Neill, Freitas, & Fals-Stewart, 1999). Although nearly half of the couples reported male-to-female violence in the year before treatment, the number reporting violence in the year after treatment was significantly lower for BCT (17%) than for individual treatment (42%).

In a second randomized study of BCT with drug-abusing clients (Fals-Stewart, O'Farrell, & Birchler, 2001), 30 married or cohabiting male clients in a methadone maintenance program were randomly assigned to individual treatment only or to BCT plus individual treatment. The individual treatment was standard outpatient drug abuse counseling for the drug-abusing partner. Results during the 6 months of treatment favored the group that received BCT on both drug use and relationship outcomes. BCT compared to individual treatment had significantly fewer drug urine screens that were positive for opiates, fewer drug urine screens that were positive for any of the nine drugs tested, and more positive relationship adjustment measured with a standard questionnaire.

A third study (Fals-Stewart & O'Farrell, 1999) randomly assigned 80 married or cohabiting men with opioid addiction to equally intensive naltrexone-involved treatments: (1) BCT plus individual treatment (i.e., the client had both individual and couple sessions and took naltrexone daily in the presence of his spouse), or (2) individual treatment only (i.e., the counselor asked the client about naltrexone compliance but there was no spouse involvement or compliance contract). In the year after treatment, BCT had significantly more days abstinent from opioids and other drugs, longer time to relapse, and fewer drug-related legal and family problems than did individual treatment.

ADDITIONAL TREATMENT CONSIDERATIONS

BCT for alcoholism and substance abuse is most often delivered in the context of other services and self-help support. In some of our studies, BCT is used as part of a comprehensive treatment package that includes individual and group therapy for the identified substance-abusing client. In other trials, BCT is used as a "stand-alone" treatment; in both situations, BCT appears to be very effective.

It should be noted that, over the last 3 decades, proponents of the disease model of substance abuse (i.e., AA and related 12-step facilitation approaches) and behavior therapy have clashed over the nature of addictive behavior and the most effective methods for its treatment (McCrady, 1994). Because the disease model is, by far, the most common treatment philosophy espoused by treatment providers and treatment programs (e.g., Fuller & Hiller-Sturmhofel, 1999), the conviction that BCT, because of its behavior therapy underpinnings, may be at odds with the treatment philosophies of many programs is a major roadblock in the widespread use of BCT in community-based settings. This concern about the compatibility of BCT and program philosophy has been raised often by treatment providers who have attended workshops and practitioner-oriented presentations that we have conducted about BCT.

However, the BCT intervention we have used in our clinical trials is far from incompatible with a disease-model treatment orientation; in fact, in all of our current studies, BCT is being provided in settings in which nearly all the BCT therapists are proponents of the disease model of addiction. Moreover, as part of the BCT intervention, we strongly encourage clients to attend Alcoholics Anonymous, Narcotics Anonymous, and other self-help support programs. Thus, in our experience, BCT and the disease-model treatment orientation can be easily integrated, with BCT typically delivered within the context of a disease model framework. Understandably, most treatment providers are more comfortable with BCT once they become aware that it is compatible with a disease-oriented treatment approach.

CASE ILLUSTRATION

To illustrate some of the procedures we have described thus far, a case example is provided, based on a couple treated by a therapist under the supervision of the first author. Although selected background data have been changed to protect these partners' confidentiality, the methods used and results obtained have not been altered. To illustrate the communication patterns we have often observed in these couples, a partial transcript of a conflict-resolution discussion between the partners is also provided.

David was 35 years old and was referred to outpatient substance abuse treatment by a local judge after being convicted of driving while under the influence of alcohol. During a psychosocial assessment, the client described an extensive history of problematic alcohol use. David reported that, in his early 20s, he drank nearly every day, usually consuming three to five beers on each occasion. By his mid-20s, he began drinking greater quantities of alcohol on weekends (i.e., eight to ten drinks on Fridays after work and Saturday evenings) and experienced occasional blackouts.

David noted that he had entered a 28-day inpatient treatment program about 5 years before the present evaluation and stayed sober for roughly 1 year after treatment. He reported that financial problems, arguments with his wife, and stress at work contributed to his relapse. He also reported that, during the last 4 years, he drank daily, but that there had been a steady increase in daily alcohol consumption over that time period. It started at two to three drinks daily but had more recently become six to eight drinks each day. David stated that he drove his car while intoxicated on "too many nights to count." David met DSM-IV criteria for alcohol dependence. Although he had used marijuana occasionally in his early 20s, David did not abuse drugs other than alcohol.

David was asked if he was willing to participate in marital assessment with his wife, Janice. Although David acknowledged that he was reluctant to participate, he stated he would if his wife agreed to participate. He signed a release of confidentiality form to allow his therapist to discuss the possibility of participation with Janice. She agreed to come to the clinic with David; the assessment procedures to be used were described to the partners. It was also emphasized that this was only an assessment and participation in this evaluation did not commit either the couple or the therapist to treatment. Both partners agreed to complete the assessment.

During the assessment, the therapist collected background data from Janice and information about the couple's marriage. Janice was 31 years old and was employed part-time as an accounts payable clerk in an apartment rental agency. She reported she had never abused alcohol or used other drugs. David and Janice married after a 1-year courtship. Janice noted she knew David drank "heavily," but was not aware of the extent of his drinking until he entered inpatient treatment.

Both partners described their relationship as unstable and had recently discussed divorce. David added that Janice would state that she wanted a divorce every time the partners had a disagreement. David's primary complaint was that Janice "is never satisfied with anything and criticizes me for any and everything." Janice reported that David spent money they "could not afford to give up" to buy alcohol, which exacerbated their financial problems. Because of limited income, the partners reported that they could not afford to have and support a child, although both wanted to have children.

Along with financial problems, Janice said she felt neglected because David spent so much time with his friends drinking. Janice added that the partners rarely spoke to each other for more than 10 minutes on a given day and had not spent time engaging in recreational activities they enjoyed (e.g., going to the movies, eating out). Neither partner reported any episodes of spousal violence.

As part of the assessment, the partners were asked to discuss a problem they both agreed existed in their relationship while the therapist observed. This discussion was scheduled to last 10 minutes and was videotaped. The topic the partners chose was "financial problems." As part of this conflict resolution task, the partners were asked to describe the problem and work toward a solution. The following is a partial transcript of the partners' discussion, occurring about 1 minute after the task was initiated:

WIFE: Why is it that your priorities are your f**king friends, bars, spending our money? It makes me sick.

HUSBAND: Can you give me a good reason why I would want to be home? When I'm there, you crack on me about my drinking and about all the s**t I've done when I've been drunk. When I'm out, you bitch. I can't win . . . which is the way you like it.

WIFE: That's not fair. I want you to care about me and stop drinking.

HUSBAND: I've tried, but even when I am sober for a few days, you just bitch at me about what I did when I was drunk.

WIFE: It is the only time I can talk to you. You come home drunk, go to sleep, we never talk, we don't have sex. . . . You come in and pass out on the couch and leave before I get up. I go days without seeing you.

HUSBAND: I know. . . . For all I know, I thought you would be happy with this.

WIFE: That's bulls**t and you know it. We never talk about anything, never go out . . . the car needs to be fixed, you need to talk to your brother. . . . I'm left to solve everything and you are judge and jury. And, by the way, I hear you say you've not been drinking, but I never believe it . . . never. . . .

HUSBAND: If you won't let me off the mat . . . if I stop drinking, you use that time to piss all over me about what I did when I drink and you don't believe I am sober anyway . . . if I drink, you don't deal with me and I will not deal with you.

WIFE: I am just so lonely. I want to move back home near my parents so at least I can talk to someone.

HUSBAND: Yeah, to talk to them about me. . . .

This exchange revealed not only significant deficits in these partners' communication patterns, but also a lack of mutual caring and a general level of interpersonal antagonism. Although the agreed topic was financial problems, they introduced several other conflict areas without addressing the problem at hand. The content of the communication sample revealed the corrosive effects of alcohol on the marriage, with David's drinking at least appearing to interfere greatly with important relationship activities (e.g., talking to each other, having sex).

The partners ultimately agreed to participate in treatment. Early sessions involved introducing and following through with a negotiated sobriety contract which included five primary components: (1) David agreed to take Antabuse (for which he was medically evaluated) while being observed by Janice; (2) the couple agreed to a positive verbal exchange at the time when David took the Antabuse (i.e., David reporting he had stayed sober during the last day and promising to remain sober for the ensuing day and Janice thanking him for remaining sober); (3) Janice agreed not to bring up negative past events concerning David's drinking; (4) David agreed to attend Alcoholics Anonymous (AA) meetings daily; and (5) the partners would not threaten to divorce or separate while at home and would, for the time being, bring these thoughts into the sessions.

The partners reported that David's use of Antabuse was very helpful to both of them; David did not consider drinking while on Antabuse and Janice, because she watched David take the Antabuse, trusted that he was not drinking and thus had much greater peace of mind. The positive verbal exchange between the partners made the daily sobriety contract a caring behavior rather than a "checking up" procedure. David said there was less stress in the home because Janice did not bring up his past drinking. David's AA involvement provided him with a support network that did not include friends with whom he drank. Janice reported she occasionally attended an Al-Anon group for wives of alcoholics, which gave her a supportive forum to discuss her marriage.

Communication skills training focused on slowing down the partners' verbal exchanges, with an emphasis on recognizing and stopping "kitchen sinking" (i.e., talking about a multitude of problems rather than focusing on a single agreed-upon topic area). Partners were trained to make positive specific requests and to use "I" statements as a way to own their feelings rather than attributing how they feel to their spouse.

Later sessions addressed identified relationship problems. Assignments such as Catch Your Partner Doing Something Nice and Shared

Rewarding Activities served to increase positive verbal exchanges and mutual caring, along with reestablishing a long-term commitment to the relationship. Toward the end of therapy, the partners reported that BCT helped them learn to "enjoy each other again." They noted their sex life had improved dramatically and, with the help of the therapist, that they had sought the services of a credit counselor to assist them with some of their financial problems.

During the 2-year posttreatment follow-up interviews, David reported he had remained sober and continued to take Antabuse. Both partners reported that they made a point of doing something fun together at least once per week. David was attending AA meetings three times weekly. Although the partners continued to have money problems, Janice received a work promotion, which helped to alleviate some of the stress.

CONCLUSION AND FUTURE DIRECTIONS

Results from multiple studies conducted over the last 2 decades indicate that behavioral couple therapy (BCT) is an effective treatment for married or cohabiting alcohol- and drug-abusing clients, both in terms of reduced substance use, reduced spousal violence, and improved relationship satisfaction. To assist clinicians who wish to use BCT with substance-abusing clients and their partners, several overviews and detailed therapist manuals are available (e.g., McCrady, 1982; O'Farrell, 1993; O'Farrell & Fals-Stewart, 2000; Wakefield, Williams, Yost, & Patterson, 1996).

However, despite a large and growing body of empirical support, BCT for substance abuse is not frequently used in community-based treatment settings (Fals-Stewart & Birchler, 2001). Given the positive effects of BCT, this is most unfortunate. Thus, even more than additional BCT research, we need to concentrate on technology transfer (i.e., moving empirically supported treatments from research settings to practice) so that clients and their families can benefit from what we have already learned about BCT for alcoholism and drug abuse. The Institute of Medicine (1998) has documented a large gap between research and practice in substance abuse treatment. BCT is one example of this gap and is a general problem in behavior therapy in particular (Hayes, 1998) and in health care overall (Ferguson, 1995).

Thus, in terms of future directions, there needs to be more involvement in BCT research activities by clinicians who practice in treatment programs, who can identify those aspects of BCT that impede its move from research settings to community-based treatment facilities. In our recent trials, we have involved and solicited extensive feedback from practicing clinicians about the BCT intervention we use with clients. Among the fundamental concerns about BCT that have been raised by these clinicians are the following:

1. BCT often involves too many therapy sessions and needs to be abbreviated.
2. BCT is typically delivered by master's-level clinicians, even though most community-based treatment programs employ bachelor's-level and paraprofessional counselors.
3. BCT has not been extensively evaluated with female substance-abusing patients, gay and lesbian couples, and dyads in which both partners use drugs or alcohol.

These concerns have pointed the way for our future research. Addressing these issues in future studies (e.g., exploring the effectiveness of an abbreviated version of BCT compared to standard BCT, examining the comparative clinical effectiveness of BCT delivered by master's- versus bachelor's-level counselors) may help BCT to continue its progress from the ivory tower, where it frequently resides, into the hands of providers who routinely treat these clients, which is where it truly belongs.

REFERENCES

Adesso, U. J. (1995). Cognitive factors in alcohol and drug use. In M. Galizio & S. A. Maisto (Eds.), *Determinants of substance abuse: Biological, psychological, and environmental factors* (pp. 179–208). New York: Plenum Press.

American Psychiatric Association. (1994). *Diagnostic and statistical manual of mental disorders* (4th ed.). Washington, DC: Author.

Azrin, N. H., Sisson, R. W., Meyers, R., & Godley, M. (1982). Alcoholism treatment by disulfiram and community reinforcement therapy. *Journal of Behavior Therapy and Experimental Psychiatry, 13,* 105–112.

Becker, J. V., & Miller, P. M. (1976). Verbal and nonverbal marital interaction patterns of alcoholics and nonalcoholics. *Journal of Studies on Alcohol, 37,* 1616–1624.

Billings, A. G., & Moos, R. H. (1983). Psychosocial process of recovery among alcoholics and their families: Implications for clinicians and program evaluators. *Addictive Behaviors, 8,* 205–218.

Birchler, G. R., & Fals-Stewart, W. (2000). Considerations for clients with marital dysfunction. In M. Hersen & M. Biaggio (Eds.), *Effective brief therapies: A clinician's guide* (pp. 391–410). San Diego, CA: Academic Press.

Bowers, T. G., & Al-Rehda, M. R. (1990). A comparison of outcome with group/marital and standard/individual therapies with alcoholics. *Journal of Studies on Alcohol, 51,* 301–309.

Brown, E. D., O'Farrell, T. J., Maisto, S. A., Boies, K., & Suchinsky, R. (Eds.). (1997). *Accreditation guide for substance abuse treatment programs.* Newbury Park, CA: Sage.

Dunn, N. J., Jacob, T., Hummon, N., & Seilhamer, R. A. (1987). Marital stability in alcoholic-spouse relationships as a function of drinking pattern and location. *Journal of Abnormal Psychology, 96,* 99–107.

Fals-Stewart, W., & Birchler, G. R. (1994). *Marital functioning among substance-abusing patients in outpatient treatment.* Poster presented at the Annual Meeting of the Association for Advancement of Behavior Therapy, San Diego, CA.

Fals-Stewart, W., & Birchler, G. R. (2001). A national survey of the use of couples therapy in substance abuse treatment. *Journal of Substance Abuse Treatment, 20,* 277–283.

Fals-Stewart, W., Birchler, G. R., & Ellis, L. (1999). Procedures for evaluating the marital adjustment of drug-abusing patients and their intimate partners: A multimethod assessment procedure. *Journal of Substance Abuse Treatment, 16,* 5–16.

Fals-Stewart, W., Birchler, G. R. & O'Farrell, T. J. (1996). Behavioral couples therapy for male substance-abusing patients: Effects on relationship adjustment and drug-using behavior. *Journal of Consulting and Clinical Psychology, 64,* 959–972.

Fals-Stewart, W., Birchler, G. R., & O'Farrell, T. J. (1999). Drug-abusing patients and their partners: Dyadic adjustment, relationship stability and substance use. *Journal of Abnormal Psychology, 108,* 11–23.

Fals-Stewart, W., & O'Farrell, T. J. (1999). *Behavioral therapy enhancement of opioid antagonist treatment: Naltrexone with supervised administration using behavioral family counseling.* Unpublished manuscript, Old Dominion University, Norfolk, VA.

Fals-Stewart, W., O'Farrell, T. J., & Birchler, G. R. (1997). Behavioral couples therapy for male substance abusing patients: A cost outcomes analysis. *Journal of Consulting and Clinical Psychology, 65,* 789–802.

Fals-Stewart, W., O'Farrrell, T. J., & Birchler, G. R. (2001). Behavioral couples therapy for male methadone maintenance patients: Effects on drug-using behavior and relationship adjustment. *Behavior Therapy, 32,* 391–411.

Ferguson, J. H. (1995). Technology transfer: Consensus and participation. The NIH Consensus Development Program. *Joint Commission Journal on Quality Improvement, 21*(7), 332–336.

Finney, J. W., Moos, R. H., Cronkite, R. C., & Gamble, W. (1983). A conceptual model of the functioning of married persons with impaired partners: Spouses of alcoholic patients. *Journal of Marriage and the Family, 45,* 23–34.

Fuller, R. K., & Hiller-Sturmhofel, S. (1999). Alcoholism treatment in the United States: An overview. *Alcohol Research and Health: The Journal of the National Institute on Alcohol Abuse and Alcoholism, 23,* 69–77.

Grant, B. F., Harford, T. C., Dawson, D. A., Chou, S. P., Dufour, M., & Pickering, R. (1994). Prevalence of DSM-IV alcohol abuse and dependence: United States, 1992. *Alcohol Health and Research World, 18*, 243–247.

Gurman, A. S., Kniskern, D. P., & Pinsof, W. M. (1986). Research on the process and outcome of marital and family therapy. In S. L. Garfield & A. E. Bergin (Eds.), *Handbook of psychotherapy and behavior change* (3rd ed., pp. 565–624). New York: Wiley.

Hahlweg, K., & Markman, H. J. (1988). Effectiveness of behavioral marital therapy: Empirical status of behavioral techniques in preventing and alleviating marital distress. *Journal of Consulting and Clinical Psychology, 56*, 440–447.

Halford, W. K., & Osgarby, S. M. (1993). Alcohol abuse in clients presenting with marital problems. *Journal of Family Psychology, 6*, 245–254.

Hayes, S. C. (1998). Dissemination research now. *The Behavior Therapist, 29*, 166–169.

Hedberg, A. G., & Campbell, L. (1974). A comparison of four behavioral treatments of alcoholism. *Journal of Behavior Therapy and Experimental Psychiatry, 5*, 251–256.

Institute of Medicine. (1998). *Bridging the gap between practice and research: Forging partnerships with community-based drug and alcohol treatment.* Washington, DC: National Academy of Sciences Press.

Jellinek, E. M. (1960). *The disease concept of alcoholism.* New Haven, CT: Hillhouse Press.

Keller, M. (1974). Trends in treatment of alcoholism. In M. Keller (Ed.), *Second special report to the U.S. Congress on alcohol and health* (pp. 145–167). Washington, DC: Department of Health, Education, and Welfare.

Kelley, M. L., Fals-Stewart, W., Clarke, E. G., Cooke, C. G., & Winters, J. J. (2000, August). *Couples treatment for drug abusers: Effects on children.* Poster presented at the 105th Annual Convention of the American Psychological Association, Washington, DC.

Maisto, S. A., O'Farrell, T. J., McKay, J., Connors, G. J., & Pelcovitz, M. A. (1988). Alcoholics' attributions of factors affecting their relapse to drinking and reasons for terminating relapse events. *Addictive Behaviors, 13*, 79–82.

McCrady, B. S. (1982). Conjoint behavioral treatment of an alcoholic and his spouse. In W. M. Hay & Nathan, P. E. (Eds.), *Clinical case studies in the behavioral treatment of alcoholism* (pp. 127–156). New York: Plenum Press.

McCrady, B. (1994). Alcoholics Anonymous and behavior therapy: Can habits be treated as diseases? Can diseases be treated as habits? *Journal of Consulting and Clinical Psychology, 62*, 1159–1166.

McCrady, B., Stout, R., Noel, N., Abrams, D., & Nelson, H. (1991). Comparative effectiveness of three types of spouse involved alcohol treatment: Outcomes 18 months after treatment. *British Journal of Addiction, 86*, 1415–1424.

McLellan, A. T., Luborsky, L., Cacciola, J., Griffith, J., Evans, F., Barr, H. L., & O'Brien, C. P. (1985). New data from the Addiction Severity Index: Reliability and validity in three centers. *The Journal of Nervous and Mental Disease, 173*, 412–423.

Moos, R. J., Finney, J. W., & Cronkite, R. C. (1990). *Alcoholism treatment: Context, process and outcome.* New York: Oxford University Press.

Nace, P. E. (1982). Therapeutic approaches to the alcoholic marriage. *Psychiatric Clinics of North America, 5,* 543–561.

Nathan, P. E. (1981). Prospects for a behavioral approach to the diagnosis of alcoholism. In R. E. Meyer, T. F. Babor, B. C. Glueck, J. H. Jaffe, J. E. O'Brian, & J. R. Stabenau (Eds.), *Evaluation of the alcoholic: Implications for theory, research, and treatment* (DHHS Publication No. ADM 81-1003, pp. 85–102). Washington, DC: National Institute on Alcohol Abuse and Alcoholism.

O'Farrell, T. J. (1993). A behavioral marital therapy couples group program for alcoholics and their spouses. In T. J. O'Farrell (Ed.), *Treating alcohol problems: Marital and family interventions* (pp. 170–209). New York: Guilford Press.

O'Farrell, T. J., & Birchler, G. R. (1987). Marital relationships of alcoholic, conflicted, and nonconflicted couples. *Journal of Marital and Family Therapy, 13,* 259–274.

O'Farrell, T. J., Choquette, K. A., Cutter, H. S. G., Brown, E. D., Bayog, R., McCourt, W., Lowe, J., Chan, A., & Deneault, P. (1996). Cost–benefit and cost-effectiveness analyses of behavioral marital therapy with and without relapse prevention sessions for alcoholics and their spouses. *Behavior Therapy, 27,* 7–24.

O'Farrell, T. J., Cutter, H. S. G., Choquette, K. A., Floyd, F. J., & Bayog, R. D. (1992). Behavioral marital therapy for male alcoholics: Marital and drinking adjustment during the two years after treatment. *Behavior Therapy, 23,* 529–549.

O'Farrell, T. J., & Fals-Stewart, W. (2000). Behavioral couples therapy for alcoholism and drug abuse. *Journal of Substance Abuse Treatment, 18,* 51–54.

O'Farrell, T. J., & Murphy, C. M. (1995). Marital violence before and after alcoholism treatment. *Journal of Consulting and Clinical Psychology, 63,* 256–262.

O'Neill, S., Freitas, T. T., & Fals-Stewart, W. (1999). *The effect of behavioral couples therapy on spousal violence among drug abusers.* Paper presented at the Annual Meeting of the Association for Advancement of Behavior Therapy, Toronto.

Pattison, E. M., Sobell, M. B., & Sobell, L. C. (1977). *Emerging concepts of alcohol dependence.* New York: Springer.

Prochaska, J. O., & DiClemente, C. C. (1983). Stages and process of self-change of smoking: Toward and integrative model of change. *Journal of Consulting and Clinical Psychology, 51,* 390–395.

Reich, J., & Thompson, W. D. (1985). Marital status of schizophrenic and alcoholic patients. *Journal of Nervous and Mental Disease, 173,* 499–502.

Stanton, M. D., & Heath, A. W. (1997). Family and marital treatment. In J. H. Lowinson, P. Ruiz, R. B. Millman, & J. G. Langrod (Eds.), *Substance abuse: A comprehensive textbook* (3rd ed., pp. 448–454). Baltimore: Williams & Wilkins.

Vanicelli, M., Gingerich, S., & Ryback, R. (1983). Family problems related to the treatment and outcome of alcoholic patients. *British Journal of Addiction, 78,* 193–204.

Wakefield, P. J., Williams, R. E., Yost, E. B., & Patterson, K. M. (1996). *Couple therapy for alcoholism.* New York: Guilford Press.

World Health Organization. (1992). *International classification of diseases and related health problems* (10th rev.). Geneva: Author.

Wulfert, E., Greenway, D. E., & Dougher, M. J. (1996). A logical functional analysis of reinforcement-based disorders: Alcoholism and pedophilia. *Journal of Consulting and Clinical Psychology, 64,* 1140–1115.

CHAPTER 8

Sexual Dysfunction

LISA G. REGEV
WILLIAM O'DONOHUE
CLAUDIA AVINA

W hat we know intuitively has been demonstrated empirically: There is a strong relationship between marital and sexual satisfaction (Barnett & Nietzel, 1979). Couples who are satisfied in their marital relationship tend to also be satisfied in their sexual relationship and vice versa. While the causal mechanisms for this association are less clear, there is a well-documented bidirectional relationship between marital satisfaction and sexual satisfaction. Sexuality and sensuality are ways in which couples share and express intimacy. Some individuals may choose to terminate a relationship due to sexual dissatisfaction and others may suspect or consider affairs in the face of sexual problems. Conversely, marital and sexual dissatisfaction may result from similar problems including lack of communication, trust, or attentiveness.

Unfortunately, researchers and clinicians have generally treated these two domains as distinct. Clinicians and researchers have generally focused on either what happens in the bedroom or out of the bedroom, rather than taking an integrative approach. Guided by the research literature, this chapter seeks to integrate these two issues. We begin by introducing the concept of sexual dysfunction.

CONCEPTUALIZATION

Sexual dysfunction is characterized by a disruption in the processes associated with the sexual response cycle or by genital pain associated with sexual activity (American Psychiatric Association, 2000). This includes problems of desire, arousal, orgasm, and genital pain. According to the text revision of the fourth edition of the *Diagnostic and Statistical Manual of Mental Disorders* (DSM-IV-TR; American Psychiatric Association, 2000), sexual problems are diagnosed if they are persistent or recurrent, cause marked distress or interpersonal difficulty, are not better accounted for by another Axis I disorder, are not due exclusively to the direct physiological effects of a substance, and are not due exclusively to a general medical condition.

Problems of desire include hypoactive sexual desire disorder and sexual aversion disorder. One is said to be suffering from low desire if he or she infrequently experiences fantasies or infrequently desires to engage in sexual activities. It is difficult to identify the "normal" frequency in which one is expected to desire sexual activity. Pridal and LoPiccolo (2000) caution against referencing an external standard when distinguishing between normal and low sexual desire in clinical practice. It is important to consider the distress level when making this determination, particularly considering the wide variability of responses on this dimension.

Sexual aversion disorder consists of "persistent or recurrent extreme aversion to, and avoidance of, all (or almost all) genital sexual contact with a sexual partner" (American Psychiatric Association, 2000, p. 542). Generally, this avoidance manifests itself as anxiety, fear, or disgust when the possibility of engaging in sexual activity arises. Clients presenting with such an aversion may indicate panic attacks and physiological reactions such as feeling faint, nauseous, and dizzy when presented with sexual stimuli. These individuals may seek to avoid sexual situations in various ways, including immersing themselves in work or other relationships or substance use.

Sexual arousal disorders include female sexual arousal disorder and male erectile disorder. These problems relate to the inability to attain or maintain until completion of the sexual activity an adequate lubrication–swelling response in women or an adequate erection in men, assuming adequate sexual stimulation. For women, this disorder may be accompanied by low desire, the inability to reach orgasm, or pain associated with intercourse. For men, this disorder may be associated with preoccupations regarding the inability to perform sexually and satisfy his partner.

Orgasmic disorders include female orgasmic disorder, male orgasmic disorder, and premature ejaculation. The first two disorders consist of delayed orgasm or the inability to reach orgasm, assuming this is preceded by a normal excitement phase. Younger women and older men are more likely to experience these problems (Laumann, Paik, &

Rosen, 1999). Women's orgasmic capacity is positively correlated with sexual experience, whereby greater sexual experience is associated with an increased likelihood of reaching orgasm.

Conversely, premature ejaculation consists of ejaculation with minimal sexual stimulation. Additionally the individual must be distressed by this and wish to prolong his period of ejaculation. This disorder is inversely related to age, whereby the younger the individual, the more likely he is to ejaculate prematurely. Additionally, the novelty of the sexual partner and recent frequency of sexual activity must be taken into account. Latency of ejaculation has been found to be inversely related to the period of abstinence from intercourse or ejaculation (Spiess, Geer, & O'Donohue, 1984).

The sexual pain disorders consist of dyspareunia and vaginismus. Dyspareunia is defined as genital pain associated with sexual intercourse in either gender. Vaginismus consists of involuntary spasms in the vagina that interfere with sexual intercourse. These disorders may result in avoidance of sexual experiences.

Recent epidemiological data indicate that 43% of women and 31% of men will experience sexual dysfunction during their lifetime (Laumann et al., 1999). More specifically, 22% of women and 5% of men will suffer from low desire, 14% of females and 5% of males will suffer from problems of arousal, 21% of males will suffer from premature ejaculation, and 7% of females will suffer from genital pain during intercourse. These data could be an underestimate considering that long-term abstainers were excluded from the study. These abstainers may be overrepresentative of the sexual desire disorders, considering that one common manifestation of the disorder is not engaging in sexual activity. Given the relational nature of these disorders, it is reasonable to surmise that practically all individuals will encounter one form of a sexual problem at some point in their lives. This may occur by experiencing the disorder themselves or in their sexual interactions with a partner. Clearly, these problems are pervasive and call for clinicians working with couples to be knowledgeable regarding assessment and treatment.

Laumann and his colleagues also found that married men and women were less likely to experience sexual problems as compared to individuals who were never married or no longer married. The authors suggest that this finding is likely due to the differing sexual lifestyles of those who are married and those who are not married. Married individuals are less likely to experience sexual stress in that they engage in sexual activity with a consistent partner. People who engage in sexual activity with a consistent partner may also be more likely to know how to sexually satisfy their partner than those who engage in activity with a new partner. Additionally, people who experienced emotional or stress-related problems were more likely to experience sexual dysfunction, including deteriorating social and economic position and prior sexual victimization. Likewise, education level was also negatively correlated with sexual problems, whereby the more educated the individual, the less likely he or she was to report sexual problems.

As noted earlier, there appears to be a strong relationship between marital and sexual satisfaction (Barnett & Nietzel, 1979). Couples who report high overall relationship satisfaction also report two to three times more frequent and more satisfying sexual relationships. In contrast, there appears to be no relationship between marital satisfaction and sexual dysfunction, with the exception of problems of desire (Morokoff & Gillilland, 1993). This is not surprising given that sexual dysfunction is not related to sexual satisfaction (Heiman, Gladue, Roberts, & LoPiccolo, 1986). In other words, couples who experience sexual dysfunction may also experience sexual as well as relationship satisfaction. In fact, couples presenting to sex therapy clinics often report being in the normal range of marital satisfaction (LoPiccolo, Heiman, Hogan, & Roberts, 1985).

As such, although sexual dysfunction may both impact and be impacted by relationship variables, couples with a strong, committed relationship need not be adversely affected by sexual dysfunction. Heiman et al. (1986) found that among couples presenting for sex therapy, sexual satisfaction and marital satisfaction were experienced independently. More specifically, they found that couples experiencing sexual problems reported being satisfied in their marital relationship. Regarding desire, however, there appears to be a negative relationship between desire to engage in sexual activity and marital satisfaction (Morokoff & Gillilland, 1993). They found that men who wanted to engage in sex more often were more likely to be dissatisfied in the relationship.

However, for couples experiencing marital problems, sexual problems may further distance them in ways that lead to loss of trust and intimacy, which may then be sought outside the relationship. Sexual aversion may leave the partner feeling rejected, unwanted, and unloved. Additionally, sexual dysfunction may have developed as a result of marital problems. Hostility toward the partner, role conflicts, and loss of attraction may lead to sexual avoidance and loss of desire. Lack of trust or fear within the couple's relationship may result in sexual dysfunction, such as vaginismus, which may result in unconsummated marriages or "infertility." Snyder and Berg (1983) found that for couples seeking sex therapy, sexual dissatisfaction was associated with two relationship variables including the partner's lack of response to sexual requests and lack of affection towards the partner.

Metz and Epstein (2002) suggest a number of possible links between relationship conflict and sexual functioning. One possibility relates to characteristics of one of the partners that lead to both sexual dysfunction and relationship distress, such as childhood sexual abuse. This history for one partner may affect the way he or she approaches both the relationship and sex, such as with a lack of trust. Another prospect includes relationship conflict and ways in which this may possibly lead to sexual dysfunction. Partners may feel "global negative emotions" which may then preclude sexual desire and arousal. Additionally, couples in conflict may seek to protect themselves, thereby precluding becoming vulnerable emotionally and sexually. Although these may be theoretically logical, more research is necessary to substantiate causal links for these various paths.

Leiblum and Rosen (1991) have identified four primary variables of the couple's relationship that may develop or maintain sexual problems, in sensual and erectile disorders in particular. These include status and dominance, intimacy and trust, sexual attraction and desire, and sexual scripts. Regarding status and dominance, they suggest that dissatisfaction with the balance of power in the relationship may result in sexual dysfunction, particularly for males. Regarding trust and intimacy, they indicate that it is difficult to maintain sexual interest or receptivity to sexual advances when feeling anger and distrust. They further suggest that these feelings may result in sexual dysfunction. The same may be true for individuals who are not sexually attracted to their partners. Lack of attraction may result in little desire to engage in sexual activity and when engaging in these activities partners may experience low levels of arousal. They also discuss ways in which differing sexual scripts may result in sexual dysfunction. "Sexual scripts define the range of sexual behaviors that are acceptable, with whom, under what circumstances, and with what motives" (p. 156). Sexual dysfunction may occur when the partners' scripts diverge considerably.

ASSESSMENT

There are a number of strategies to consider when determining what domains to assess for a given disorder. Generally, it is important to assess variables that may be influencing the problem, particularly variables that can be manipulated in treatment. The following section discusses various approaches of assessment, including assessment based on symptomatology as delineated in DSM-IV-TR (American Psychiatric Association, 2000) and etiological and maintaining factors. Currently the primary way in which clinicians collect this information is through self-report and partner report of the problem. This may include conducting an interview, using questionnaires, and asking clients to chart their sexual behavior using a behavioral record. The *Handbook of Sexuality-Related Measures* (Davis, Yarber, Bauserman, Schreer, & Davis, 1998) provides interested readers with information regarding many of the self-report measures available to assess sexual functioning, including psychometric properties of these instruments. Unfortunately, most of these instruments do not have sufficient psychometric information to justify their clinical use.

As noted earlier, the DSM delineates four categories of sexual dysfunction including problems of desire, arousal, orgasm, and genital pain. Assessment based on this nosological system would require collecting data regarding each of these possible problems. Overall, it is also important to identify the presence and degree of distress caused by the sexual problem, for the individual as well as the interpersonal relationship. Additionally, it is important to rule out another Axis I disorder that may be etiologically related to the dysfunction, such as depression, obsessive–compulsive disorder, and posttraumatic stress disorder. The use of substances (such as street drugs, prescription medications, and alcohol) and a general medical condition (such as diabetes) may interfere with sexual functioning as well. To rule out an organic cause for the disorder, it is generally prudent to refer individuals to a primary care physician, a gynecologist, or urologist for a medical examination. Likewise, it is important to determine when the problem began (e.g., is it lifelong or acquired?), whether it occurs with a specific partner or more generally, and is it due to psychological factors or combined psychological and medical problems. Answers to these questions guide treatment decisions, including whether to treat the relationship or the sexual dysfunction.

When measuring desire, it is important to assess subjective factors of desire such as fantasies and urges to engage in sexual activity. This is in contrast to simply inquiring about the frequency of sexual activity, which may be influenced by pressure from the sexual partner or guilt about not satisfying the partner. Additionally, avoidance of genital contact must be assessed. Because frequency of desire may be influenced by the individual's age and other factors in the person's life (including relationship factors), it is important to take these factors into account prior to reaching a diagnostic decision.

Regarding arousal, it is necessary to assess the woman's lubrication–swelling response and the presence and degree of the man's erection until completion of the sexual activity. When seeking to diagnose arousal disorders, it is important to inquire about the adequacy of sexual stimulation. Problems that may present as deficits of arousal may be due to inadequate time spent on foreplay or differing notions regarding what constitutes foreplay. There is an old joke that states the reason women fake orgasm is because men fake foreplay. For example, being awakened by demands for immediate sexual activity often does not result in sexual excitement.

Assessment of orgasmic disorders includes asking about the presence of orgasm, the amount of time elapsed prior to reaching orgasm, the presence of a normal sexual excitement phase, the type and intensity of stimulation, and contextual factors such as age, novelty of the sexual partner, sexual experience, and stress level. Assessment of the pain disorders includes inquiring about the presence of genital pain, degree of lubrication, presence of involuntary spasm of the musculature of the outer third of the vagina, and degree of interference with coitus.

It is important to inquire as to when the dysfunction began and the circumstances surrounding this time. Additionally, it is important to assess relationship factors including attraction to the partner, overall relationship satisfaction, and the couple's ability to communicate sexual preferences. Asking detailed questions regarding a specific recent sexual encounter may assess other possible factors (Regev, 2001). By asking about how the interaction was initiated, time spent on individual activities, thoughts and feelings during the interaction, and how the interaction ended, important maintaining variables may be uncovered. Generally, thoughts and feelings experienced during the sexual encounter can influence the presence or absence of sexual problems. For example, thoughts involving monitoring one's genital arousal (called spectatoring) will likely diminish genital arousal (Barlow, 1986). Feeling rushed or pressured during a sexual interaction may have similar effects.

TREATMENT

There are numerous variables that may play a role in sexual problem maintenance. Assessment plays a central role in uncovering the problems to be addressed in treatment. The way in which a therapist treats a given client depends on the reason the problem persists. Two people suffering from the same disorder may be treated differently, depending on circumstantial factors. For example, two people suffering from low desire may benefit from very different treatments. One individual may be experiencing low desire as a result of relationship distress and the other may simply not enjoy sexual interactions but is very satisfied in the relationship. Although these two individuals fit the same DSM diagnostic category, they will likely benefit most from different treatments, as will be discussed below. To make matters more complicated, two people suffering from different disorders may benefit most from the same treatment. For example, a male client may have difficulties maintaining an erection when being intimate with his partner. A female may experience genital pain while engaging in intercourse with her partner. Both of these individuals may be treated similarly if assessment indicates that problematic thinking contributes to both dysfunctions.

Although clients may be treated individually for a given sexual problem, if the client has a partner who is willing and able to participate, it is very beneficial for the partner to participate in treatment. This may take one of two forms: One is to engage the couple in couple therapy; the other is to treat the sexual problem in a way that engages both partners, also referred to as partner-assisted treatment. These treatments, including their theoretical rationale and empirical findings regarding treatment efficacy, will be discussed below. For those interested in a more extensive review of the empirical literature, see reviews by O'Donohue and colleagues (O'Donohue, Dopke, & Swingen, 1997; O'Donohue, Swingen, Dopke, & Regev, 1999).

Couple Therapy

The quality of the relationship may play a significant role in maintaining sexual problems. Deficits in communication skills, problem resolution, emotional intimacy, and trust have been found to be associated with low desire in women (Stuart, Hammond, & Pett, 1987). Other sexual problems may result from relationship difficulties. For example the sexual demands that one partner places on the other may result in sexual dysfunction, such as tracking the time it takes for one partner to reach orgasm or expecting that nonsexual affection always leads to intercourse.

To date, we know little regarding the efficacy of general couple therapy when treating sexual dysfunction. Research suggests that: (1) sex therapy, primarily consisting of sensate focus, is comparable to communication therapy in primary and secondary anorgasmic women (Everaerd & Dekker, 1981); (2) couples receiving couple therapy in addition to sex therapy demonstrate more pronounced and comprehensive treatment gains, including significantly more intense experiences of sex and sexual desire (Zimmer, 1987); and (3) sex therapy positively influences both sexual and marital problems, whereas general couple therapy appears to facilitate only marital problems (Hartman & Daly, 1983).

Jacobson and Margolin (1979) provide guidelines for couple therapists treating clients presenting with relationship and sexual problems.

The determination of which problem to treat first should depend on (1) whether relationship problems preceded or resulted from sexual problems; (2) the willingness and eagerness of the couple to address the identified problem; and (3) which intervention will likely "provide the quickest benefits and have the more profound overall effect on the relationship" (p. 292). In a review of the empirical data regarding couple interventions for sexual dysfunction, Baucom, Shoham, Mueser, Daiuto, and Stickle (1998) concluded that direct focus on the couple's sexual interactions is important when treating sexual dysfunction, as opposed to using couple therapy to treat the sexual problems indirectly. They also indicated that it is not necessarily true that severe marital complaints should be addressed prior to addressing sexual problems. Additionally, their findings suggest that including the male partner in treatment of women's sexual dysfunction yields better outcomes.

Because of the paucity of specific information about how to treat interrelated sexual and relationship problems, the therapist must use general clinical problem solving skills. The therapist should consider (1) the couple's priorities; (2) the probability of each problem being successfully treated; (3) any "ripple effect" in which a successful treatment of one problem will improve others; (4) finding and focusing on core problems that are the basis of both marital and sexual difficulties, such as communication problems; and (5) creatively combining these two therapies either within sessions or in some alternating pattern.

The remainder of this section focuses on treatments of sexual dysfunction that may be administered either individually or with the assistance of a partner. By including the partner, the couple may learn to apply techniques learned in couple therapy, including communication skills and problem-solving skills, to their sexual problem. For example, helping couples openly communicate sexual preferences may be one way to integrate these two therapies. This may provide the couple with an opportunity to work toward the common goal of improving their sexual relationship, while imparting communication techniques that generalize to other areas of their relationship and enhance their overall functioning. Sex therapy treatments that may be implemented with the assistance of the partner include psychoeducation, environmental factors, directed masturbation, sensate focus, orgasm consistency training, and the squeeze technique.

Psychoeducation

Providing an individual or couple with information regarding sexuality is an important component of treatment. This information helps correct myths and misunderstandings that may negatively impact sexual functioning. These myths may include the notion that a man should not initiate sexual activity before being erect or that it is common for women to experience multiple orgasms. These myths may prevent couples from initiating sex or feeling satisfied with their sexual relationship. Zilbergeld's (1992) and Heiman and LoPiccolo's (1988) self-help books provide examples of common myths and discuss more accurate portrayals of human sexuality. Psychoeducation is generally one component of the treatment package for all of the sexual dysfunctions. Moreover, Jacobson and Margolin (1979) recommend that all couples be provided with education regarding sexual functioning to enhance their sexual relationship, which they suggest will likely have a positive impact on the relationship as a whole. Markman, Floyd, Stanley, and Storaasli (1988) found this to be true by incorporating a "sensual/sexual education and relationship enhancement" component in their Prevention and Relationship Enhancement Program (PREP) in addition to communication skill and problem-solving training. At the 4-year follow-up, they found that couples who underwent PREP were less likely to become dissatisfied in their marital and sexual relationship.

Environmental Factors

The setting and circumstances in which sexual interactions take place may play an important role in the etiology or maintenance of sexual problems. The possibility of onlookers, a boss in the next room, and children screaming on the other side of the door may interfere with sexual functioning. It is important to help couples presenting with sexual dysfunction to establish a pleasant, relaxing environment that will facilitate sexual expression.

Directed Masturbation

LoPiccolo and Lobitz's (1972) directed masturbation program is effective in treating women who have difficulty reaching orgasm (Ersner-Hershfield & Kopel, 1979). The program consists of education and self-exploration, directed masturbation, sexual fantasy and imagery, and sensate focus. Women begin this process on their own and are then instructed to include their partner in sensate focus and in sharing effective masturbatory techniques with their partner. Incorporating the partner both facilitates progress throughout the program and teaches the partner to bring the woman to orgasm. This program is also available in bibliotherapy form. The book and video entitled *Becoming Orgasmic* (Heiman & LoPiccolo, 1988) provide women with an affordable and private method of learning to reach orgasm with their partner.

Sensate Focus

Sensate focus is a widely used technique to help the individual or couple to develop a heightened awareness of sensations and decrease focus on sexual performance (Masters & Johnson, 1970). This approach seeks to focus the individual or couple on the immediately achievable goal of experiencing pleasure through the senses as opposed to focusing on the anxiety-provoking goal of erection, reaching orgasm, or controlled ejaculation. The couple is coached to be affectionate with each other and learn to receive pleasure through homework assignments encouraging them to engage in sexually related exercises.

The homework assignments begin with nongenital pleasuring, whereby both partners engage in nongenital touching while clothed. The next step usually involves genital touching; the couple is encouraged to gently caress each other's genitals and breasts while discouraging them from focusing on performance-related goals. Once the couple is comfortable with these exercises, sexual intercourse may resume. This last step is typically broken down into a number of steps as well. First, the couple may engage in "containment without thrusting," thus again not focusing on reaching orgasm as the goal. The goal is simply to contain the penis in the vagina. Additionally, during these steps, the couple is asked to disengage in the task if, for example, an erection is achieved, thereby stressing that erection is not the goal. Once both partners are comfortable with the sexual procedures thus far and accept that erection, orgasm, or controlled ejaculation are not the goal, the couple is permitted to engage in intercourse with thrusting. Few controlled studies have demonstrated the effects of this approach by itself. This technique is usually one component of a broader treatment package.

Orgasm Consistency Training

Teaching women to consistently reach orgasm is effective in teaching those who experience low desire to engage in sexual activity (Hurlbert, White, Powell, & Apt, 1993). The rationale for this stems from the idea that people will want to engage in activities they find enjoyable and one possible reason some women do not want to engage in sexual activity is that they do not find it enjoyable. Therefore, if women are helped to consistently reach orgasm, they will want to engage in sex more often. This technique incorporates directed masturbation, sensate focus, and techniques involving teaching voluntary male self-control and timing of male orgasm. Additionally, couples are directed to have the woman reach orgasm first, prior to the male reaching orgasm and prior to sexual intercourse. Finally, couples are taught to reach orgasm using the coital alignment technique, as described by Eichel, Eichel, and Kule (1988). This position places the couple in the traditional missionary position, with the exception of the male being farther forward such that the penis shaft presses against the woman's mons veneris while both partners move their pelvises together in short, rocking strokes. Hurlbert et al. (1993) found that this technique was effective in increasing women's desire, particularly when women were treated with their partners. The authors suggest treating sexual problems in the context of the relationship because these problems are likely to affect both partners and it is in the interest of both to work toward the common goal of improving their sexual relationship.

Squeeze Technique

For males suffering from premature ejaculation, the squeeze technique is used to help teach ejaculatory control (Masters & Johnson, 1970). The male is instructed to masturbate to a point prior to ejaculation. At this time he should stop masturbating and firmly squeeze the head of his penis by placing two fingers on the top and his thumb on the bottom of the coronal ridge. He is instructed to repeat this process at least three times prior to ejaculation. Each time he is to pay attention to and attempt to enjoy the sensations and identify the various levels of arousal that he experiences. A similar technique is the "start–stop" or "pause" technique whereby he is to stop masturbating for 10 seconds and resume without squeezing his penis. Alternatively, in order to incorporate his partner in treatment, the partner would squeeze the head of his penis when instructed to do so by the male just prior to ejaculation.

ADDITIONAL TREATMENT CONSIDERATIONS

The following are additional interventions that should be considered when presented with an individual suffering from a sexual dysfunction. These treatments focus primarily on the individual including cognitive restructuring, systematic desensitization, insertion of dilators, and surgical procedures and medication.

Cognitive Restructuring

Some clients experience thoughts during a sexual encounter that interfere with sexual expression. These thoughts may influence arousal level, ability to reach orgasm, and desire to engage in sexual activity.

Treatment primarily consists of identifying interfering thoughts and reducing the occurrence of these thoughts, such as by providing alternative images on which to focus during sexual activity. Dobson's (2001) *Handbook of Cognitive-Behavioral Therapies* provides more information on cognitive restructuring.

Systematic Desensitization

Some individuals experience anxiety or fear in relation to sex, as in sexual aversion disorder and male erectile disorder. This may result from a traumatic experience such as rape, or from an irrational belief regarding their sexuality. Systematic desensitization helps clients habituate to the stimulus they previously feared (Wolpe, 1958). Treatment consists of teaching relaxation and gradually exposing the client to the anxiety-provoking stimuli. By reducing the client's anxiety relating to sex, he or she may be more likely to engage in sexual activity, focus on pleasurable aspects during sex, and thereby enhance sexual arousal.

Insertion of Dilators

For women suffering from vaginismus, the seemingly uncontrollable spasms of the outer-third of the vaginal wall, the insertion of graduated dilators (or fingers) is likely the most common treatment approach (Masters & Johnson, 1970). Women are taught to relax and gradually insert dilators while relaxed so as to help prevent spasms during insertion. To date, there are no controlled treatment outcome studies demonstrating the effectiveness of this technique.

Surgical Procedures and Medication

Dyspareunia, acute genital pain associated with intercourse, may result from a variety of sources. Little is known regarding effective treatments for this dysfunction. Vestibulectomy, a minor day surgery involving the excision of the vestibular area, is effective for women suffering from dyspareunia resulting from vulvar vestibulitis (see Binik, Bergeron, & Khalife, 2000). With respect to male erectile disorder, sildenafil (Viagra) promotes corporal smooth muscle relaxation and increased blood flow to the penis, which is necessary to maintain an erection. Viagra does not cause an erection in the absence of sexual stimulation. Instead, it has been found to successfully maintain the erection in response to sexual stimulation. Interested readers are referred to Rosen (2000) for more information on medical interventions for erectile dysfunction.

Additional Resources for the Individual and Couple

The private nature of sexuality has inspired numerous self-help books for couples to access anonymously. These provide couples with discreet help for a problem they may be embarrassed to discuss with others. Efficacy studies suggest that individuals can be treated effectively using bibliotherapy (see Marrs, 1995). This is particularly true when minimal therapist contact is incorporated into treatment to help motivate the client to comply with treatment and to clarify misunderstandings.

As such, self-help books can be a cost-effective alternative for clients presenting with sexual problems. Heiman and LoPiccolo's (1988) book and video on *Becoming Orgasmic* teaches women about their body and effectively helps them learn to become orgasmic. Men presenting with erectile problems may be referred to *The New Male Sexuality* (Zilbergeld, 1992).

Resources for the Couple Therapist

There are a number of useful resources for therapists as well. As indicated above, Davis et al. (1998) provide clinicians and researchers with information regarding the contents and psychometric properties of numerous sexuality-related measures, including measures of sexual dysfunction. Wincze and Carey (2001) provide clinicians with a step-by-step procedural book for treating clients presenting with sexual dysfunction. Weeks and Hof (1987) seek to integrate sex and couple therapy in their clinical guide. O'Donohue and Geer (1993) and Leiblum and Rosen (2000) provide clinicians with valuable handbooks for sex therapy.

In addition to these books noted above, there are a number of sexological organizations that offer supplementary information and annual conferences presenting the latest research. These include the International Academy of Sex Research, the Kinsey Institute (*www. indiana.edu/~kinsey/*), the Society for the Scientific Study of Sexuality (*www.ssc.wisc.edu/ssss/*), and the Society for Sex Therapy and Research.

CASE ILLUSTRATION

Amy and Frank were a married couple in their early 30s who self-referred to a mental health clinic after a brief temporary separation. They had been married 7 years and had a 2-year old child. The couple reported that they argued about financial issues and household responsibilities. Generally, Amy would not tell Frank that they were behind on payments until they were on the verge of dire consequences such as having utilities shut off or receiving an eviction notice. They stated that their problems began 2 years previously when Frank became depressed after losing his job as an electrician.

During the first session, Frank reported feeling very depressed without suicidal ideation. He scored 40 on the Beck Depression Inventory (BDI-II), indicating severe depression. Amy scored 19, indicating moderate depression. Frank and Amy obtained distressed scores of 70 and 67, respectively, on the Dyadic Adjustment Scale (DAS). Those items mutually endorsed included "never calmly discussing something," "occasionally discussing divorce, separation, or terminating the relationship," "always disagreeing about household tasks," and "always disagreeing on major decisions." They also endorsed "being too tired for sex" and "not showing love" during the weeks prior to their visit.

The initial assessment indicated the following treatment targets: communication around financial and domestic matters, trust (since Amy had not been forthcoming about their financial status), intimacy, and satisfaction. During the first and second session, the couple was asked to monitor the frequency of their arguments, level of depression, amount of time spent together, and to rate intimacy and satisfaction.

During the second session the clients' ratings were reviewed. They reported a large amount of time spent together but low ratings of intimacy and satisfaction. They both stated that they wanted to engage in more productive activities than watching TV and going out to see movies. The therapist inquired about endorsed items on the DAS regarding problems with sex and affection. Frank said that he felt that he was "inadequate" because he could not maintain an erection long enough to make Amy reach orgasm during intercourse.

These statements prompted the therapist to assess the latency of Frank's orgasm, the latency of Amy's orgasm, erectile status, the quality and frequency of the sexual activity, and the overall context in which sexual activity was initiated. The assessment revealed that Amy was able to experience an orgasm in response to clitoral stimulation, oral stimulation, digital penetration, and had previously experienced orgasms during intercourse with Frank. The couple also indicated that Amy typically initiated the sexual activity and that Frank either stated that he was too tired or else only participated in activities where Amy likely reached orgasm (e.g., clitoral stimulation).

During her change in employment, Frank experienced a decreased ability to control his orgasms. At the time of the assessment, Frank would ejaculate immediately after penetrating the vagina or following one or two thrusts. Amy said that she typically assured Frank that she had been sexually satisfied, but that he would withdraw from her, apologize, or make jokes. She said that this in turn made her feel angry and frustrated.

Amy and Frank indicated that the communication problems and the sexual difficulties were equally important issues. The therapist proceeded with the treatment by spending half of each session discussing more general domestic problems (e.g., financial matters, household chores) and communication regarding intimacy, and targeting sexual dysfunction during the other half. Sex therapy included psychoeducation, cognitive restructuring, relaxation training, sensate focus, and the squeeze technique.

The first two sessions of treatment involved psychoeducation. The couple was taught about normal sexual functioning and likely outcomes. The purpose of this component was to dispel myths that Frank and Amy had about sexuality (e.g., "Well-functioning couples have intercourse daily," "My partner should know when and how I want to engage in sexual activity"). This component was equally relevant to both partners because neither was knowledgeable about these issues. The couple was also coached in making accurate disclosures by employing "I" statements and discussing their experiences in a nonjudgmental and nonpejorative manner. The therapist asked that Amy and Frank begin discussing recent conflicts in session and coached them in using these communication skills.

The next four sessions involved cognitive restructuring for both partners, which allowed for further modification of harmful myths about sexual functioning. More specifically, the therapist addressed Frank's beliefs that Amy would not be satisfied unless she reached orgasm and that she was dissatisfied when he ejaculated early. The couple was instructed to engage in sexual activity other than intercourse (this was the first segment of sensate focus). The clients and the therapist problem solved around the most frequent arguments. Because Frank frequently became angry when Amy was not honest about their financial situation, the couple scheduled a time during each week when they could discuss household finances together so that each was aware of what was paid and due.

Two sessions were spent on relaxation training for Frank. Through the tensing and releasing of specific muscle groups, Frank was taught how to achieve a state of relaxation on demand. The couple was instructed to continue with sensate focus by taking turns stimulating one another through massaging, stroking, or kissing any of their partner's body except breasts or genitals. Frank was instructed to use relaxation techniques during these interactions. These sexual interactions provided opportunities for each partner to attend to the immediate sexual experience in an environment where they were assured that intercourse would not take place.

The therapist and Amy completed a chain analysis of the most recent incidents in which she did not advise Frank that they were behind on their bills. Amy and the therapist identified several opportunities for Amy to intervene and respond more effectively. The therapist and the couple problem solved on how to bring Amy in contact with the multiple negative consequences of her behavior, including problems in their relationship, poor credit ratings, and the termination of services.

The next three sessions continued to focus on effective communication and problem solving, sensate focus excluding intercourse, and teaching the squeeze technique. Clients should not be encouraged to proceed to touching breasts and genitals until they feel comfortable engaging in nongenital sexual activity. The therapist coached Frank to communicate when he was close to ejaculating and either squeeze the head of his penis himself or have Amy do it. It was important to assess each partner's willingness to engage in these behaviors. In this case, Amy was very comfortable in carrying out this role and was able to do so in a nonjudgmental manner. The therapist also reviewed sexual interactions occurring during the previous weeks in order to coach the couple in using more effective communication and techniques. The therapist continued to instruct Frank to use relaxation skills during sexual interactions when appropriate.

In the final three sessions of treatment, Amy and Frank were instructed to use these techniques (e.g., relaxation skills, squeeze technique) while engaging in intercourse. Throughout the treatment the therapist inquired about cognitive distortions, unreasonable outcome expectancies, and myths about sexual functioning. The therapist addressed these through psychoeducation and cognitive restructuring. The couple was instructed to increase the frequency of pleasurable activities that they enjoyed together. The therapist also worked individually with Frank on increasing the frequency of participation in pleasant social activities.

Amy and Frank were motivated to solve their relationship problems and their difficulties with their sex life. Despite articulating that they were committed to the treatment, they did not always complete their homework assignments. For instance, both individuals would at times feel too depressed to engage in pleasurable activities. This would result in more severe depression and diminished relationship satisfaction. Also, sometimes they would not engage in sufficient sexual activity to practice new techniques (e.g., they would not engage in any sexual activity or would not employ the squeeze technique) or else not meet at their specified time to go over their bills. Because it was integral to the treatment that both partners were able to competently carry out steps and complete their homework assignments, the therapist would problem solve with them when they attended sessions without accomplishing assigned tasks. The couple discontinued treatment after significant improvements were made.

CONCLUSIONS

There appears to be a strong relationship between marital and sexual satisfaction. Problems in one of these domains may influence the other domain. Relationship problems may spill over into the bedroom. Problems in the bedroom may result in relationship distress. Therefore, it is essential that therapists treating couples be adept in assessing these problems and identifying what form of treatment would likely yield the most favorable results. Unfortunately, research has generally divided these two domains and treated them as distinct from one another. Clinicians treating relationship distress must be familiar with treating sexual problems as well. Sex is often a vital part of the couple's relationship and should not be neglected when determining appropriate treatment.

REFERENCES

American Psychiatric Association (2000). *Diagnostic and statistical manual of mental disorders* (4th ed., text rev.). Washington, DC: Author.

Barlow, D. H. (1986). Causes of sexual dysfunction: The role of anxiety and cognitive interference. *Journal of Consulting and Clinical Psychology, 54,* 140–148.

Barnett, L. R., & Nietzel, M. T., (1979). Relationship of instrumental and affectional behaviors and self-esteem to marital satisfaction in distressed and nondistressed couples. *Journal of Consulting and Clinical Psychology, 47,* 946–957.

Baucom, D. H., Shoham, V., Mueser, K., Daiuto, A. D., & Stickle, T. R. (1998). Empirically supported couple and family interventions for marital distress and adult mental health problems. *Journal of Consulting and Clinical Psychology, 66,* 53–88.

Binik, Y. M., Bergeron, S., Khalife, S. (2000). Dyspareunia. In S. Leiblum & R. Rosen (Eds.), *Principles and practice of sex therapy* (3rd ed., pp.154–180). New York: Guilford Press.

Davis, C., Yarber, W., Bauserman, R., Schreer, G., & Davis, S. (Eds.). (1998). *Handbook of sexuality-related measures.* Thousand Oaks, CA: Sage.

Dobson, K. (Ed.) (2001). *Handbook of cognitive-behavioral therapies* (2nd ed.). New York: Guilford Press.

Eichel, E. W., Eichel, J. D., & Kule, S. (1988). The technique of coital alignment and its relation to female orgasmic response and simultaneous orgasm. *Journal of Sex and Marital Therapy, 14,* 129–141.

Ersner-Hershfield, R., & Kopel, S. (1979). Group treatment of pre-orgasmic women. *Journal of Consulting and Clinical Psychology, 47,* 750–759.

Everaerd, W. & Dekker, J. (1981). A comparison of sex therapy and communication therapy: Couples complaining of orgasmic dysfunction. *Journal of Sex and Marital Therapy, 7,* 278–289.

Hartman, L. M., & Daly, E. M. (1983). Relationship factors in the treatment of sexual dysfunction. *Behavior Research and Therapy, 21,* 153–160.

Heiman, J. R., Gladue, B. A., Roberts, C. W., & LoPiccolo, J. (1986). Historical and current factors discriminating sexually functional from sexually dysfunctional married couples. *Journal of Marital and Family Therapy, 12,* 163–174.

Heiman, J., & LoPiccolo, J. (1988). *Becoming orgasmic: A sexual and personal growth program for women* (rev. ed). New York: Prentice-Hall.

Hurlbert, D. F., White, L. C., Powell, R. D., & Apt, C. (1993). Orgasm consistency training in the treatment of women reporting hypoactive sexual desire: An outcome comparison of women-only groups and couples-only groups. *Journal of Behavior Therapy and Experimental Psychiatry, 24,* 3–13.

Jacobson, N. S., & Margolin, G. (1979). *Marital therapy: Strategies based on social learning and behavior exchange principles.* New York: Brunner/Mazel.

Laumann, E.O., Paik, A., & Rosen, R.C. (1999). Sexual dysfunction in the United States: Prevalence and predictors. *Journal of the American Medical Association, 281,* 537–544.

Leiblum, S. R, & Rosen, R. C. (1991). Couples therapy for erectile disorders: Conceptual and clinical considerations. *Journal of Sex and Marital Therapy, 17*(2), 147–159.

Leiblum, S. R., & Rosen, R. C. (Eds.) (2000). *Principles and practice of sex therapy* (3rd ed.). New York: Guilford Press.

LoPiccolo, J., Heiman, J. R., Hogan, D. R., & Roberts, C. W. (1985). Effectiveness of single therapists versus cotherapy teams in sex therapy. *Journal of Consulting and Clinical Psychology, 53,* 287–294.

LoPiccolo, J. & Lobitz, W. C. (1972). The role of masturbation in the treatment of orgasmic dysfunction. *Archives of Sexual Behavior, 2,* 163–171.

Markman, H. J., Floyd, F. J., Stanley, S. M., Storaasli, R. D., (1988). Prevention of marital distress: A longitudinal investigation. *Journal of Consulting and Clinical Psychology, 56,* 210–217.

Marrs, R. W. (1995). A meta-analysis of bibliotherapy studies. *American Journal of Community Psychology, 23,* 843–870.

Masters, W., & Johnson, V. (1970). *Human sexual inadequacy.* Boston: Little, Brown.

Metz, M. E., & Epstein, N. (2002). Assessing the role of relationship conflict in sexual dysfunction. *Journal of Sex and Marital Therapy, 28,* 139–164.

Morokoff, P. J., & Gillilland, R. (1993). Stress, sexual functioning, and marital satisfaction. *Journal of Sex Research, 30,* 43–53.

O'Donohue, W. T., Dopke, C., & Swingen, D. (1997). Psychotherapy for female sexual dysfunction: A review. *Clinical Psychology Review, 17,* 537–566.

O'Donohue, W. T., & Geer, J. (Eds.). (1993). *Handbook of sexual dysfunctions: Assessment and treatment*. Needham Heights, MA: Allyn & Bacon.

O'Donohue, W. T., Swingen, D., Dopke, C., & Regev, L. (1999). Psychotherapy for male sexual dysfunction: A review. *Clinical Psychology Review, 19,* 591–630.

Pridal, C. G., & LoPiccolo, J. (2000). Multielement treatment of desire disorders: Integration of cognitive, behavioral, and systemic therapy. In S. Leiblum & R. Rosen (Eds.), *Principles and practice of sex therapy* (3rd ed., pp. 57–81). New York: Guilford Press.

Regev, L. G. (2001). *Determining the effectiveness of the training protocol for administering the sexual functioning interview*. Unpublished master's thesis, University of Nevada, Reno.

Rosen, R. C. (2000). Medical and psychological interventions for erectile dysfunction. In S. Leiblum & R. Rosen (Eds.), *Principles and practice of sex therapy* (3rd ed., pp. 276–304). New York: Guilford Press.

Snyder, D. K., & Berg, P. (1983). Determinants of sexual dissatisfaction in sexually distressed couples. *Archives of Sexual Behavior, 12*(3), 237–246.

Spiess, W. F., Geer, J. H., O'Donohue, W. T. (1984). Premature ejaculation: Investigation of factors in ejaculatory control. *Journal of Abnormal Psychology, 93,* 242–245.

Stuart, F. Hammond, D., & Pett, M. (1987). Inhibited sexual desire in women. *Archives of Sexual Behavior, 16,* 91–106.

Weeks, G. R., & Hof, L. (Eds.). (1987). *Integrating sex and marital therapy: A clinical guide*. New York: Brunner/Mazel.

Wincze, J. P., & Carey, M. P. (2001). *Sexual dysfunction: A guide for assessment and treatment* (2nd ed.). New York: Guilford Press.

Wolpe, J. (1958). *Psychotherapy by reciprocal inhibition*. Stanford, CA: Stanford University Press.

Zilbergeld, B. (1992). *The new male sexuality: The truth about men, sex, and pleasure*. New York: Bantam.

Zimmer, D. (1987). Does marital therapy enhance the effectiveness of treatment for sexual dysfunction? *Journal of Sex and Marital Therapy, 13,* 193–209.

CHAPTER 9

Physical Aggression

AMY HOLTZWORTH-MUNROE
AMY D. MARSHALL
JEFFREY C. MEEHAN
UZMA REHMAN

TYPES, PREVALENCE, AND CONSEQUENCES OF PHYSICAL AGGRESSION IN COUPLES

Physical aggression in intimate relationships is a heterogeneous phenomenon that can be differentiated into at least two types (Johnson, 1995; O'Leary, 1993). One type, labeled "severe physical aggression" or "patriarchal terrorism," is probably what most people picture when they think of "battering." This level of violence is found among batterers entering domestic violence treatment programs and battered women seeking assistance at shelters. It is characterized by severe husband violence, with less severe wife violence or severe wife violence primarily in self-defense, and by a high risk of wife injury and a high degree of wife fear. This aggression is believed to function to control and dominate the wife. Most experts in the field agree that couples experiencing this level of violence are inappropriate candidates for conjoint couple therapy.

The second type of aggression, labeled "mild physical aggression" or "common couple violence," is often studied among newlywed, community, or marital therapy samples. It is characterized by more bidirectional aggression (i.e., both spouses engage in physical aggression) that is mild to moderate in severity and frequency. It is believed to be less likely to cause fear in, or to endanger, the wife and may be less likely to be used to control her. Clinical experience suggests that this type of physical aggression will be seen more often than the first type among couples seeking marital therapy. Thus, the focus of this chapter is on this type of aggression, and our therapy recommendations are geared toward these couples.

Unfortunately, this second type of aggression is a relatively common problem among heterosexual couples. Data from nationally representative samples suggest that, each year, one out of every eight husbands engages in physical aggression against his wife, with most of this aggression being "mild" (e.g., push, grab, shove, or slap; Straus & Gelles, 1990). The figures are even higher among couples seeking marital therapy. In such samples, over 50% of couples have experienced husband-to-wife physical aggression in the past year (Holtzworth-Munroe, Waltz, et al., 1992; O'Leary, Vivian, & Malone, 1992).

Women also engage in physical aggression in their intimate relationships, in proportions equal to, or slightly higher than, men (Archer, 2000). Among marital therapy clinic samples, as much as 86% of partner aggression is reciprocal, with both partners engaging in primarily low levels of aggression (Cascardi, Langhinrichsen, & Vivian, 1992). Although the rates of female and male physical aggression are comparable, husband violence has more negative consequences for women than vice versa. Men are more likely than women to physically injure their partners (Archer, 2000). For example, among couples presenting for marital therapy, Cascardi et al. (1992) found that although most violence was reciprocal, wives were more likely to sustain severe injuries. Thus, although couples presenting for therapy often will report that both partners have engaged in physical aggression, we argue that it is particularly important for therapists to focus on husband violence and its possible consequences.

In addition to injury, husband violence is associated with negative psychological outcomes for women and children. For example, among couples seeking marital therapy, relative to women in nonaggressive relationships, women in aggressive relationships are more likely to report clinical levels of depressive symptoms (Cascardi et al., 1992). Similarly, in a study of newlyweds, Quigley and Leonard (1996) found that wives who experienced husband physical aggression over the first 3 years of marriage reported more depressive symptoms than women whose husbands were consistently nonviolent or who desisted from violence. Empirical evidence also indicates that, just as children from homes with marital conflict are at risk, children from homes with intense conflict (e.g., marital physical aggression) are at risk for behavior problems, emotional distress, and impaired social and academic functioning (for a review, see Margolin, 1998).

The presence of physical aggression in a marriage also predicts relationship deterioration. In a study of newlyweds, O'Leary, Barling, Arias et al. (1989) found that, over time, individuals who were married to stably aggressive spouses (i.e., aggressive at more than one point in time) were less satisfied with their marriages than individuals married to stably nonaggressive spouses. In the same sample, Heyman, O'Leary, and Jouriles (1995) found that husbands' premarital aggression longitudinally predicted wives' steps toward divorce and lower marital adjustment. Similarly, Quigley and Leonard (1996) found that the presence of stable husband physical aggression in the first 3 years of marriage was associated with declines in the wife's marital satisfaction, and Rogge and Bradbury (1999) found that physical aggression among newlyweds predicted relationship dissolution.

Increasingly, researchers also are examining the problem of husband-to-wife psychological aggression. Psychological aggression is a correlate of physical aggression; Cascardi, O'Leary, Lawrence, and Schlee (1995) reported that, relative to nonabused women, women who had experienced husband violence and were seeking marital therapy reported their husbands to be significantly more coercive and psychologically aggressive. In addition, psychological aggression predicts the onset of physical aggression; Murphy and O'Leary (1989) found that husbands' use of psychological aggression at 18 months after marriage predicted physical aggression 30 months after marriage.

Given the prevalence of physical aggression among couples, most couple therapists, at some point, will treat a violent couple even if they do not specialize in the treatment of marital violence. Unfortunately, however, many therapists have not received formal training regarding the problem and may not be well prepared to address this issue. We hope that the present chapter will provide part of that training.

THEORIES OF HUSBAND VIOLENCE AND RELATED DATA ON THE CHARACTERISTICS OF MARITALLY VIOLENT MEN

Theories of husband violence are often divided into three groups, based on their level of analysis: those focusing on the intrapersonal, interpersonal, or sociocultural causes of violence. Here, we present a few of the many available theories, along with some supporting data for each. Our focus is on theories and data suggesting the potential usefulness of couple therapy alone or combined with cognitive-behavioral approaches in treating husband physical aggression.

Intrapersonal Theories

Intrapersonal theories assume that characteristics of the individual increase one's risk of engaging in physical aggression. For example, Bandura (1973) outlined a social learning theory of aggression that has been applied to husband violence (e.g., Dutton, 1995). This theory argues that aggressive behavior is acquired (e.g., through observation of interparental aggression in the family of origin), activated (e.g., particular stimuli gain aggression-eliciting functions through association with differential consequences), and maintained (e.g., through pairing of aggression with reinforcers) through learning. Consistent with this theory, across many studies comparing violent and nonviolent men's retrospective reports of violence in their families of origin, the findings are fairly consistent: for men, exposure to violence in the home as a child is a correlate of later adult engagement in intimate partner aggression (Sugarman & Hotaling, 1989). Using this theory, therapists would do well to regard relationship violence as a learned behavior and to examine and change the stimuli eliciting aggression and the balance of positive to negative consequences received for aggression.

The social information-processing model, as applied to husband violence (Holtzworth-Munroe, 2000), another interpersonal model, proposes three steps in the processing of social information. In the first step, decoding, one must perceive and interpret the relevant social stimuli in a situation. Misconstrual of social stimuli may occur due to interference from factors such as inattention, faulty attributions, anger, or alcohol use. Indeed, in tests of the decoding stage, relative to nonviolent men, violent husbands have been found to attribute more hostile intent to their wives' actions; such attributions may help a husband to justify his own aggression as a form of retaliation against his supposedly hostile wife. In the second step, response generation and selection, one must consider possible responses to this situation and choose one. Our studies have demonstrated that, when presented with hypothetical conflict situations, violent men provide less competent, more aggressive responses than nonviolent men. In addition, when asked what would be the "best" thing to do in these situations, violent men still provide less competent responses, suggesting that either they do not know or do not care. In the third step, enactment, one must carry out the chosen response and monitor it to see if it has the expected impact. In a recent study, we asked men to enact a competent response to conflict situations; violent husbands' enactments were rated as less competent than those of nonviolent husbands, suggesting that something in their behavior undermined their ability to enact a competent response. Incompetent responses may escalate a conflictual situation, increasing the risk of violence. Thus, this model and our research suggest that a focus on conflict resolution skills is an appropriate intervention target for maritally violent men.

Other intrapersonal theories focus on the individual's psychological problems. For example, personality disorders, particularly antisocial (e.g., Magdol et al., 1997) and borderline (e.g., Dutton & Golant, 1995) personality, are more commonly found among men who perpetrate relationship violence than among nonviolent men. Violent husbands also are more likely than nonviolent husbands to have drinking problems (e.g., Kaufman Kantor & Straus, 1987; Magdol et al., 1997), and alcohol intoxication is involved in many incidents of intimate aggression. In fact, husbands' premarital alcohol use predicts future husband aggression in newlywed samples (Heyman et al., 1995; Leonard & Senchak, 1996). Some theorists suggest that men who are highly dependent upon, or anxiously attached to, their wives are jealous and hypervigilant to any threats to the relationship, using violence in a rage when they fear the loss of the wife (Dutton & Golant, 1995). Indeed, violent husbands have been found to score higher than nonviolent men on measures of jealousy, dependency on their wives, and fearful and preoccupied attachment (e.g., Holtzworth-Munroe, Stuart, & Hutchinson, 1997). As a final example, relative to nonviolent men, violent husbands have higher levels of general and spouse specific (i.e., directed at the wife) anger and hostility (Holtzworth-Munroe, Rehman, & Herron, 2000), which may provide a motivation for aggression. These findings suggest the need to screen carefully for such psychological problems and suggest the potential usefulness of substance abuse treatment and anger management training with aggressive husbands.

Interpersonal Theories

Interpersonal theories of husband violence focus on marital interaction patterns. In family systems theory, the marriage is a system defined by repetitious patterns in spousal interactions. As events occur, it is hypothesized that the marital relationship system works to maintain a state of homeostasis or balance; thus, the theory assumes that marital violence is a product of all the interdependent parts of a relationship. Marital violence is, therefore, viewed as a product of dysfunctional interactions in which both spouses contribute to an escalation of tension.

Although numerous characteristics of battering relationships have been hypothesized, marital communication patterns have been the subject of the most empirical research. Across studies, the findings are consistent. During discussions of marital problems, relative to their nonviolent counterparts, violent husbands display more extreme negative and hostile behaviors (e.g., contempt, belligerence, blame); violent couples engage in more negative reciprocity and, for them, this pattern lasts longer; and violent couples engage in both more demanding and withdrawing behavior, particularly husband demand–wife withdraw communication (e.g., Holtzworth-Munroe, Smutzler, & Stuart, 1998; Jacobson, Gottman, Waltz et al., 1994; Margolin, Burman, & John, 1989). These high levels of negativity may also characterize other types of marital discussions; in one study of discussions of wives' personal (i.e., not relationship) problems, relative to nonviolent men, violent husbands displayed more negative behavior and provided less social support (Holtzworth-Munroe, Stuart, Sandin, Smutzler, & McLaughlin, 1997). Such data suggest the potential usefulness of communication and problem-solving training in couple therapy.

Sociocultural Theories

The broadest level of theoretical analysis is that of sociocultural theories. Feminist theories, for example, maintain that marital violence exists because violent and patriarchal societies allow, and even encourage, violence as a means of dominating women (e.g., Dobash & Dobash, 1979). Such theories suggest that violence against women is caused by a social organization in which men possess greater power and privilege, as well as a concomitant ideology that legitimizes this organization. Contributing to male dominance are men's economic advantage and adherence to traditional gender roles. Husband violence is assumed to be supported by society through factors such as peer support, lack of police response to domestic violence, and minimal criminal sentences for domestic violence offenders.

As reviewed in Gelles and Straus (1979) and Bersani and Chen (1988), other sociocultural theories of violence have been proposed. For example, it has been suggested that the uneven distribution of violence in society is a function of differential cultural norms concerning violence and related issues (e.g., values regarding masculinity, the worth of life, the meaning of honor). Others suggest that when resources (e.g., status, income) are lacking, violence may be used as a resource to maintain dominance or may be due to the frustration associated with few opportunities for achievement, power, or prestige. This notion is consistent with data demonstrating that the groups at highest risk for husband violence include young couples, unemployed and low-income couples, and couples who are members of socially disadvantaged ethnic groups.

Although theories at this level of analysis may have few direct implications for therapy with couples, they can be useful in the therapist's conceptualization of husband violence. For example, the therapist may wish to view physical aggression in the context of the gendered power difference found in most marriages (Vivian & Heyman, 1996) or consider the subculture in which the couple lives and the stressors they confront in their lives.

Subtypes of Maritally Violent Men

Above, we highlighted general differences between maritally violent and nonviolent men. Recent research, however, has made it clear that samples of maritally violent men are heterogeneous. Based on a review of previous batterer typologies, Holtzworth-Munroe and Stuart (1994) suggested that batterer subtypes can be identified using three descriptive dimensions: (1) severity/frequency of husband violence; (2) generality of husband violence (i.e., family only or extrafamilial also); and (3) the husband's psychopathology or personality disorders. Using these dimensions, we proposed that three subtypes would be identified. First, family-only men would engage in the least marital violence, the least violence outside the home, and evidence little or no psychopathology. Second, dysphoric/borderline batterers would engage in moderate to severe wife abuse, but their violence would be primarily confined to the wife; this group would be psychologically distressed and evidence borderline personality characteristics. Finally, generally violent/antisocial batterers would engage in the highest levels of marital violence and extrafamilial violence and evidence characteristics of antisocial personality disorder.

In a developmental model of these differing types of violence, Holtzworth-Munroe and Stuart (1994) predicted that family-only men would evidence the lowest levels of risk factors for violence. The violence of family-only men was proposed to result from a combination of stress (personal and/or marital) and low-level risk factors (e.g., lack of relationship skills), such that, on some occasions during escalating marital conflicts, these men engage in physical aggression. Following such incidents, however, their low levels of psychopathology, combined with their relatively positive attitudes toward women and negative attitudes toward violence, lead to remorse and help prevent their aggression from escalating. In contrast, dysphoric/borderline batterers were hypothesized to come from a background involving parental abuse and rejection. As a result, these men have difficulty forming a stable, trusting attachment with an intimate partner. Instead, they are highly dependent upon, yet fearful of losing, their wives, and are very jealous. When frustrated, their borderline personality organization, anger, and insecure attachment lead to violence against the adult attachment figure (i.e., the wife). Finally, generally violent/antisocial batterers were predicted to resemble other antisocial, aggressive groups, with high levels of many risk factors (e.g., impulsivity, few social skills). Their marital violence was conceptualized as one part of their general antisocial and aggressive behavior.

Recent batterer typologies have provided support for our typology (e.g., Holtzworth-Munroe, Meehan, Herron, Rehman, & Stuart, 2000). Although researchers have not yet studied the question of how different batterer subtypes fare in conjoint couples therapy, we have hypothesized that family-only men may be the only group for whom conjoint treatment is appropriate. Family-only men are the least violent and have the fewest risk factors for violence, and the risk factors that do characterize them (e.g., social skills deficits) may be amenable to conjoint therapy. In the Holtzworth-Munroe et al. study, the family-only group did not differ significantly from a comparison group of nonviolent, maritally distressed men on any measure except that of marital violence, suggesting that family-only men resemble nonviolent/distressed husbands (who are usually the target of conjoint therapy) in many ways.

ASSESSMENT OF PHYSICAL AGGRESSION

As discussed above, over half of couples seeking couple therapy have experienced husband physical aggression in the past year. However, therapists may easily fail to detect the presence of physical aggression, as couples usually do not spontaneously report it as a presenting problem. For example, O'Leary et al. (1992) found that only 6% of wives reported violence as a presenting problem on an intake form. Yet, during individual interviews that included direct questioning about marital violence, 44% of these wives reported the presence of husband physical aggression. This figure increased to 53% when the wives were asked to complete a self-report behavior checklist measure, the Conflict Tactics Scale (CTS; Straus, 1979). Also suggesting that a behavioral checklist may reveal more aggression than an interview, Ehrensaft and Vivian (1996) found that about half of spouses reporting mild husband physical aggression on the CTS had failed to mention this aggression during an interview, and approximately one-quarter of spouses reporting severe husband violence on the CTS had not mentioned the violence during an interview. Ehrensaft and Vivian asked the couples why they had not reported the violence at intake. The most common reasons given were that the violence was not considered a problem, it was considered unstable or infrequent, or the couple perceived the violence to be a secondary problem that would resolve once primary relationship problems were addressed.

These data clearly indicate that to increase the likelihood of detecting husband violence, a structured instrument such as the CTS should be routinely administered to all couples seeking therapy. We find that the most efficient way to assess for relationship violence is to administer the CTS to both partners, asking them to complete it individually and with privacy from one another. On the CTS, each person reports the occurrence and frequency of various behaviors, including psychological and physical aggression. Because spouses often provide incongruent reports regarding the occurrence of specific violent behaviors, either partner's report of violence should be accepted as valid and assessed further.

Although the CTS is the most widely used measure of relationship violence, it suffers a number of shortcomings. It only assesses violent behaviors that occur during conflicts, yet husband violence can occur in other situations, and it only assesses a limited set of violent behaviors. Also, the CTS does not assess the context of violence (e.g., precipitating events, sequence of events, aggressor's intentions, partner's responses, consequences of the violence).

To assess such issues, we recommend conducting separate interviews with each spouse, so that both partners, particularly wives, can be honest. We assure couples of the confidentiality of these interviews but also work with each person to allow us to share information with their partner, particularly if safety issues are involved. Ultimately, however, we view a battered woman as being in the best position to judge whether or not such information can safely be shared with her partner. This assessment should also focus on issues to help determine whether conjoint treatment is appropriate for a couple. For example, the therapist should assess the level of the woman's fear for her safety and each partner's motivation to enter conjoint treatment and to remain in the relationship. In addition, therapists should assess the level of each partner's willingness to acknowledge that physical aggression is a problem and to take responsibility for his or her own violent actions. Previous attempts to deal with the aggression also should be assessed.

If severe or frequent violence is reported, the potential lethality of the situation should be assessed immediately. The therapist must ask about the presence of guns or other weapons in the home, recent escalations in violence, direct and indirect threats of lethality, level of the wife's fear, and whether substance use is associated with the violence. If the therapist determines that the likelihood of continued violence and/or lethality is present, he or she should immediately, and individually, discuss safety planning and resource mobilization with both partners. The discussion with the husband should focus on the seriousness of the problem, developing emergency plans that he can take to prevent his use of violence (e.g., time outs; calling the therapist or a crisis line), and understanding the need for safety planning on the part of his wife. Discussion with the wife should include developing a detailed and individualized safety plan for responding to dangerous situations. Such discussions should cover practical issues such as how she can get herself and any children out of the home, a safe place where they can go (e.g., a relative's home or a shelter), and having quick access to items such as car keys, money, and important documents. The wife should also be informed of appropriate local resources, including shelters and social service agencies, as well as legal options (e.g., protective or restraining orders).

DECIDING WHETHER OR NOT
CONJOINT THERAPY IS APPROPRIATE

After completing a thorough assessment and dealing with any necessary safety planning, therapists must decide whether to proceed with conjoint therapy or refer the individual partners to gender-specific treatments (GST; i.e., men's and women's groups). GST is the treatment format most commonly used for husband violence, with men being seen in batterer treatment programs. Indeed, many state standards for the treatment of men court ordered to treatment recommend that batterers be treated in groups of men and indicate that conjoint treatment of the couple is inappropriate. For example, Section 4.5 of the Massachusetts state standards states, "Any form of couples or conjoint counseling or marriage enhancement weekends or groups are inappropriate initially . . . couples counseling shall not be considered a component of batterer treatment" (Massachusetts Guidelines and Standards, 1994, p. 13). Such guidelines have developed, in part, because the use of a conjoint treatment format with husband violent couples is considered controversial.

Potential Disadvantages and Advantages to Conjoint Treatment

Indeed, there are potential disadvantages to the conjoint format. There is concern that seeing both partners in therapy and focusing on such issues as a couple's communication patterns may imply that the husband's violence is caused by both partners, rather than being the batterer's sole responsibility. An additional concern is that the wife may not feel comfortable expressing herself in the presence of the batterer (e.g., may not be able to be fully honest about such issues as the level of violence, her level of fear, or her desire to end the relationship), as she may fear further violence from her partner if she is honest. Also, there is concern that the process of discussing difficult relationship problems could increase anger and conflict, such that the therapy itself could increase the risk of violence (for further discussion of such issues, see O'Leary, Heyman, & Neidig, 1999).

In contrast, there are some potential advantages to the conjoint treatment format. One is the ability to obtain a more accurate picture of the violence (i.e., the husband's and wife's reports may differ significantly). In addition, therapists can ensure that both partners understand the therapist's conceptualization of the violence and how techniques should be implemented. In our experience, some interventions go more smoothly when both partners are present to hear the rationale and procedures (e.g., both partners will understand what an appropriate, versus an inappropriate, time-out involves), and a husband may be less likely to use therapy to further abuse his wife when his wife has also heard what the therapist says (e.g., in batterers' treatment, some men go home and tell their wives, "My therapist told me that it's your fault I'm violent"). Conjoint therapy also allows couples to postpone volatile discussions until the therapy sessions, thus helping them to avoid escalating arguments at home until they are trained to discuss such problems.

There are additional rationales for using conjoint treatment. First, because physical aggression often occurs in the context of an argument between partners (O'Leary et al., 1999), direct intervention to decrease negative communication in conjoint treatment may decrease violence by changing the interactional patterns that precede it. Second, most couples presenting for couple therapy have experienced bidirectional violence, and self-defense accounts for less than 20% of these cases (Cascardi & Vivian, 1995), suggesting that both partners may benefit from learning to control their use of physical aggression. Moreover, although husband violence often can have severe physical and psychological effects, many women seeking couple therapy have not experienced that level of violence and are not fearful of participating in conjoint treatment (O'Leary et al., 1999). Indeed, in many cases, these wives are seeking conjoint therapy and wish to remain in their relationship.

Guidelines for Deciding Whether or Not Conjoint Treatment Is Appropriate

Unfortunately, no available research provides empirically based rules for deciding whether or not conjoint treatment is appropriate. Three research groups, however, have examined the efficacy of conjoint therapy with violent couples (all are reviewed below) and an examination of these studies may provide ideas for guidelines (Brannen & Rubin, 1996; Harris, Savage, Jones, & Brooke, 1988; O'Leary et al., 1999). In all of these studies, the wife had to report, in an individual interview, that she was willing to participate in conjoint therapy and did not feel endangered by her partner's knowledge that she had discussed his violence with a counselor. One research group (O'Leary et al., 1999) additionally screened out couples in which the wife had sustained an injury requiring medical attention and required, for participation, that the man admit the perpetration of at least one act of physical aggression. All of the research groups excluded couples if either spouse evidenced severe psychopathology likely to interfere with treatment (e.g., psychotic symptoms), and two of the three studies excluded men with untreated substance abuse problems. Each research team helped wives to construct individualized safety plans and provided them with information about community resources for battered women and emergency phone numbers.

Most experts in the field agree that conjoint treatment is only appropriate for low to moderate levels of aggression and only if the wife is not perceived to be in danger of imminent physical harm. Related to this, the wife must not fear the husband, must feel comfortable in therapy with him, and must not feel so intimidated or dominated by him that she is unable to be honest in therapy. In addition, both partners must be interested in staying in the relationship. A conjoint format is inappropriate if one partner does not acknowledge the existence or problematic nature of the violence or is not willing to take steps to reduce it (e.g., removing weapons from home, drug/alcohol treatment, temporarily separating).

ALTERNATIVES TO CONJOINT THERAPY

If it is determined that conjoint therapy is inappropriate, then both the husband and wife should be provided with referrals to other sources of help. We explain such referrals by telling a couple that we are very concerned about the level of violence they have experienced: it is too severe to begin conjoint treatment (e.g., concerns about safety and the possible escalation of violence if difficult issues were addressed in therapy). We also clearly convey our belief that each partner is responsible for his or her own behavior (i.e., the abused partner did not "provoke" the violence) and thus must take steps to end it. We usually offer to reevaluate the appropriateness of conjoint therapy once each has sought appropriate help elsewhere and after the husband has completed a violence treatment program.

For women, referrals to support groups for battered women and advocacy services are important, because a battered woman often is not able to begin considering her long-term options or dealing with the trauma she has experienced (i.e., more traditional psychotherapy) until she has obtained adequate support and resources (e.g., housing, legal protection, and childcare; Sullivan & Bybee, 1999). Therapists should refer the husband to gender-specific therapy (GST). Referring the husband to GST gives both spouses the clear message that he is responsible for his violence and for learning to become nonviolent. It also is often a test of a man's willingness to change, providing his wife with information about the level of his willingness to work to become nonviolent. In some cases, after a thorough assessment and discussion of the violence, we have seen wives decide to leave their violent husbands when it becomes clear that they have not followed our recommendation to seek GST. Many communities offer batterer treatment programs, and there are numerous examples of GST in the literature (e.g., Dutton & Golant, 1995). Unfortunately, the effectiveness of gender-specific treatments for husband violence has not been clearly established (e.g., Dunford, 2000). Nonetheless, we recommend referral of a violent husband (who is judged to be an inappropriate candidate for conjoint treatment) to such a program, given a lack of any empirically demonstrated effective alternatives and our hope that referring the man to a program designed for this problem and staffed by experienced therapists may be effective.

CONJOINT TREATMENT PROCEDURES

Therapy Goals and Contracts

Before beginning conjoint treatment with a couple experiencing physical aggression, the partners need to be made aware of the therapist's expectations and treatment goals. Specifically, couples should be clearly informed that cessation of husband violence is one of the primary goals of treatment. Despite our careful assessment of aggression during intake procedures, many couples still are surprised by our concern regarding their aggression and wish to dismiss it as excessive.

Thus, in an effort to motivate couples to change, we review the reasons for our concern. We note that while the current level of aggression may be low, any level of physical aggression always carries with it a risk of injury, and we give examples of relevant cases (e.g., a man who pushed his wife with no intent to hurt her, but, because the floor was wet that day, she slipped and hit her head on the kitchen counter, suffering a concussion). We also explain that whereas some couples cease their aggression or maintain low levels of aggression, many couples escalate their levels of aggression and, unfortunately, the current data do not allow us to predict which couples are at risk for continuing or escalating aggression. Thus, to be conservative, we must assume that every aggressive couple we work with is at risk for escalating violence. If during the assessment, we have discovered that a couple has risk factors for violence (e.g., psychological aggression, excessive substance use, violence in the family of origin), we present these as factors that make us concerned that their aggression may escalate, explaining the relevant research. To further motivate the couple, we discuss any possible negative consequences of the aggression that have occurred. For example, often couples are concerned about their children's awareness of their fights. Finally, we explain that without a direct focus on ending the aggression, there is a risk that the therapy itself may escalate the aggression, because the couple will be asked to discuss difficult topics likely to engender anger and frustration. Indeed, with some couples, the assessment reveals that one way the couple avoids aggression is to avoid the discussion of sensitive topics, but now the therapist is going to ask them to address these issues. Thus, we must ensure that aggression won't occur in the course of such discussions.

Related to this concern, we explain that treatment will focus first on helping the partners to control their behavior when angry. Then, once anger management skills are learned, they will be in a safer position to engage in problem solving regarding their major presenting problems. We find that following such a discussion, most couples are willing, though some are not enthusiastic, to agree to a treatment plan that will initially focus on anger management and controlling aggression.

In many couples, both partners have used physical aggression. Thus, we acknowledge that both parties must take responsibility for their own aggression and any consequences of it. We discuss the fact that we believe violence is a learned behavior and a choice and, accordingly, each person must take responsibility for stopping his or her aggression. In most cases, however, we also emphasize that because husband violence carries greater risk (e.g., physical injury, negative psychological effects), it will be a particular target of treatment.

If it has not already been done, it is important to consider safety plans with both partners. Among couples accepted for conjoint therapy (e.g., less severe violence), detailed planning may not be necessary. There still, however, should be a conversation with the woman about safety (e.g., places to go if a fight is escalating; relevant local resources). In addition, both partners should be asked to consider steps they could take to prevent further perpetration of physical aggression (e.g., discussing heated issues only in public or in therapy sessions) and lessen the risk of injury (e.g., removing weapons from the home, refraining from drinking).

Both persons should be asked to make a "no violence" contract, either written or verbal, with the therapist. In doing so, the couple should agree to report any incidents of physical aggression to the therapist. To remove the burden on (or danger to) either person bringing up such events, the therapist should explain that he or she will regularly ask about the occurrence of any physical aggression. The therapist should explain that further occurrences of aggression will lead to a reexamination of the level of danger, the reasons the treatment plan is not working, and the appropriateness of the treatment plan. In some cases, continuing or worsening violence will be grounds for termination of conjoint treatment and referral of the partners to GST. This message is an important motivator, demonstrating to couples how concerned the therapist is about their aggression.

We use a cognitive-behavioral approach to conjoint treatment. Thus, in our approach, the therapist explains that therapy involves a "two-pronged" approach; most of the therapy time will be dedicated to two modules: (1) anger recognition and management; and (2) communication and problem solving skills. These sections parallel, to a large extent, the treatment protocols for other existing conjoint treatment programs for relationship aggression (e.g., Geffner, Mantooth, Franks, & Rao, 1989; Heyman & Neidig, 1997).

Anger Management

Because intimate aggression frequently occurs during an argument as part of an escalation of angry feelings, the first set of skills introduced involves anger management. We explain to couples that the term "anger management" is a misnomer, because anger is a natural emotion; we are actually trying to help spouses manage their behavior (i.e., aggression or abuse) when angry. In most cases, given the lower levels of aggression among the couples we accept into conjoint therapy, we find that one to three full therapy sessions devoted to anger management, followed by some attention to these skills in subsequent therapy sessions, provides adequate coverage. Our procedures are borrowed from previous programs for anger management (e.g., Novaco, 1975), batterer treatment (e.g., Hamberger & Hastings, 1988), and conjoint therapy for relationship aggression (e.g., Heyman & Neidig, 1997).

Recognition of Anger

To adequately manage and control their anger, partners must first be able to identify it. Thus, the therapist should solicit examples from each person regarding how they experience anger, helping partners to identify the physical, cognitive, and behavioral cues that accompany their anger. Physical cues include physiological changes (e.g., flushing, tenseness, rapid heart beat, sweating). Cognitive cues are described as "hot thoughts" or "anger up statements"; they can be broken into categories such as labeling ("She's so stupid"), hostile attributions ("She did that just to spite me"), catastrophizing ("Now my whole life is ruined"), and "should" statements ("She should have known better than to do that"). Behavioral cues consist of the ways in which anger is expressed through facial expression, verbalizations, and motor behavior (e.g., tapping fingers, slamming doors, or violence). It is important to point out how anger (a feeling) differs from aggression (a behavior).

Next, the therapist asks each person to construct a personalized anger continuum from the least to most extreme anger they experience, using a line marked from 1 to 10. To facilitate an appreciation for the different intensities of anger, the therapist helps the clients to label key anchor points along the line (e.g., "frustrated," "angry," "furious," "no longer in control of behavior and in danger of using aggression"). The therapist should guide the discussion so that physical, cognitive, and behavioral signs of anger are listed for each of these key points along the continuum.

Anger logs are introduced as an ongoing homework assignment. On the anger log, each person reports the details of one or more episodes during the week when they felt angry. The client records the situation, the intensity of the anger (on the 1–10 scale), and the physical, cognitive, and behavioral anger cues experienced. Partners are instructed to keep these anger logs and, across situations and weeks, to look for patterns in their anger (e.g., when, and with whom, they are angry; how they know they are angry), perhaps helping them to identify high risk situations for arguments and aggression. For example, one couple discovered, after completing anger logs for several weeks, that their major fights always occurred when the husband was running late as they prepared to go out as a couple.

Time-Outs

Time-outs are the first skill taught for managing behavior when angry to prevent aggression. We find that some couples have a difficult time accepting time-outs, because this procedure (i.e., leaving a fight) runs counter to many common cultural beliefs (e.g., one should never walk away from a fight; it is good to hash out an issue until insight or resolution is reached). In such cases, the therapist must help the couple to weigh the risk of continued aggression against the temporary suspension of the discussion of a heated issue. In other cases, couples may have been avoiding the discussion of issues and there is a danger that time-outs can be used to continue such a pattern. In either situation, it is important that both parties understand that a time-out does not permanently end the discussion of a problem; they will be asked to discuss the issues, calmly, after the time-out or, if this is impossible, to bring the issue to therapy for eventual discussion. Many couples initially respond negatively to the term "time-out," having heard it applied to the discipline of children. In contrast, we introduce the procedures using analogies to time-outs taken during sporting events (e.g., a chance to regroup and collect yourself before making a costly mistake that could lose the game).

Time-outs have several components. First, each individual must recognize his or her anger and take responsibility both for acknowledging it and for taking a time-out. They need to inform the partner of these facts, saying, "I am beginning to feel angry and I need to take a time-out." Each part of that statement is discussed in detail: using an "I" statement to take responsibility for one's feelings; acknowledging the anger without blaming their partner; calmly announcing a time-out rather than just leaving the discussion. We have implemented a rule that neither person can tell the other when to take a time-out, as this quickly becomes another weapon of abuse ("You need to take a time-out"). However, given that some women report that they fear their husband's anger but he is not taking time-outs, we have implemented another version of time-out, in which either person can take a time-out for any negative feeling that is likely to make further discussion of an issue unproductive (e.g., "I am beginning to feel frightened and need to take a time-out").

The time-out statement includes another important component: notifying the partner of when one will return. This is necessary to prevent abuse of time-outs (e.g., a man who left home for 3 days and nights during a "time-out"). Men in batterer treatment programs often need 1–3 hours to calm down. With couples in couple therapy, partners often need less time (e.g., 15 minutes–1.5 hours). Thus, we usually ask couples to try a ½-hour period initially, to see if this is too long or too short. The full time-out statement becomes, "I am beginning to feel angry and I need to take a ½-hour time-out."

After announcing the time-out, the individual leaves the area where the argument was occurring. Ideally, they should leave the house or apartment, because some individuals may get angrier as they listen to their partner in another room (e.g., "How can she be calmly watching TV after what she just said to me?") or begin to interrupt each other's time-outs. In some situations (e.g., a woman taking a time-out late at night), this rule needs to be modified. Couples should be asked to consider how to take time-outs in various problematic situations (e.g., a fight in the car or in public). During a time-out, partners are encouraged to engage in techniques aimed at decreasing anger, such as meditation and relaxation techniques or physical exercise. Also helpful are "cool thoughts" or "anger down statements" that can be used to deescalate angry thoughts. Activities to be avoided during a time-out include things that may further escalate the anger or be dangerous in an angry state, such as alcohol and drug use, aggressive exercising (e.g., chopping wood), driving, and ruminating about the argument.

At the end of the specified time, the person taking the time-out must either return or contact the partner and take another time-out (e.g., "I am still angry and need to take another ½-hour time-out"). After the time-out is over, the couple should try to discuss the problem. They are encouraged to take another time-out if needed or to suggest another time (including therapy) in which to continue discussing the problem.

The act of taking a time-out can be awkward for many couples, and it is helpful to have them practice taking time-outs in session and at home. Using a time-out log, clients should write down incidents in which they used a time-out, including the argument that led to the time-out, how the time-out was implemented, and what happened after the time-out. Therapist debriefing of these incidents often can pinpoint problems in the use of time-outs, as well as identify problem areas in the relationship that may be amenable to problem solving.

We find it very useful to ask couples to take time-outs during therapy sessions in which they become angry (*in vivo* training). Usually the therapist must initially suggest that they take a time-out (usually a 10 minute one); later, couples will be able to call a time-out on their own or with minimal prompting (e.g., the therapist asks, "This conflict is escalating. What might be a good thing to do now?"). One person makes the time-out statement and leaves the room. The therapist also should leave the room and go to a neutral place, so as not to get drawn into an alliance with either partner. Both the partner leaving the room and the therapist should return at the agreed upon time. At that point, the therapist can help review the time-out from both partners' perspectives. What steps did the person taking the time-out use to calm down? How did their partner who didn't take the time-out feel (e.g., abandoned, angry that the conversation was cut short)? Such discussions often help elucidate potential problems with time-outs, allowing the couple and therapist to brainstorm methods for handling such issues.

Other Anger Management Skills

Although many methods of managing anger are covered in the time-out procedure, it is often necessary to further develop these methods. Such discussions should focus on learning to manage the three components of anger discussed during anger recognition: physical (e.g., relaxation, slow breathing, exercise), cognitive (e.g., self-statements), and behavioral (e.g., communication skills). Once these skills are taught, the weekly anger logs should be modified to include an additional section regarding what steps either person took to manage each of the three components of anger. Anger logs and time-out logs can be combined and should be monitored for many weeks and, in some cases, for the entire course of therapy.

Communication and Problem-Solving Skills

Once couples are managing their anger more appropriately and have not engaged in further aggression, it is appropriate to begin communication and problem-solving skills training (e.g., paraphrasing, feeling expression, use of a structured problem-solving format). The couple is often eager to do so, because attention to their presenting problems may have been delayed for the few weeks of anger management training. At this point, we generally use techniques derived from behavioral couple therapy (BCT; e.g., Jacobson & Margolin, 1979). Given that such methods are well outlined in other places, we will not present them here. Rather, we will briefly discuss some issues that, in our experience, are particularly important to address when teaching these skills to couples experiencing physical aggression.

Expressing Feelings

We find that maritally violent men often have difficulty with feeling expression. First, some physically aggressive men claim not to know when they are angry until it is "too late" and they are engaged in destructive behavior. By completing anger management prior to communication training, this usually is not an issue. Second, other aggressive men often express only vague feelings (e.g., "good" or "bad") or are only comfortable expressing angry feelings. We have found that it is useful to discuss "softer" feelings that may underlie anger (e.g., hurt, rejection) and to provide men with a list of feeling words to be used as a guide. In some cases, therapists may want to discuss how men may have more difficulty with this exercise than women, because women usually are explicitly socialized to pay attention to and express their feelings. Otherwise, the husband may become frustrated and embarrassed as his wife acquires these skills more quickly than he does.

Problem Solving

Informally, some of our colleagues have told us that they no longer rigidly adhere to the formal problem-solving structure originally used in BCT (Jacobson & Margolin, 1979). We, however, have found it necessary to do so with physically aggressive couples. Clients should be informed that the problem-solving structure will seem artificial and stilted, and we know that it does not resemble the naturalistic problem discussions of happily married couples. We don't know how to make distressed couples interact like happy couples (in part due to the large variety in communication styles across happily married couples). We do know, from observational studies, however, the mistakes that distressed and aggressive couples make when discussing problems, and the problem-solving format is designed to eliminate these destructive behaviors. Specifically, the structure of problem solving can prevent the escalation of arguments and can keep couples on task.

Consistent with data on the communication patterns of violent couples, we have found that physically aggressive couples often hold the belief that it is necessary to discuss an issue *ad nauseum* (by definition, they have discussed some issues to the point of violence), and both partners may alternately play the roles of demander and withdrawer. Thus, we warn physically aggressive couples that they may find problem solving frustrating. Specifically, we predict that, when in the role of the demander, that person will find it difficult to stick to the structured and brief problem definition format, instead preferring to list many examples of the problem, thoroughly examine possible causes of the problem, express all of their feelings about the problem, etc. We remind the couple of the negative outcomes (e.g., violence) of such past discussions and of the need to learn a new problem-solving style to avoid further aggression. We also predict that, when in the role of the withdrawer, that person may find it difficult to engage in the process, having learned to escape past negative interactions by avoiding them. We note that the structured format should make the discussion process less aversive and thus allow engagement in problem solving.

Clients should be informed that a collaborative approach to problem solving is critical (e.g., being willing to accept responsibility for one's contributions to the problem and to change one's behavior). Part of this collaboration involves being able to overlook the short-term personal costs in a solution for the long-term gains of an improved relationship. Additionally, problems should be thought of as mutual problems, not just a problem for just one person or the other. This is difficult for some aggressive couples, given their past pattern of hurting one another and not resolving major issues. To deal with this, we sometimes find ourselves resorting to the implementation of additional problem-solving rules and structure. For example, when defining the problem, for some couples we ban "anger" words in the problem definition, instead insisting that they identify softer feeling words, because such feeling statements can generate sympathy in spouses. As another example, given a tendency for violent couples to blame one another, we have established a rule that, during the brainstorming phase of problem solving, the first proposed solution offered by each partner must involve something that he or she can personally do to change the problem (e.g., "I could . . ." rather than "You could . . .").

We also find that, with violent couples, the problem solution contract should be as specific as possible (who will be doing what and when). Contracts should also include a time when the couple will review the contract, evaluate how well the problem solution has worked, and make adjustments, as necessary. This step is useful because one spouse is often resistant to agree to a solution unless guaranteed that the solution can be changed if it isn't working. The problem contract phase should also include troubleshooting, which entails thinking about potential problems that might arise when implementing the contract. For instance, if a contract specifies who is to make dinner on a given night, the therapist and spouses should ask questions such as what would happen if one spouse is sick or out of town? Couples should write ideas for how to handle potential problems into the contract.

Other Interventions

Once couples have learned problem solving, the remaining therapy sessions involve applying these methods to their major presenting problems. In addition, at this point in therapy, other interventions or methods may be considered to address problems. We find that many aggressive couples benefit from some sessions of parent training, learning to discipline their children in nonaggressive ways.

On a regular basis (e.g., every four to five sessions), the therapist and couple jointly review the progress they have made on presenting problems and new problems identified during the course of therapy. They then adjust the therapy plan to make sure that all of these problems are addressed before termination. Once violence has been eliminated, the major issues have been addressed, and the skills taught are being successfully applied, the therapist moves to less frequent meetings (e.g., every other week and then once per month), serving as a consultant to a couple who is now managing their problems on their own and helping them to anticipate upcoming stressors or major life changes.

CASE ILLUSTRATION

Bill and Judy responded to a newspaper advertisement offering "low-cost couple therapy" in our training clinic. They were a couple in their late 20s, with two preschool children. They had met in high school and married shortly after high school graduation. Both had high school and technical school degrees. Judy worked part-time at an office; Bill had recently been laid off from his job. When both were working, the children stayed with Judy's parents.

In their first therapy session, a conjoint meeting, they listed their problems, including being unable to resolve problems, "nit-picking" at each other all the time, and fighting about finances and what Judy perceived to be Bill's "laziness" (i.e., not yet having gotten a new job). In addition, Judy was concerned that Bill had begun drinking too much since being laid off. During that session, the therapist asked them to describe their worst fight ever. They disagreed on which fight that was. Judy reported a fight that had occurred 5 years before, in which Bill had pushed her into a hot water heater, which had become unattached and the water had spilled out, luckily not burning them. Bill reported a recent fight in which, he reported, Judy had slapped him; upon further probing, Bill admitted that he had pushed her so hard that she had fallen over a chair before she had slapped him; he also acknowledged being drunk during this fight. They both stated that those had been their only two fights involving physical aggression.

The therapist had them arrive early for the next session and, in separate rooms, complete a series of questionnaires, including the CTS. On the CTS, they did not report any further violence. In individual sessions, neither reported being afraid of the other and each reported having sustained only red marks that did not require medical attention. However, while claiming not to fear Bill, Judy did report being "bothered" by the fact that sometimes, when they were arguing, he would pick up his gun and polish it in front of her. Judy was asked about safety planning. Her family lived nearby and she said that she sometimes went there after bad marital fights and that Bill had never followed or harassed her there. She did worry about whether Bill would let her take the children with her and said that she would find it hard to leave for a safe place if she couldn't take the kids. She agreed that the therapist could discuss these issues with Bill. She also was given more information on safety planning and information on the local battered women's support group and shelter. She was encouraged to call the shelter or police should further violence occur.

Whereas Bill had little more to add about the violence in his individual session, the therapist did assess his level of drinking and was concerned that Bill was beginning to abuse alcohol. They discussed this issue at length and Bill agreed to seek help for his alcohol use. Specifically, he said that he would attend an Alcoholics' Anonymous meeting that week, because AA had been helpful to him several years before when he also had been drinking heavily.

In the third therapy-planning session, the therapist expressed serious concern about the couple's violence. Judy didn't need much convincing that it was a problem, but Bill seemed embarrassed and tried to laugh it off. For example, he said that cleaning his gun during a fight was "a joke" and that he would never hurt Judy. However, the hot water heater incident provided the therapist with a wonderful example of a situation that could have (i.e., if the water had been hot) led to very serious consequences. Bill was informed that for therapy to commence, he would have to remove his gun from the house for the course of therapy; he agreed, saying that he could store it at his parents' house for a while. In addition, Bill agreed to continue attending AA and had already stopped drinking in the past week; indeed, he did not drink again during the course of therapy. The therapist gave him much reinforcement for having taken this step. The issue of safety planning was also discussed and, after some discussion, he agreed that Judy could take the children with her to her parents' house if she left during a fight. He was happy to hear that the therapist did not approve of her use of aggression either and would be teaching them both to use anger management to avoid violence perpetration. Both spouses understood the rationale for addressing anger management first, so that they could stop their destructive fights and feel comfortable with one another when the time came to solve other problems in therapy. At first, however, Bill refused to sign a no-violence contract, as he said it was "silly and unnecessary." The therapist reexplained the reasons for her concern and said that therapy could not continue unless he signed the contract, and offered to give him the week to decide. Instead, he chose to sign the contract in the session.

The therapist then proceeded to explain the time-out procedure to them and encouraged them to take practice and, as needed, real time-outs before the next session. The following week, the couple reported that they had three fights but had only tried a time-out once and it had not gone well. First, the therapist reviewed the two fights in which they had not used time-outs and developed, with the couple, ways to remember to call a time-out when they were fighting. For them, this primarily involved the need to call a time-out earlier in the process, before they were too angry to want to take a break. They then debriefed the time-out that hadn't gone well and found that Judy had told Bill that he needed to take a time-out but he had disagreed, so she had stomped out of the room and purposefully banged dishes in the other room. The basic rules of time-out and the rationales for each (e.g., you can't tell someone else to take a time-out, you announce a time-out, you leave the house) were reviewed.

The following week, the couple reported no fights and no real time-outs, but had each remembered to take one "practice" time-out, which they said "felt stupid"; the reasons for practice were reviewed. During the session, the couple started to argue and Bill was becoming visibly angry. The therapist suggested that this would be a good time to practice time-out, and coached Bill through the time-out statement. The therapist and Bill left the room for 10 minutes, going to separate areas. Upon their return, they found that Judy was furious about "being left"; she was so noncollaborative that she decided that she should take a time-out. After her 5-minute time-out, the therapist helped the couple to debrief the time-outs. Judy's feelings of "being left" were discussed. She developed a plan to keep herself busy and distracted, rather than ruminating about the fight, when Bill was taking a time-out. The discussion with Bill focused on why he hadn't recognized the need for a time-out himself and how he could do so at home.

In the next session, the couple reported that Bill had taken two time-outs and Judy had taken one, in response to Bill's. These had been successful, and during Bill's second time-out, Judy had been able to stop ruminating and hadn't needed to take her own time-out. During these weeks, therapy sessions had also focused on anger recognition and management. Judy reported that the relaxation tape they had been given was very useful to her. Although not always using it in angry situations, she was using it each night before bed to calm down for the evening; she found that it helped to distract her from ruminating about their problems. Bill found that going for walks and cognitive restructuring were the most helpful to him in managing his anger. In particular, he focused his thoughts on not wanting to repeat his parents' marital patterns (i.e., they had engaged in violent fights and had divorced when he was young) and remembering to control himself so that his children would see a better role model. Their anger logs had not revealed particular high-risk situations for fights, although Bill's job search was the topic of many of the situations reported on their anger logs.

The following week, the couple had taken two successful time-outs. They had also had one failed time-out, when they had fought in the car and neither wanted to leave the car, given that it was a rainy night. Other ways of handling these situations were discussed, including a temporary ban on any discussion until they got to their destination and could take a proper time-out. Given their progress, the therapist moved onto communication training at this time.

The couple spent one session learning basic communication skills and three sessions learning the structured problem-solving format; part of each of these sessions was also devoted to reviewing time-outs and anger logs and anger management skills. Over the course of the next seven sessions, they applied the problem-solving format to their own problems. During the session devoted to solving the problem of Bill's job search, they became angry enough that they had to take two time-outs in the session. Eventually, they did problem solve their major issues.

The therapist then offered to provide them with parent training, because they had realized that they often got angry with their children and were worried that their discipline was too harsh (i.e., yelling and spanking but not to the level of reportable child abuse). On their own, they had been using some anger management strategies when dealing with their children, but they seemed to benefit substantially from a series of five sessions of additional training in positive reinforcement, including use of time-outs with children.

Therapy was almost complete when they decided to end a few weeks early, because Bill's new job required him to be out of town for most of the week. They came to one booster session a month later and reported that things were going well. They spent the session problem solving issues that had arisen given Bill's absences from home for his job. They both reported that therapy had been very helpful and that while it wasn't as consistent as "it should be," they were still both using time-outs and were occasionally using the problem-solving techniques.

RESEARCH EXAMINING THE EFFECTIVENESS OF CONJOINT THERAPY FOR COUPLES EXPERIENCING HUSBAND PHYSICAL AGGRESSION

To our knowledge, only three research teams have published studies of the effectiveness of conjoint therapy with couples experiencing husband violence. All compared conjoint treatment to gender-specific treatment (GST), using random assignment of couples to treatment condition. In all three studies, the couple treatment was designed to address husband violence as the primary problem.

Harris et al. (1988) recruited over 70 couples requesting therapy at a family service agency. Thirty-five percent of the sample never began treatment, and many additional couples did not complete it (i.e., attrition was 67% in the couples conditions, 16% in the gender specific condition). At the 6- to 12-month follow-up assessment, only 28 women were interviewed. Given the severe limitations imposed by this high level of attrition, we nonetheless note that the data indicated that the two treatment conditions were equally effective in reducing the husbands' physical violence (based on wife report) and in improving participants' sense of psychological well-being.

Brannen and Rubin (1996) recruited couples referred to batterers' treatment by the court system that had indicated a desire to remain in their relationship. Forty-two of the 49 couples that began treatment completed it; six of the seven batterers who dropped out of treatment were in the GST condition. Six-month follow-up data showed no significant differences between the two groups in levels of recidivism; approximately 90% of the subjects reported that they were violence-free. These researchers also assessed, on a weekly basis, any ongoing abuse. Over the course of treatment, six instances of physical and emotional abuse were reported; two involved couples in conjoint treatment, while four were among couples in GST, suggesting that women in couple treatment were not in more danger than women in GST.

O'Leary et al. (1999) recruited 75 couples with a newspaper ad offering free therapy to couples experiencing low levels of physical aggression. Thus, it is not clear how generalizable these study findings are to couples seeking marital therapy that usually do not report violence as a presenting problem. Only 37 couples completed treatment; dropout rates did not differ significantly across the treatment conditions. Although both treatment approaches resulted in statistically significant changes in men's violence, neither appears to have been particularly effective because over 70% of the men engaged in physical aggression during the follow-up period. Comparing the two treatment formats, there were no differences in rates of husbands' physical and psychological aggression, wives' depressive symptoms, or wives' marital adjustment. Husbands' marital adjustment was higher for husbands in the conjoint therapy condition. Finally, based on regular checks, it was found that women in the conjoint treatment did not report fearing their husbands during therapy and did not report that therapy discussions led to physical aggression.

Thus, across the three available studies, no difference in outcome favored either GST or conjoint therapy. Given that all of the studies involved couples that were interested in remaining together and willing to enter conjoint therapy, these samples may resemble couples likely to be seen by couple therapists. However, whereas the study couples were seeking help for husband violence, most couples seeking therapy don't report violence as a presenting problem, thus potentially limiting the generalizability of the finding to couples seeking therapy. In addition, in all of the studies, a specialized couple treatment, with a primary focus on the man's violence, was used; in two of the studies (Brannen & Rubin, 1996; O'Leary et al., 1999), a group format was used for the couple therapy. Thus, these data do not support the use of standard marital therapy, applied to individual couples, in reducing male violence. Finally, two of the studies had high attrition rates, suggesting that a large number of couples experiencing husband violence may not complete treatment.

SUMMARY

Physical aggression is a common problem among couples seeking therapy. Most therapists, if they screen for violence, will find that over half the couples seeking help have experienced husband aggression in the past year. Familiarity with theories of husband violence and research on the correlates of such aggression can help therapists to assess potentially important aspects of the problem and to understand better the potential causes and consequences of violence for each aggressive couple they treat. Assessments sensitive to such issues will help therapists decide whether or not conjoint treatment is appropriate for a given couple. Current data suggest that conjoint therapy with a direct and specific focus on eliminating husband violence may be as effective as the more widely utilized gender specific treatments, although the current data are mixed regarding how effective such interventions will be. In general, we suggest a cautious and informed approach, focusing on anger management and communication skills, to help couples end the violence in their relationship.

REFERENCES

Archer, J. (2000). Sex differences in aggression between heterosexual partner: A meta-analytic review. *Psychological Bulletin, 126,* 651–680.

Bandura, A. (1973). *Aggression: A social learning analysis.* Englewood Cliffs, NJ: Prentice-Hall.

Bersani, C. A., & Chen H. T. (1988). Sociological perspectives in family violence. In V. B. Van Hasselt, R. L. Morrison, A. S. Bellack, & M. Hersen (Eds.), *Handbook of family violence* (pp. 57–86). New York: Plenum Press.

Brannen, S. J., & Rubin, A. (1996). Comparing the effectiveness of gender-specific and couples groups in a court-mandated spouse abuse treatment program. *Research on Social Work Practice, 6,* 405–424.

Cascardi, M., Langhinrichsen, J., & Vivian, D. (1992). Marital aggression: Impact, injury, and health correlates for husbands and wives. *Archives of Internal Medicine, 152,* 1178–1184.

Cascardi, M., O'Leary, K. D., Lawrence, E. E., & Schlee, K. A. (1995). Characteristics of women physically abused by their spouses and who seek treatment regarding marital conflict. *Journal of Consulting and Clinical Psychology, 63,* 616–623.

Cascardi, M., & Vivian, D. (1995). Context for specific episodes of marital violence: Gender and severity of violence differences. *Journal of Family Violence, 10,* 265–293.

Dobash, R. E., & Dobash, R. P. (1979). *Violence against wives.* New York: Free Press.

Dunford, F. W. (2000). The San Diego Navy experiment: An assessment of interventions for men who assault their wives. *Journal of Consulting and Clinical Psychology, 68,* 468–476.

Dutton, D. G. (1995). *The domestic assault of women: Psychological and criminal justice perspectives.* Vancouver, Canada: University of British Columbia Press.

Dutton, D. G., & Golant, S. K. (1995). *The batterer: A psychological profile.* New York: Basic Books.

Ehrensaft, M. K., & Vivian, D. (1996). Spouses' reasons for not reporting existing physical aggression as a marital problem. *Journal of Family Psychology, 10,* 443–453.

Geffner, R., Mantooth, C., Franks, D., & Rao, L. (1989). A psychoeducational conjoint therapy approach to reducing family violence. In P. L. Caesar & L. K. Hamberger (Eds.), *Therapeutic interventions with batterers: Theory and practice* (pp. 103–133). New York: Springer.

Gelles, R. J., & Straus, M. A. (1979). Determinants of violence in the family: Toward a theoretical integration. In W. R. Burr, R. Hill, F. I. Nye, & I. L. Keiss (Eds.), *Contemporary theories about the family* (Vol. 1, pp. 549–581). New York: Free Press.

Hamberger, L. K., & Hastings, J. E. (1988). Skills training for treatment of spouse abusers: An outcome study. *Journal of Family Violence, 3,* 121–130.

Harris, R., Savage, S., Jones, T., & Brooke, W. (1988). A comparison of treatments for abusive men and their partners within a family-service agency. *Canadian Journal of Community Mental Health, 7,* 147–155.

Heyman, R. E., & Neidig, P. H. (1997). Physical aggression couples treatment. In W. K. Alford & H. J. Markman (Eds.), *Clinical handbook of marriage and couples interventions* (pp. 589–617). Chichester, UK: Wiley.

Heyman, R. E., O'Leary, K. D., & Jouriles, E. N. (1995). Alcohol and aggressive personality styles: Potentiators of serious physical aggression against wives? *Journal of Family Psychology, 9,* 44–57.

Holtzworth-Munroe, A. (2000). Social information processing skills deficits in maritally violent men: Summary of a research program. In J. P. Vincent & E. N. Jouriles (Eds.), *Domestic violence: Guidelines for research-informed practice* (pp. 13–36). London: Jessica Kingsley.

Holtzworth-Munroe, A., Meehan, J.C., Herron, K., Rehman, U., & Stuart, G. L. (2000). Testing the Holtzworth-Munroe and Stuart (1994) batterer typology. *Journal of Consulting and Clinical Psychology, 68,* 1000–1019.

Holtzworth-Munroe, A., Rehman, U., & Herron, K. (2000). General and spouse specific anger and hostility in subtypes of maritally violent men and nonviolent men. *Behavior Therapy, 31,* 603–630.

Holtzworth-Munroe, A., Smutzler, N., & Stuart, G. L. (1998). Demand and withdraw communication among couples experiencing husband violence. *Journal of Consulting and Clinical Psychology, 66,* 731–743.

Holtzworth-Munroe, A., & Stuart, G. L. (1994). Typologies of male batterers: Three subtypes and the differences among them. *Psychological Bulletin, 116,* 476–497.

Holtzworth-Munroe, A., Stuart, G. L., & Hutchinson, G. (1997). Violent versus nonviolent husbands: Differences in attachment patterns, dependency, and jealousy. *Journal of Family Psychology, 11,* 314–331.

Holtzworth-Munroe, A., Stuart, G. L., Sandin, E., Smutzler, N., & McLaughlin, W. (1997). Comparing the social support behaviors of violent and nonviolent husbands during discussions of wife personal problems. *Personal Relationships, 4,* 395–412.

Holtzworth-Munroe, A., Waltz, J., Jacobson, N. S., Monaco, V., Fehrenbach, P. A., & Gottman, J. M. (1992). Recruiting nonviolent men as control subjects for research on marital violence: How easily can it be done? *Violence and Victims, 7,* 79–88.

Jacobson, N. S., Gottman, J. M., Waltz, J., Rushe, R., Babcock, J., & Holtzworth-Munroe, A. (1994). Affect, verbal content, and psychophysiology in the arguments of couples with a violent husband. *Journal of Consulting and Clinical Psychology, 62,* 982–988.

Jacobson, N. S., & Margolin, G. (1979). *Marital therapy: Strategies based on social learning and behavior exchange principles.* New York: Brunner/Mazel.

Johnson, M. P. (1995). Patriarchal terrorism and common couple violence: Two forms of violence against women. *Journal of Marriage and the Family, 57,* 283–294.

Kaufman Kantor, G., & Straus, M. A. (1987). The "Drunken Bum" theory of wife beating. *Social Problems, 34,* 213–230.

Leonard, K. E., & Senchak, M. (1996). Prospective prediction of husband marital aggression within newlywed couples. *Journal of Abnormal Behavior, 105,* 369–380.

Magdol, L., Moffitt, T. E., Caspi, A., Newman, D. L., Fagan, J., & Silva, P. A. (1997). Gender differences in rates of partner violence in a birth cohort of 21-year-olds: Bridging the gap between clinical and epidemiological approaches. *Journal of Consulting and Clinical Psychology, 65,* 68–78.

Margolin, G. (1998). Effects of domestic violence on children. In P. K. Trickett & C. J. Schellenbach (Eds.), *Violence against children in the family and the community* (pp. 57–101). Washington, DC: American Psychological Association.

Margolin, G., Burman, B., & John, R. S. (1989). Home observations of married couples reenacting naturalistic conflicts. *Behavioral Assessment, 11,* 101–118.

Massachusetts Guidelines and Standards for Certification of Batterers' Treatment Program. (1994, May revision).

Murphy, C. M., & O'Leary, K. D. (1989). Psychological aggression predicts physical aggression in early marriage. *Journal of Consulting and Clinical Psychology, 57,* 579–582.

Novaco, R. W. (1975). *Anger control: The development and evaluation of an experimental treatment.* Lexington, MA: Lexington Books.

O'Leary, K. D. (1993). Through a psychological lens: Personality traits, personality disorders, and levels of violence. In R. J. Gelles & D. R. Ioseke (Eds.), *Current controversies in family violence* (pp. 7–29). Newbury Park, CA: Sage.

O'Leary, K. D., Barling, J., Arias, I., Rosenbaum, A., Malone, J. & Tyree, A. (1989). Prevalence and stability of marital aggression between spouses: A longitudinal analysis. *Journal of Consulting and Clinical Psychology, 57,* 263–268.

O'Leary, K. D., Heyman, R. E., & Neidig, P. H. (1999). Treatment of wife abuse: A comparison of gender-specific and couples approaches. *Behavior Therapy, 30,* 475–505.

O'Leary, K. D., Vivian, D., & Malone, J. (1992). Assessment of physical aggression against women in marriage: The need for multimodal assessment. *Behavioral Assessment, 14,* 5–14.

Quigley, B. M., & Leonard, K. E. (1996). Desistance of husband aggression in the early years of marriage. *Violence and Victims, 11,* 355–370.

Rogge, R. D., & Bradbury, T. N. (1999). Till violence does us part: The differing roles of communication and aggression in predicting adverse marital outcomes. *Journal of Consulting and Clinical Psychology, 67,* 340–351.

Straus, M. A. (1979). Measuring intra family conflict and violence: The Conflict Tactics (CT) scales. *Journal of Marriage and the Family, 41,* 75–88.

Straus, M. A., & Gelles, R. J. (1990). *Physical violence in American families: Risk factors and adaptations to violence in families.* New Brunswick, NJ: Transaction.

Sugarman, D. B., & Hotaling, G. T. (1989). Violent men in intimate relationships: An analysis of risk markers. *Journal of Applied Social Psychology, 19,* 1034–1048.

Sullivan, C. M., & Bybee, D. I. (1999). Reducing violence using community-based advocacy for women with abusive partners. *Journal of Consulting and Clinical Psychology, 67,* 43–53.

Vivian, D., & Heyman, R. E. (1996). Is there a place for conjoint treatment for couple violence? *In Session: Psychotherapy in Practice, 2,* 25–48.

PART III

Adapting Couple Therapy to Individual Problems

The chapters in this section focus on conceptual and clinical issues for working with couples in which mental or physical health problems are present but for which specific couple-based interventions have not yet been developed or empirically validated. In some cases, as in the application of emotionally focused couple therapy to posttraumatic stress, the treatment strategy or specific components of that approach have received empirical support but have not been intensively examined in application to the specific disorder advocated here. In other cases, as in the treatment of narcissistic disorder, chapters describe the adaptation of a particular approach to couple therapy to a specific disorder recognized by the therapist, but unlikely to be acknowledged by both partners as an individual or relationship problem. Other chapters, such as those addressing physical illness and bereavement, emphasize basic principles of adapting couple therapy to such issues largely separate from any particular theoretical modality. Independent of the extent of empirical findings underlying the specific guidelines they offer, each of the authors contributing to this part brings extensive experience and clinical wisdom to treating couples in which one or both partners have mental or physical health problems.

By definition, personality disorders comprise enduring and pervasive patterns of behavior that disrupt functioning across a broad interpersonal spectrum, including not only the couple's own relationship but typically partners' relationship with their therapist as well. Often such disorders fundamentally compromise the therapeutic alliance on which subsequent interventions depend. In his chapter on paranoia,

Terkelsen emphasizes not only the importance of pharmacological interventions in more severe expressions of paranoia but also describes clinical strategies for establishing and maintaining a therapeutic alliance with less impaired individuals still predisposed to heightened mistrust of others. Managing the therapeutic alliance also comprises an important aspect of the chapter by Scharff and Bagnini on applying object-relations therapy to couples in which one or both partners exhibit a narcissistic disorder. Their chapter highlights the interactive nature of partners' and therapists' emotional responses and offers suggestions to therapists for attending to their own internal reactions, as both an assessment and therapeutic strategy. Building on previous research regarding dialectical behavior therapy with individuals suffering a borderline personality disorder, Fruzzetti and Fruzzetti describe an extension of this approach to couples in which one or both partners exhibit features of a borderline personality disorder. Although empirical studies of their approach for borderline disorders might warrant inclusion of this chapter in Part II, we include it instead in Part III given the less extensive research more generally regarding couple-based interventions for personality disorders.

Posttraumatic stress disorders (PTSD) are commonly observed among couples in therapy. For many couples, particularly among women partners, PTSD relates to physical, sexual, or severe emotional abuse in the individual's childhood; for other couples, the trauma are more recent, whether from violence, natural disaster, or related to work. In their chapter on posttraumatic stress, Johnson and Makinen emphasize the interpersonal nature of most trauma and the adverse consequences for attachment bonds in the couple's own relationship. Their description of emotionally focused couple therapy with trauma survivors highlights the basis of this approach in attachment theory and draws on emerging empirical investigations of this specific application to distressed couples. By comparison, McCarthy and Sypeck's chapter on childhood sexual trauma emphasizes the impact of such trauma on both the individual's and couple's sexual functioning. They underscore the need to integrate individual-, traditional couple-, and more focused sex-therapy interventions; they also highlight potential iatrogenic effects of focusing on emotional reprocessing of childhood abuse issues to the neglect of more current relationship issues.

Few of us escape confronting at some time in our lives such challenges as physical health problems in ourselves or others, difficulties of aging and related physical and mental decline, or the burdens of death and bereavement. Nevertheless, therapists often receive limited training for addressing such difficulties among the couples they treat. In their chapter on physical illness, Osterman, Sher, Hales, Canar, Singla, and Tilton emphasize the reciprocal influence of health problems and relationship difficulties, as well as ethical challenges in continually reconceptualizing the "client" as couples transition through progressive stages of terminal illness. Qualls addresses similar issues in working with couples in which one partner exhibits cognitive difficulties due to aging or similar neurological impairments. Both Qualls, as well as Osterman and her colleagues, emphasize the value of working within an interdisciplinary approach and the importance of addressing changing roles for partners confronting physical decline or death. Often the loss that partners face is not their own or each other's decline but the death of someone outside the relationship who is dear to one or both partners, such as a parent or child. In his chapter on bereavement and complicated grief, Wills draws on the individual treatment literature in providing explicit guidelines for conceptualizing, assessing, and intervening with loss and bereavement from a couple perspective. Similar to other authors, he offers specific suggestions for selecting among individual, couple-based, and combined treatment modalities. Drawing on his experiences both as an ordained minister as well as a mental health professional, Wills notes the role of individuals' faith and spirituality as potential resources in the grieving and coping process.

Collectively, the chapters in this part emphasize two themes. The first involves the advantages of working with couples from a theoretical perspective best-suited to the specific emotional or behavioral problems characterizing the individual partners and their relationship. These chapters suggest that some theoretical approaches lend themselves particularly well to conceptualizing specific characteristics of partners' difficulties and tailoring interventions from the approach most likely to be effective. A second theme involves the advantages of adopting an interdisciplinary approach to treating difficult couples. Particularly complex couples, such as those described in these chapters, often require skillful integration of individual interventions emphasizing intrapersonal issues, pharmacotherapy addressing biological components of a partner's disorder, couple-based treatments targeting partners' interactions, and system-based interventions addressing the broader social, medical, legal, and faith communities in which individuals' lives and relationships are embedded.

CHAPTER 10

Borderline Personality Disorder

ALAN E. FRUZZETTI
ARMIDA R. FRUZZETTI

Dialectical behavior therapy (DBT) with couples is a treatment in development for extreme presenting problems for which no treatment has yet demonstrated efficacy. DBT with couples has its roots in individual DBT for borderline personality disorder (BPD; Linehan, 1993a, 1993b), which has a strong empirical base (e.g., Fruzzetti, 2002; Koerner & Dimeff, 2000). DBT is predicated on a model that maintains that emotion dysregulation is the core problem of borderline personality and related disorders, and that balancing acceptance and change strategies is at the core of treatment. Furthermore, both acceptance and change behaviors (of self and the partner) are treatment targets. Both acceptance-oriented and change-oriented intervention strategies have accrued considerable empirical support in couple therapy. The dialectical integration (or synthesis) of these approaches, in particular vis-à-vis treating both severe individual and couple distress, will be emphasized in this chapter.

Although full BPD may not be especially common in couples that seek therapy, certain borderline features such as emotion dysregulation are quite common in very distressed couples. We will briefly explicate the characteristics of borderline personality and related disorders and the transactional model for the development and maintenance of BPD, and then describe the many ways that BPD, or even a subset of BPD features, affect couple relationships. We will also discuss how particular partner responses and couple interactional styles may create or maintain the problem behaviors of borderline personality and related disorders. We will then provide an overview of the hierarchy of treatment targets and a range of intervention strategies, along with some specific guidelines for managing special problems and issues in this client population.

UNDERSTANDING BORDERLINE PERSONALITY AND RELATED DISORDERS

Definitions, Prevalence, and Comorbidity

Borderline personality disorder is the most common personality disorder and overlaps significantly with other personality disorders and Axis I disorders (Widiger & Rogers, 1989). BPD is characterized by a "pervasive pattern of instability in interpersonal relationships, self-image, and affects, and marked impulsivity" (American Psychiatric Association, 1994, p. 654). Linehan (1993a) has reorganized the specific criteria into multiple areas of *dysregulation*. Specifically, emotion dysregulation includes emotional lability and problems with anger; interpersonal dysregulation includes chronic fears of abandonment and interpersonal chaos; behavioral dysregulation includes suicidal behaviors and other impulsive or "out-of-control" behaviors; self-dysregulation includes feelings of emptiness; and cognitive dysregulation includes transient paranoia and difficulties in thinking. Reorganizing the criteria this way allows the problem behaviors that define the disorder to be identified as specific treatment targets in a theoretically consistent way. DBT itself is then organized to teach and strengthen skills to self-manage each of these areas of dysregulation.

It is difficult to know accurately how common BPD or significant borderline features are among those couples seeking therapy. However, it is estimated that 10–15% of outpatients (individual treatment) and upwards of 20% of inpatients meet full criteria for BPD (Linehan & Heard, 1999). Obviously, using less stringent criteria such as "significant borderline features" results in much higher estimates of the prevalence of these kinds of presentations. Moreover, clients with less severe problems, whose borderline characteristics primarily affect their romantic relationships, are not included in these prevalence rates. In our own clinic, approximately half of couples seeking therapy have at least one partner with significant borderline features (at least three criteria being met).

Similarly, it is unknown what proportion of borderline individuals experience significant relationship distress. However, when an individual with BPD is in treatment, the likelihood is high that the client's individual relationship is significantly distressed. For example, among female clients in our individual DBT program who have partners, more than 80% report that their relationship is distressed on standard measures, and nearly 100% report significant problems within their relationship at some point in the course of one year of individual treatment.

Transactional or Biosocial Model for the Development and Maintenance of BPD

Borderline personality is considered to result from a *transaction* between an individual's level of *vulnerability to negative emotion* and the social environment's *invalidating* responses that likely began in the individual's family of origin and likely continue in present couple or family relationships. In a transactional model factors exert mutual influence, and thus this model is quite compatible with both traditional behavioral and family systems models.

Emotional Vulnerability and Emotion Dysregulation

Vulnerability to negative emotional experiences and emotion dysregulation is the core of the individual factor in this model. Emotion vulnerability has three parts: (1) high sensitivity to emotional stimuli; (2) high reactivity to emotional stimuli; and (3) a slow return to baseline following emotion dysregulation (Linehan, 1993a). Negative emotional arousal per se is not equivalent to emotion *dysregulation,* which occurs when emotional arousal becomes high enough to disrupt effective self-management, and leads to problematic and often destructive actions (to self, other, or the relationship). Thus, high emotional arousal is better considered ordinary emotional "upset" whereas emotion dysregulation gets in the way of effective living or general life satisfaction.

Invalidating Family Environment

The other factor in the biosocial/transactional model is the invalidating family environment. An *invalidating* person or family (or other social contact) *pervasively* invalidates (demeans, criticizes, punishes, ignores, responds inconsistently, pathologizes, etc.) the *valid* behaviors of the individual, including her or his wants or desires, emotions, thoughts, and other responses. An invalidating family environment is, in some sense, a mismatch between an individual and her or his partner or other family members (Hoffman, Fruzzetti, & Swenson, 1999). The effects of criticism, contempt, and other negative partner reactions on individuals are well documented (cf. Fruzzetti, 1996). Defining and identifying specific behaviors that are specifically invalidating, rather than simply negative, allows us to examine the impact on individual functioning in specific domains and to develop interventions that are useful for the individual with BPD, her or his partner, and their relationship.

Impact on Couple Functioning

Borderline problems can have a particularly acute presentation in couple therapy. For example, some clients with BPD vacillate between extreme attachment and dependence on a partner and detachment, anger, or contempt with the same partner. Moreover, such transitions can occur very quickly, leaving partners confused or angry in return. Similarly, the emotional sensitivity and reactivity of borderline clients can result in frequent outbursts in response to what might normatively seem like small transgressions. Of course, once a couple's interactions become reciprocally negative, things can get intensely destructive very quickly.

Jealousy also may be quite common, given clients' histories of abandonment, subsequent fears of abandonment, pervasive sense of shame, and low self-worth. Such fears are often expressed ineffectively as anger, aggression, or entitlement if the individual has learned a lot of escape conditioning (e.g., learned to respond with anger in situations of fear), or has poor emotion identification, labeling, or modulation skills, all hallmarks of clients with BPD.

Chronic suicidality and other chronic impulsive actions of one partner can be a particularly difficult problem with couples. Not only are these problems taxing for the suicidal or impulsive individual, they are also very difficult for her or his partner. Partners may intermittently reinforce these kinds of behaviors by providing soothing and nurturance at the "wrong" times. The difficult therapeutic task often becomes finding ways for the partner to provide soothing without reinforcing escalation or dysfunction.

Finally, severely distressed borderline clients may also exhibit transient paranoia or other stress-related cognitive difficulties. Thus, normative couple conflict situations can elicit extreme responses, resulting in the experience of "walking on eggshells" that many family members describe. Of course, if normative conflict is avoided or remains unresolved, relationship and other life problems grow, resulting in escalating distress.

Dialectics in Couples

Dialectical principles in DBT with couples reflect those of individual DBT and were adapted from both Western contemplative and Eastern meditative practices, informed by dialectical philosophy (Linehan, 1993a; Pinkard, 1988). These principles are particularly compatible with couple work. There are several central dialectics, or apparent contradictions or polarities, that need to be resolved (synthesized) in successful treatment with couples: (1) closeness versus conflict; (2) partner acceptance versus change; (3) one partner's needs and desires versus the other's; (4) individual versus relationship satisfaction; and (5) intimacy versus autonomy. A dialectical philosophy allows these apparent polarities to be targeted for synthesis. In each of these pairs the dialectical treatment target is to achieve *both* poles despite the fact that they lie in apparent opposition (e.g., achieving both intimacy *and* autonomy rather than sacrificing one for the other). "Trading off" or compromising would not be a dialectical synthesis.

It is important not to pathologize clients' positions on any of these dimensions. For example, a client with BPD might want a lot of closeness with her partner while he desires less intense emotional intimacy. Dialectics allow the therapist to validate her desire for more and his desire for less without pathologizing either partner. The treatment target is *synthesis:* To find ways of being with each other that are intense enough for her without overwhelming him.

The model of "chaotic" couples (Fruzzetti, 1996) may be particularly salient when one or both partners have borderline features. Specifically, chaotic couples may have periods of intense and satisfying closeness, but their intimacy may be quite fragile, as one or both partners may be highly sensitive or reactive to any diminished closeness (conflicts about intimacy). Similarly, in chaotic couples one or both partners may have difficulty expressing their emotions and desires or may lack the skills to stay emotionally regulated during ordinary negotiations such that destructive conflict may erupt quickly and intensely. Consequently, finding intervention strategies that synthesize or transform conflict into closeness and utilize desired closeness to manage conflict constructively are important aspects of DBT with couples.

Treatment Strategies

Dialectics also provide the foundation for therapist strategies and interventions, communication style, and the approach to serious dysfunctional behaviors such as suicidal and aggressive behaviors (cf. Linehan, 1993a). The central dialectic in DBT is that of acceptance and change, which provides the organizing principle for treatment targets: accepting the legitimate or valid parts of a situation, emotional reaction, or partner behavior while also focusing on changing the parts that are ineffective or problematic. Thus, the therapist utilizes the acceptance and change dialectic both as a treatment strategy to maximize outcomes and as a model for how partners may more effectively manage themselves and their relationship.

Overview of Modes and Functions of Treatment

DBT with couples can involve more than one mode of intervention, just as individual DBT includes multiple concurrent intervention modes. For example, it is common for one partner in a couple simultaneously to be in couple therapy along with individual treatment for suicidal behaviors, which may in turn include both individual psychotherapy and group skill training. With nonsuicidal/nonviolent clients, partners may be in a couple skill group and couple therapy, or all aspects of the treatment may be delivered in conjoint format. Regardless of format, five different *functions* must be delivered if DBT is to be considered "comprehensive" (Fruzzetti, 2002; Linehan, 1993a): (1) skill acquisition or enhancement; (2) skill generalization; (3) client motivation/behavior change; (4) therapist capability enhancement and motivation; and (5) structuring the environment.

Skill Acquisition or Enhancement

Skill enhancement or skill training is an essential part of DBT with couples (Fruzzetti & Iverson, in press; Hoffman et al., 1999). The assumption of the model is that borderline clients have psychological and relationship skill deficits and that their partners, even if not deficient in emotion skills, need to learn more individual emotion regulation skills to support the borderline person, and need to learn relationship skills to alleviate distress and improve their relationship. Skill training for individual skills follows the guidelines presented in Linehan's skill train-

TABLE 10.1. Individual DBT Skills and Treatment Targets

Individual skill	Targets
Mindfulness	Attention control; awareness of self and others.
Emotion regulation	Identify and label emotions accurately; reduce vulnerability and suffering associated with negative emotion; change negative emotions.
Distress tolerance	Counterbalance impulsiveness; tolerate emotions without engaging in dysfunctional behaviors.
Interpersonal effectiveness	Achieve interpersonal objectives without damaging their relationship or the person's self-respect.

TABLE 10.2. Couple DBT Skills and Treatment Targets

Couple skill	Targets
Relationship mindfulness	Awareness of one's partner and relationship without judgment or criticism; awareness of the interactions and interaction patterns between self and partner.
Validation	Accurate and effective self-expression; respond effectively to the "valid" points made by one's partner; enhance self-disclosure/validation reciprocity (and reduce negative escalation).
Problem management	Resolve problems in a dialectical manner either by solving a problem or understanding it differently and accepting it (at least temporarily).
Acceptance and closeness	Let go of negative emotional reactivity and resolve intimacy and autonomy conflicts; achieve mutually desired levels of closeness and intimacy while preserving or enhancing individual well-being.

ing manual (1993b), which are summarized in Table 10.1. Relationship skill targets are summarized in Table 10.2. Helping couples to acquire necessary skills is a core of this treatment. Thus, skills are taught overtly with explicit handouts (Fruzzetti, Hoffman, & Linehan, 2002), practiced in session and at home, and the abilities and motivation of partners to use skills when needed (especially in difficult or incendiary situations) are regularly assessed.

Skill Generalization

Direct attention to the transfer of skills from the therapy situation to the couple's life at home and in the world is required, and thus skill generalization is another essential function of DBT with couples. The combination of planning (homework or practice outside sessions) plus the use of occasional telephone coaching can be particularly effective. Because distressed couples in general and borderline partners in particular are often quite emotionally reactive, the therapist may re-create some of the conditions under which clients have problematic reactions and teach or strengthen self-management or relationship skills in that specific context to maximize generalization.

For example, Bob and Carole would often come to session after an argument having "solved" the problem in each of their heads and would proceed from there. However, their arguments were full of rage and did significant damage to their relationship and each other. The therapist helped them to remember the hurtful things the other had said, allow themselves to get emotionally escalated, and then begin the argument again. The therapist was then able both to assess specifically their emotional reactivity *in vivo* and coach them on the skills they needed to use to steer their argument toward a more fruitful conclusion. Having identified the steps, they were able to write them down and practice them successfully (one skill at a time at first, then chained together) at home. Similarly, Maria and José were able to discuss effectively in session how to handle parenting issues with their 2-year-old, Christina. However, when Christina was tired, crying, interrupting, and so on at home, each would begin to react with strong emotion, blame the other, and escalate their argument. The therapist instructed them to call the next time this situation emerged, and coached each of them briefly (for about 2 minutes each) on the skills they had been practicing (being mindful of collaboration goals, letting go of judgments of the other, specific emotion reregulation skills) and then to reengage in their discussion. This brief phone intervention effectively interrupted their negative pattern enough for them to work through the rest of the disagreement.

Behavior Change and Motivation

This component of treatment addresses those factors necessary to achieve important behavior change (including both changes in overt behaviors and changes in thoughts and feelings). Such behavior change might include more acceptance and validation or specific changes in partner responses. The therapist and clients collaborate to identify and modify the conditions (antecedents and consequences) that create or maintain dysfunctional behaviors, or that inhibit, punish, or fail to reinforce more functional and skillful alternative behaviors. This is described more fully below (see "chain analysis").

Therapist Motivation and Skills

All DBT treatments require therapists to acquire necessary treatment skills and maintain a high level of motivation (Fruzzetti, Waltz, & Linehan, 1997), typically through an ongoing treatment consultation team. Participating in treatment consultation teams is common in family systems work, but is much less so in cognitive and behavioral couple and family therapy. However, ongoing consultation is of particular importance with this population because borderline, suicidal, violent, emotionally reactive, or multiproblem clients can be difficult to treat and often evoke intense reactions from treatment providers. A peer consultation team that meets regularly facilitates: (1) therapists enhancing their own skills; (2) keeping the therapist in "balance" via alternate perspectives and support; and (3) communication among multiple treatment providers to enhance efficiency and to prevent conflict among treatment providers (often called "splitting" with borderline clients).

Structuring the Environment

Finally, structuring the client's treatment or family environment may be necessary to achieve acceptable outcomes. The point of structuring the environment is to increase the likelihood that when clients make progress neither their families nor the treatment environment will punish their improved behaviors. For example, if it became clear that a suicidal client only received soothing and emotional support from her husband when emotionally dysregulated and suicidal, and that he largely ignored her when she was not dysregulated, changing his responses to her would be an important treatment target.

In addition, treatment programs (including, for example, third-party payers) sometimes construct or maintain barriers to improvement as well. For example, if a third-party payer has a rule that limits treatment sessions unless an individual is suicidal, there may be a real disincentive for improvement for that client (whether they are aware of it or not). Structuring the environment in this example would involve trying to change the reimbursement rules so that: (1) the client and couple could continue in treatment (so long as other criteria were met demonstrating improvement), or (2) treatment could be provided for a fixed length of time (and therefore not be dependent on *not* making progress).

ASSESSMENT

There are multiple functions of assessment with any complex case, and assessing multiproblem individuals in distressed relationships presents many obstacles. Both individual and relationship functioning must be assessed initially to (1) know whether to accept into treatment or refer elsewhere; (2) develop treatment targets; and (3) to measure progress and outcome.

The most common assessments for BPD are the Structured Clinical Interview for DSM-IV Axis II Personality Disorders (First, Gibbon, Spitzer, & Williams, 1995), the Revised Diagnostic Interview for Borderlines (Zanarini, Gunderson, Frankenburg, & Chauncey, 1989), or an unstructured (but comprehensive) clinical interview using the DSM-IV criteria. Although reliability is often only modest, these are the best available methods to date for assessing the presence or absence of BPD. It is very important to do this painstaking assessment and not to rely on someone else's diagnosis. BPD is frequently misdiagnosed as something else in some clients (e.g., bipolar II disorder, attention deficit disorder, substance abuse, depression, posttraumatic stress disorder) and often missed entirely in others (especially male clients).

Diary Cards

Treatment targets are very specifically defined in DBT, and daily diary cards or self-monitoring sheets are the means by which they are assessed. Partners monitor both individual behaviors (e.g., drinking, suicidal urges, self-injury, thoughts of aggression, mood ratings) and relationship targets (time together, criticism of partner, thoughts about leaving the relationship, expressing love). Diary cards include current targets, both as a reminder to the client to work on specific improvements and as a means to organize the next therapy session. Targets that are achieved (e.g., accurate self-expression) or are no longer relevant (e.g., the client no longer has suicidal thoughts) are dropped from the sheet. Regular monitoring via the diary card allows the therapist to assesses individual and relationship functioning since the last session and set an agenda for the present session simply by going over the diary sheet with the partner(s).

Chain Analysis of Target Behaviors

Assessment of treatment targets does not only occur at the beginning of treatment and does not stop with simple measurement of frequency or severity. Careful behavioral or *chain analyses* are conducted in virtually every session to understand the present causes of problem behaviors and to identify factors that inhibit the use of new, more functional alternatives. These, of course, become the targets for treatment. Identifying antecedents and consequences of target behaviors also identifies specific behaviors of both partners that can be a focus of treatment (cf. Fruzzetti & Levensky, 2000 for a detailed example of a chain analysis of partner violence).

For example, Ruth and Aaron both reported on their diary cards a lot of conflict and misery on the previous Wednesday, which culminated in each cursing at the other and threatening divorce, then not talking to each other for almost 2 days. Through direct questioning, the chain of behaviors that led to this outcome was explicated. Some of the more skillful alternatives to their escalating behaviors that the therapist would target in session are noted in brackets. This episode likely started Tuesday night when Ruth went to bed early, without inviting Aaron to join her. He reported feeling somewhat rejected [could have described this, asked if she'd like him to join her, or asked her to just sit and cuddle for a couple of minutes first]. Ruth reported having been very tired and had assumed it was too early for Aaron to want to go to bed [could have been mindful of his feelings and desires to be close]. Aaron then stayed up late, becoming increasingly upset [could have acted opposite to his fears and gone to bed and cuddled with her, self-validated and planned to initiate a constructive conversation in the morning about his feelings, or self-validated his feelings while also being mindful of alternative interpretations of Ruth's going to bed early]. The therapist helped him identify this "upset" as sadness by noticing just the emotion (not the judgmental thoughts he was having), even though he had initially described himself as angry at Ruth [he could have focused on his sadness at their distance instead of his anger in response to his judgments about it]. In the morning, he slept in later than usual (getting up after Ruth left for work), so they didn't speak again until arriving home from work that night [he could have used "willingness" skills to get up with her or to check in with her during the day; she could have been more mindful of his staying in bed late and related emotions and checked in with him and validated his feelings while clarifying her own]. Aaron was very irritable [he could have regulated his emotions prior to coming home and engaged in a constructive, mutually validating discussion], and Ruth started out trying to "validate that he had a bad day" [she could have been more validating, asking about his feelings and validating them], which just provoked Aaron further (she "wasn't acknowledging that she had made me miserable" [he could have let go of his judgments and negative assumptions, been more self-validating by noticing the original sadness and that his irritability would not get him the closeness he wanted]). Ruth felt worried and annoyed, and began criticizing Aaron for being hostile [she could have been more mindful of her worry about Aaron and described that in a validating way]. Aaron criticized Ruth for being cold and distant and uncaring [at this point both could have been more mindful that they were past the point of being effective and taken a time out to regulate their own emotions], and within seconds they were both screaming at each other, bringing into the conversation many past criticisms and judgments.

It is not necessary to go through each step of the chain each time. Rather, the essence is to identify key, repetitive problem behaviors (e.g., escalating emotional reactions, judgments, or incendiary behaviors) or the absence of skillful behaviors (e.g., not noticing certain emotions in oneself; not being mindful of the broader context of the other's behavior, not validating the other). Once a couple's pattern has been identified through a few comprehensive chain analyses, going directly to the key point(s) and treating those problem behaviors (or absence of functional ones) becomes the focus.

Direct Assessment of Communication

There is no substitute for assessing couples in conversation directly (live or via videotape). Such assessments should be completed at the beginning of treatment and subsequently at regular intervals (e.g., weekly or monthly, or as indicated clinically). A videotaped sample, although often underutilized in clinical practice, can be viewed repeatedly by the clinician and by the peer consultation team, affording an opportunity to identify interaction patterns or rate partner behaviors informally according to specified target criteria. If rated in a valid way, pre- and post-treatment samples (live or videotaped) provide an important measure of specific outcomes (e.g., improvements in partner validation) not biased by demand characteristics or clinician heuristics. Videotaping can also augment client descriptions of their emotional reactions for a chain analysis by re-presenting each other's behaviors later, on tape, when partners are less negatively emotionally aroused. In addition, the tape can be used in treatment as a means of feedback to the couple to help them learn multiple skills (see case illustration later in this chapter).

It may be particularly useful to observe the couple's target behaviors relevant to whatever stage of treatment they are in: invalidation of emotions or reinforcement of dysfunction in stage 1; problematic self-disclosures or invalidation in stage 2; problem management skill deficits and engage-distance interaction patterns in stage 3; or problems with reciprocated vulnerability and intimacy in stage 4 (Fruzzetti et al., 2002; Heyman, 2001).

INTERVENTION

Stages of Treatment, Treatment Targets, and Intervention Strategies

Treatment targets in DBT with couples are organized into an explicit hierarchy that requires more severe or out-of-control behaviors to be resolved (in control) before less severe behaviors are addressed. The overarching goal of all applications of DBT is to help clients create and maintain a life worth living according to their own core values, and a couple or family in which the relationships support individual well-being and are themselves satisfying. Consequently, treatment targets are arranged hierarchically according to how severely they interfere with a client's or couple's quality of life. For example, if a couple presents with multiple complaints including violence, conflicts about money, sex, emotional distance, household chores, and so on, violence would be stopped first and then the other problems would be addressed in each stage, with relevant skills used to resolve or manage issues and achieve greater understanding and closeness over time.

Pretreatment Stage of Treatment

DBT with couples requires a clear orientation of the patient to the nature of the treatment and any available alternatives. Partners are informed of how the treatment is conducted and evaluated, how their presenting problems will be organized in a treatment target hierarchy, what assessment procedures will be conducted, how long treatment will last (at least initially), and what factors might result in any change in the treatment "contract." The "pros and cons" of entering DBT with couples versus other available treatments should be evaluated by the client and therapist.

During this stage, partners complete all pretreatment assessments, begin to complete daily self-monitoring sheets, and try to reduce or resolve factors that are likely to interfere with active participation and commitment to the treatment program. Pretreatment typically may last from two to three sessions and, once assessment is complete and an agreement or contract is reached, treatment moves to stage 1 targets.

Stage 1

The main targets in this stage are behaviors that are out of control. In particular, behavioral safety and stability across three domains are paramount: (1) life-threatening behaviors, including suicidal and self-injurious behaviors, aggression and violence (as a perpetrator or victim), and child abuse and neglect; (2) therapy-interfering behaviors (e.g., client does not come to session, is not collaborative, or does not adhere to agreed-upon between-session practice targets); and (3) severe quality of life-interfering behaviors, such as maintaining an ongoing affair, severe drug abuse or debilitating depression, criminal activity that might lead to incarceration, or other out-of-control behaviors that severely limit quality of life.

Treatment in this stage focuses on achieving individual and relationship stability by teaching clients self-management skills, strengthening those skills, and helping them to generalize new skills to their natural environment. Similarly, treatment may also help clients to change their environments to make them safer, more stable, and more compatible with skillful living (Fruzzetti et al., 2002; Hoffman et al., 1999). It is not uncommon for depressed, borderline women to try new skills with their partners only to be met by severe invalidation or criticism that might precipitate another suicidal crisis or self-injurious act. In such cases the relationship between the female's attempt at a new behavior, her partner's criticism, and the subsequent chain of emotions, actions, and thoughts would be carefully explicated. The partner might be oriented to this sequence, and asked to notice and reinforce new skills instead of punishing them. For example, Ellen worked hard in her individual treatment to describe her emotions and her wants more accurately and assertively; her husband, Frank, had said that her obsequiousness "drove [him] crazy" and wanted to know what she wanted, felt, and thought. But when she expressed frustration or disagreement, Frank yelled at her and told her she was "self-centered," and she quickly stopped expressing herself to him. When this sequence was identified, Frank practiced listening and validating Ellen for her expression, reinforcing her new skills instead of punishing them.

Life-threatening behaviors (suicide attempts or self-harm; partner aggression or violence; and child abuse or neglect) require individual DBT, at least until they are under behavioral self-control. For DBT applications to problems of suicidality, see Linehan (1993a, 1993b); for DBT applications to aggression and violence, see Fruzzetti and Levensky (2000). However, couple interventions may simultaneously be used during stage 1 to augment individual treatment, with the target of reducing and eliminating life-threatening behaviors.

Couple Interventions to Augment Individual Outcomes

When one or both partners have serious individual distress, it may be enormously taxing on both the other partner and on the relationship. The first target in DBT with couples is to facilitate individuals getting their own seriously dysfunctional behaviors under control. Safety for oneself and others is the paramount goal and must be achieved before other targets should be considered. Thus, couple interventions augment individual treatment and include: (1) psychoeducation for both partners, especially regarding borderline personality, emotion dysregulation, and the nonblaming model for BPD that highlights the roles of both emotion vulnerability and invalidation; (2) reducing invalidation of the identified patient (and reducing her or his invalidation of the partner), which might include reducing judgments and criticisms (using mindfulness and relationship mindfulness) and teaching brief time-outs, distress tolerance or other skills to truncate escalation that might lead to self-harm or aggression; and (3) stopping any reinforcement of dysfunctional behaviors.

For example, Maureen complained that her husband Jeff was aloof and distant most of the time, "preferring the Internet to me." However, when Maureen became suicidal or self-injured, Jeff quickly became solicitous, warm, and caring. Jeff explained that following these episodes he felt very "burned out and afraid," and turned to his own escape behaviors to cope. Jeff agreed to spend 30–60 minutes every day being attentive to Maureen (including getting support for himself from Maureen). Maureen agreed not to seek support from Jeff when suicidal, but instead to get support for self-managing her suicidal thoughts and urges from her treatment team. Both partners followed through and Maureen's suicidality virtually disappeared.

Stage 2

The main individual difficulty in the second stage is severe emotional misery, and the relationship difficulties are both the presence of destructive conflict (aversive and escalating or the avoidance of conflict) and problems with closeness. One of the core issues in BPD is related to deficits in self and self-expression. In particular this may involve problems experiencing emotion (discriminating emotional experiences, accurate labeling, or accurate expression). In order to experience and express emotions effectively, anyone must have the necessary emotion skills and have a supportive or validating partner to support or reinforce effective expression (Fruzzetti, 2002).

Accurate labeling of emotions is quite difficult for clients with BPD. Clients' reactions and expression often go quickly to anger in situations where other emotions might be more normative or effective. In DBT we call the "legitimate" or normative emotion in a situation a person's *primary* emotion, and subsequent reactions *secondary* emotions. Many clients with BPD suffer a great deal with secondary emotions such as shame, sadness, or anger, and can be very enigmatic to partners or others in large measure because they fail to identify the primary emotion in many situations. Thus, considerable effort is expended to help clients accurately identify and express primary emotions while ignoring or redirecting away from secondary ones.

Thus, in stage 2, awareness of oneself (especially emotions and desires) and awareness of one's partner are taught via mindfulness and relationship mindfulness skills. The skills of self-disclosure, labeling emotions, and expressing them descriptively without self-judgment or criticism of the partner are practiced (cf. Linehan, 1993b; Fruzzetti et al., 2002). For example, Dom and Julie's interactions were characterized by escalating verbal attacks on each other, and only anger was expressed. However, with skills coaching each partner was able to identify other emotions that seemed to get lost in rapid angry outbursts. They were coached simply to describe their own emotions (using mindfulness and emotion regulation skills) without attacking their partner, while being mindful of their partner's reaction. Thus, "I'm pissed because you are always on my case about everything!" became "I feel so lonely and sad because we seem to be misunderstanding each other again." This latter expression was ripe for partner validation and mutual disclosure.

Validation skills (Fruzzetti et al., 2002; Hoffman et al. 1999) focus on how to understand the other person and communicate that understanding genuinely, and reinforce accurate expression. Validation may take many forms: (1) basic attention and active listening; (2) reflecting back the other's emotions or disclosures; (3) noticing what the other person is feeling or wanting even when they are not articulating it themselves; (4) in the face of partner "problem" behaviors, putting her or his behavior in context to lessen its negative valence (i.e., understanding the behavior given the partner's history or current level of functioning); (5) "normalizing" behavior (e.g., "of course you'd feel that way—anyone would"); (6) treating the partner as an equal, not as fragile; and (7) reciprocating vulnerability, often by reciprocating self-disclosures of vulnerability.

Chaotic couples may have experienced such high rates of aversive behavior in their relationship that they have increasingly withdrawn from each other, with little companionship and few opportunities for pleasant interactions. Thus, relationship activation is also a target in stage 2. Although not specific to BPD couples, it is important for couples to spend time doing enjoyable, mutually satisfying things (together and alone) that can provide a broader relationship context than their recent distress. For example, despite longing for more closeness, Joe and Linda had been arguing so often and so destructively that they mostly avoided each other, and were on "hair-trigger" alert when they did interact. In stage 2 they first focused on being more aware of present circumstances and present mutual commitments and less on past transgressions (relationship mindfulness), while beginning to engage mindfully (noticing the pleasant parts) in nonprovocative time together such as going for a walk, watching television together, or just sitting in the same room at the same time while reading. They then practiced easier self-disclosures and validating responses (e.g., discussing neutral topics), before moving on to more difficult topics. With a clear commitment to validating each other, both partners were more willing to be honest, but descriptive and nonjudgmental. Instead of trying to show Linda why she "shouldn't feel that way," Joe instead worked on validating her growing feelings of sadness and abandonment as he spent more time working late, and gently correcting misperceptions by accurately self-disclosing (he told her that he was afraid of more fighting, which he hated, so worked more to avoid the conflict, not to avoid her). Linda was then able to understand and validate his feelings (fear) and his behavior ("If he hates conflict that much, working late to avoid it makes some sense"), in part because the context of this discussion was so much slower and less reactive. They were able to see that what they wanted from each other was quite similar.

Finally, histories of physical or sexual trauma during childhood or adolescence are common among clients with BPD (e.g., Herman, Perry, & van der Kolk, 1989). Borderline clients with PTSD or PTSD-like problems in individual DBT typically go through exposure and response prevention treatment (see Foa & Rothbaum, 1998, for an example of this treatment) in stage 2, after achieving safety and stability in stage 1. Engaging the partner to support this work can be a very important adjunct to individual trauma treatment (Riggs, 2000). For example, after exposure therapy sessions on Tuesday afternoons Carmen came home exhausted and sad. Going over her sexual abuse involved a lot of pain as she slowly and repeatedly imagined and described the events exposure without dissociating or using alcohol to escape. Because Rick was oriented to these procedures, he expected Carmen to be tired and made Tuesday nights "quiet nights at home" in which she could tell him a little bit about her session or just hang out together. He also understood that Carmen might have diminished interest in sexual activity for a while, and got a lot of support from the therapist to be accepting of this temporary change. In these ways, Rick provided much needed support for Carmen over the 8 weeks that this part of treatment continued, and she was able to significantly reduce her traumatic stress responses.

Stage 3

The main targets in stage 3 are resolving both individual life problems and relationship problems. By this point in treatment, safety and stability should have been achieved, and partners should be involved in some prorelationship time and have the ability to engage reciprocally in self-disclosure and validation cycles. Thus, in stage 3 partners should be less reactive and more able to turn their attention to problem solving or

management, and modifying the conflict patterns that they may have
fallen into over time.

Problem/Conflict Management

Problem management builds on successful problem solving approaches
to working with distressed couples (e.g., Jacobson & Margolin, 1979),
but weaves the other skills already learned (relationship mindfulness,
accurate expression/self-disclosure, and validation) into the process. In
addition, at various points in the problem management process partners may choose to change the focus from trying to find a solution to
the target problem that requires one or both to change, to instead "accept" the situation or behavior in question. Fuller understanding and
validation, along with less reactivity, may render the "problem" no
longer problematic.

Modifying Dysfunctional Interaction Patterns

Distressed borderline couples, along with other severely distressed couples, often have adopted very dysfunctional interaction patterns such as
rapid negative escalation or engage–distance (or demand–withdraw).
One target in stage 3 is to alter these patterns. The use of videotaped
feedback may be especially useful both to identify the problem pattern itself and to help partners see the pattern and the necessity for a different
response from each of them. Mindfulness and relationship mindfulness
skills are used to slow down the interaction and keep clients focused on
their larger goals. Distress tolerance and emotion regulation skills are
used to minimize one's own negative reactivity, and accurate or mindful
self-disclosure/expression and validation are used to minimize partner
reactivity. Conflict topics can be discussed simply for understanding and
to enhance closeness, or may be the subject of problem management.

The therapist's roles are those of teacher, coach, and traffic cop,
helping partners to learn and use the skills; identifying, encouraging,
and cheerleading progress; and interrupting reactive or invalidating responses. Over time, partners take on all of these roles themselves.

Partners often come into treatment after years of quick-escalating,
highly aversive, and invalidating reactions to each other, which can
make them reluctant to express vulnerability. Their therapist, however,
can set and enforce clear guidelines limiting their responses to only validating ones. Until each is able to respond with validation, the therapist
can validate and reinforce disclosures and vulnerability and model how
to do it. With practice, partners learn to provide this validation and reinforcement themselves, and that function transfers back to them.

Stage 4

In this last stage of treatment, the individual target involves "incompleteness," or the recognition that after significant or even ordinary life problems have been resolved, many people still struggle with finding meaning, overcoming isolation, and achieving genuine intimacy. Thus, the relational targets are the synthesis of intimacy and autonomy to achieve healthy partners who can function at a high level independently as well as a close and intimate relationship that supports the individuals in it.

Synthesizing Closeness and Conflict

In the early stages of treatment, DBT with couples focuses somewhat separately on enhancing intimacy and on resolving conflict. In stage 4, the first treatment target is to transform conflict into closeness. Specifically, clients learn how to: (1) use distress tolerance and "turning the mind" (Linehan, 1993b) skills regarding the "problem behaviors" of their spouse or partner that, at least in the near term, are not likely to change; (2) use mindfulness to understand the putative problem behavior in context so that they become aware of how their critical focus actually both exacerbates the very behavior they don't like and introduces negativity into their relationship insidiously; and (3) practice "radical acceptance" of their partners' foibles, recontextualizing their partner and relationship by using mindfulness to broaden the context of the "problem behavior." These skills are augmented by using relationship mindfulness (being in the present moment) and validation to enhance closeness. In this manner, thematic conflict topics can be transformed into opportunities for emotional intimacy.

Synthesizing Intimacy and Autonomy

Struggles over this issue may be the hallmark of both individuals with BPD and their relationships. As clients learn accurate self-disclosure that is validated by their partners, learn how to self-manage negative emotion and how to seek appropriate support for self-management, and reduce reactivity collaboratively, they are simultaneously strengthening both partners' autonomy and the intimacy in their relationship. In stage 4 these ongoing processes are joined together; that is, couples learn how increased closeness (e.g., more genuine self-disclosure and vulnerability met with validation and support) actually results in each partner being stronger and more autonomous. Similarly, being capable of independent thoughts and activities can enrich the relationship, bringing new ideas and activities to the relationship to share. Many borderline clients have been pathologized for wanting intense closeness, and often fear that enhancing individuality would not only be painfully difficult but also would threaten the already less-than-optimal levels of intimacy in their relationship. Similarly, partners of borderline partners often report fears of "engulfment" or being overwhelmed by their partners, often fearing that their own individuality is threatened. Recognizing that the idea that "intimacy is in opposition to independence" is a false dichotomy can be very liberating and motivating for partners. The target becomes using one part to enhance the other: getting support for individuality and using intimacy as a motivating force for taking individual risks (a sort of relational safety net), while using individuality to enhance closeness, sharing what each partner brings to the relationship table.

For example, although George and Martha had made considerable progress in treatment over many months, they continued to have conflict around closeness and intimacy. George was afraid of being "suffocated" by Martha and that she would "lose herself." She was afraid that if she stopped engaging him that he would just become more and more distant over time. Consequently, George would push Martha to do things without him (with friends, by herself), and Martha would bristle at these suggestions, seeing them as attempts to push her away. However, they both seemed to want to be close and almost always enjoyed their time together. The therapist identified certain kinds of arguments that, upon analysis, revealed this theme early in the chain, and coached them both on acceptance and closeness skills (Table 10.2). The target was to resolve this apparent conflict between intimacy and independence by getting the couple to share and reinforce each other's independent activities. Both partners worked on accepting each other's perspective according to these three skill steps: (1) tolerating statements and actions to which they previously would have reacted; (2) becoming mindful of how, despite not saying anything, being critical and judgmental of the other increased distance and decreased feeling close and loving; and (3) transforming the previously "negative" behavior into something neutral or positive by putting the behavior in a broader context. George stopped telling Martha to go out with friends, and radically accepted that she might be happy, and not subservient, even if she sometimes wanted to just sit in the same room with George. Martha increasingly shared her independent activities with George, who learned that Martha actually had many more competencies that he had realized; he was proud and much less afraid of her "melting down" in the future. They were increasingly able to enjoy time with each other.

Generalization and Relationship Self-Management

The last target is the generalization of all of these skills to achieve sustained relationship self-management. Typically, this may be accomplished by clients' taking a month off from treatment and tracking their "stuck" points (difficulties that they could not manage on their own), and returning briefly to treatment to figure out what skills they could have used, and going back out on their own again. This may take several months but only a few visits to achieve.

CASE ILLUSTRATION

Amy and Michael had been married for 5 years, which they described as "crazy and chaotic." She was 33 and he was 35 years old, and they agreed that when their relationship was good it was wonderful, "as close as two people can get, intensely satisfying." But when their relationship was difficult, which it had become increasingly, it was destructive and "unbearable."

Amy had been in and out of treatment for more than 18 years. She was diagnosed at various times with depression, substance abuse, bulimia, bipolar II disorder, dependent personality disorder, and BPD. At presentation for individual DBT 6 months prior to coming in for couple therapy, Amy met criteria for binge eating disorder, depression, and BPD. Although she did not meet criteria for substance abuse, she did report drinking to excess several times per month. A recent suicide attempt (overdosing on prescription medications) led to her starting DBT. Michael had not been in treatment before. At the time they presented for couple therapy he did not meet criteria for any DSM disorder, but did report some depressive behaviors (trouble sleeping, difficulty concentrating) and a long history of substance use. By the time they began couple therapy, Amy had made some substantial gains in individual therapy, reporting many fewer suicidal thoughts, no binge eating, and reduced substance use.

On standard measures of relationship satisfaction they both reported high dissatisfaction. Videotaped samples of their conversations showed a pattern of rapid negative emotional escalation and criticality on Amy's part, to which Michael responded with decreased emotional expression (flatter affect) and a lot of "logical" talk that was explicitly critical of Amy and invalidated her emotions and desires (e.g., "I didn't say I *wouldn't* go with you to your sister's house, I only said that I don't want to. You did it again, assuming that I will let you down and getting all upset over nothing. You're unbelievable. I don't think your medications or your therapy are helping very much."). Not surprisingly, Amy reported a lot of fear that Michael would "get sick" of her and leave her, and vacillated between feeling intense shame about her own behavior ("I shouldn't be so needy, I'm driving him crazy") to intense hurt and anger (e.g., "How dare you! You certainly did imply that you weren't coming with me! You're such an asshole! I'd probably be better off without you!").

Because Amy had achieved individual safety and stability by the time they entered couple therapy, they began in stage 2, focusing on relationship mindfulness, accurate and effective self-disclosure, validation, and companionship activation. Amy was already familiar with mindfulness from her individual DBT skill training, but for both partners learning relationship mindfulness was both satisfying and effective. They began to spend some focused relationship time with each other every day (e.g., taking a walk, eating dinner together) and each practiced paying attention to his or her own experience, noticing the other, and letting go of judgments and nascent negative reactions. Also during this time they practiced accurate self-disclosure and in particular, sorting primary emotions from secondary emotions. Amy found that her anger often was in response to her own fears about their future together in general or about how Michael might react to her in the moment, rather than in response to his actual behavior. Michael found similarly that his own anger and withdrawal often built up in anticipation of what Amy *might* do or say (and not anything she had actually done or said in the present conversation), which became a self-fulfilling prophecy of sorts when she reacted to his anger and emotional distance. By being mindful of what she actually did and mindful of his own primary emotion (e.g., fear or sadness) he was able to increase his validation of Amy and his own self-disclosures, which Amy increasingly validated as they learned validation skills.

However, they did continue to have explosive arguments, albeit less frequently. Collaboratively, the therapist and both partners went over the details of the early stages of these arguments and performed detailed chain analyses. One example of their negative escalation went as follows: Michael denied he was frustrated with anything after dinner one night (despite communicating this in his facial expressions and voice tones); Amy assumed she had done something "wrong" again and was self-critical; Amy also felt invalidated because Michael obviously was feeling something and was denying it, resulting in her feeling more distant from him; noticing the emotional distance, she felt fear; but she expressed anger that he was "lying" to her, which led him, in turn, to feel hurt and attacked, and to attack back quickly. Using different skills, they slowed down this cycle by focusing on clarity and genuineness of expression and validation, staying descriptive without criticality or judgment. They found that if they took just a few minutes to read a recent note from the other or look at photographs from loving times they had had together, they were able to focus on the other person in the moment more, and on fears and assumptions less.

In stage 3 this work continued and integrated problem management. At first they had a lot of difficulty taking conflicts slowly, one step at a time. But after just two sessions in which they were able to negotiate previously difficult thematic conflicts, they became highly motivated. For example, they had a long history of conflict and distance around time spent with her family. Amy's father (now deceased) had been physically and sexually abusive of her, and Michael was very angry with Amy's mother and two brothers for "allowing this to happen." Amy's family members were also critical of her. Consequently, he did not like to visit her family and when he did he was often unpleasant. More importantly, when Amy sought support from Michael after being verbally criticized, his typical response was simply to tell her, "What do you expect? I've told you a thousand times you should just stay away from them." Michael had defined the problem as Amy's (that she refused to sever her relationship with them), whereas Amy had defined the problem as Michael's (that he was so not supportive of her and was so unforgiving of her family).

In treatment they were able to redefine these problems. Michael was able to understand that Amy got some important needs met from her family, and agreed to support her in these; Amy was able increasingly to assert herself with her family members such that they became somewhat less critical. Furthermore, Michael was able to see beyond his anger at her family for Amy's prior abuse, and feel sad with her and validate the emotional sequelae of her abuse. In turn, Amy was able to manage these feelings without becoming out of control, making it possible for Michael to be vulnerable in these situations over time.

Consistent with these kinds of interventions, they also focused on reducing their engage–distance interaction pattern. By watching a tape of their own discussions with the therapist, both partners were able to see how their own reactions led, paradoxically, to getting less of what they wanted. As Amy increasingly wanted more closeness and feared losing Michael, she became more angry and critical, pushing him away. Similarly, as Michael increasingly feared being overwhelmed and sought "safe" distance, he reinforced Amy's worst fears and she was more likely to "overwhelm" him. They practiced acting in opposite ways. When Michael wanted "space" he worked on describing accurately his experiences, and Amy felt closer and supported his desires (which were for rather minimal changes); when Amy experienced a lot of emptiness or fears, she used some of her own skills to manage her emotion independently before talking with Michael, who in turn was much more likely to validate or appropriately reassure her.

Finally, stage 4 focused on the partners letting go of their respective fears regarding intimacy and independence. They worked on enjoying their time together and their time apart, drawing opportunities for emotional closeness from both. Of course, there were many behaviors that still carried a negative valence for each other. Nevertheless, they both worked hard to focus only on actual problems and to do so in constructive ways, always targeting intimacy along with conflict resolution. They used mindfulness skills to enjoy their time together and to stay focused and deliberate when trying to resolve conflict.

Overall, treatment included 30 sessions spread out over a year. Amy had completed her individual treatment about halfway through their couple treatment, and maintained her stability. At the end of treatment both partners reported high levels of satisfaction in their marriage but requested the option of returning to treatment if needed. They did return for two sessions 8 months later following an argument that had left them not speaking to each other for several days. However, they had largely resolved the situation by the time they came in for their first follow-up session, and used the time to recommit to using the skills and strategies that had worked for them in the past. A follow-up phone call 6 months later found them continuing to report high relationship satisfaction and high individual well-being.

CONCLUSION

DBT with couples is a promising new treatment for couples with a partner with BPD in particular, and for very distressed couples with emotionally dysregulated partners in general. Although DBT has proven effective in treating individual clients with BPD in many studies, and preliminary evidence supports the efficacy of this work with couples, considerably more research is needed. However, the skills and strategies described here may be of use to clinicians working specifically with borderline clients in couple therapy or working more generally with difficult couples.

REFERENCES

American Psychiatric Association. (1994). *Diagnostic and statistical manual of mental disorders* (4th ed.). Washington, DC: Author.

First, M. B., Gibbon, M., Spitzer, R. L., & Williams, J. B. W. (1995). *User's guide for the Structured Clinical Interview for DSM-IV Axis II Personality Disorders (SCID-II).* Washington, DC: American Psychiatric Press.

Foa, E. B., & Rothbaum, B. O. (1998). *Treating the trauma of rape.* New York: Guilford Press.

Fruzzetti, A. E. (1996). Causes and consequences: Individual distress in the context of couple interactions. *Journal of Consulting and Clinical Psychology, 64,* 1192–1201.

Fruzzetti, A. E. (2002). Dialectical behavior therapy for borderline personality and related disorders. In T. Patterson (Ed.), *Comprehensive handbook of psychotherapy: Cognitive behavioral approaches* (Vol. 2, pp. 215–240). New York: Wiley.

Fruzzetti, A. E., Hoffman, P. D., & Linehan, M. M. (2002). *Dialectical behavior therapy with couples and families.* Unpublished manuscript.

Fruzzetti, A. E., & Iverson, K. (in press). Acceptance and "individual" psychopathology in couples. In S. C. Hayes, M. M. Linehan, & V. M. Follette (Eds.), *Acceptance, mindfulness, and relationship: The new behavior therapies.* New York: Guilford Press.

Fruzzetti, A. E., & Levensky, E. R. (2000). Dialectical behavior therapy for domestic violence: Rationale and procedures. *Cognitive and Behavioral Practice, 7,* 435–447.

Fruzzetti, A. E., Waltz, J. A., & Linehan, M. M. (1997). Supervision in dialectical behavior therapy. In C. E. Watkins, Jr. (Ed.), *Handbook of psychotherapy supervision* (pp. 84–100). New York: Wiley.

Herman, J. L., Perry, J. C., & van der Kolk, B. A. (1989). Childhood trauma in borderline personality disorder. *American Journal of Psychiatry, 146,* 490–495.

Heyman, R. E. (2001). Observation of couple conflicts: Clinical assessment applications, stubborn truths, and shaky foundations. *Psychological Assessment, 13,* 5–35.

Hoffman, P. D., Fruzzetti, A. E., & Swenson, C. R. (1999). Dialectical behavior therapy–family skills training. *Family Process, 38,* 399–414.

Jacobson, N. S., & Margolin, G. (1979). *Marital therapy.* New York: Brunner/Mazel.

Koerner, K., & Dimeff, L. A. (2000). Further data on dialectical behavior therapy. *Clinical Psychology: Science and Practice, 7,* 104–112.

Linehan, M. M. (1993a). *Cognitive-behavioral treatment of borderline personality disorder.* New York: Guilford Press.

Linehan, M. M. (1993b). *Skills training manual for treating borderline personality disorder.* New York: Guilford Press.

Linehan, M. M., & Heard, H. L. (1999). Borderline personality disorder: Costs, course, and treatment outcomes. In N. Miller & K. Magruder (Eds.), *The cost-effectiveness of psychotherapy: A guide for practitioners, researchers and policymakers.* New York: Oxford University Press.

Pinkard, T. (1988). *Hegel's dialectic: The explanation of possibility.* Philadelphia, PA: Temple University Press.

Riggs, D. S. (2000). Marital and family therapy. In E. B. Foa, T. M. Keane, & M. J. Friedman (Eds.), *Effective treatments for PTSD* (pp. 280–301). New York: Guilford Press.

Widiger, T. A., & Rogers, J. H. (1989). Prevalence and comorbidity of personality disorders. *Psychiatric Annals, 19,* 132–136.

Zanarini, M. C., Gunderson, J. G., Frankenburg, F. R., & Chauncey, D. L. (1989). The revised diagnostic interview for borderlines: Discriminating BPD from other Axis II disorders. *Journal of Personality Disorders, 3,* 10–18.

CHAPTER 11

Paranoia

KENNETH G. TERKELSEN

The expectation of being harmed through the conspiring and evil intent of others places unique burdens on intimate relationships and family life. These burdens sometimes lead to a referral for couple therapy. Alternatively, other difficulties lead to referral and paranoia is discovered during evaluation or as treatment proceeds. Either way, it is imperative for couple therapists to understand paranoia and associated phenomena.

Even though paranoia has a marked influence on the course of couple therapy, there is almost no empirical work relating to its influence on intimate relationships or on the treatment of paranoia in couple therapy. Reviewing the literature of the last 25 years, couple therapy search terms ("marriage," "marital," "divorce," and "couple therapy") yielded 21,701 citations and paranoia search terms ("paranoia," "paranoid," and "paranoid disorders") yielded 6,855 citations. Among papers indexed for couple therapy in the title, only three were also indexed for paranoia, and only one of these was relevant to couple therapy. Birtchnell (1986) described the impact of events in the life of one spouse on the other, an early reference to the burden of psychiatric illness on marriage. A broader check of 97 citations indexed for both couple therapy and paranoia turned up no additional relevant reports.

With so few empirical data on the subject, the approach taken here is to develop a clinical model from empirical reports on paranoia and on couple therapy in other major psychiatric disorders. Fundamental characteristics of paranoia are described and pertinent topics are reviewed including demographics of paranoia in marriage, diagnosis and differential diagnosis of underlying mental disorders, assortative mating and *folie à deux* in marriage, and comorbid phenomena such as substance abuse, pathological jealousy, and domestic violence. Couple adaptations to paranoia and stressors aggravating paranoia are described. Then clinical issues are addressed including alliance formation in couples with a paranoid partner and adaptations of psychoeducational and behavioral approaches. Finally, risk management issues including treatment dropout, suicide, legal entanglements, and danger to the couple therapist are addressed.

CONCEPTUALIZATION AND RELATED FEATURES

Because paranoia signals the presence of a serious condition, the symptoms of paranoia, its diagnosis and differential diagnosis, and other mental conditions frequently found in association with paranoia are covered here.

Clinical Presentations and Demographics

Historically, the term "paranoia" has been used to refer to both delusions and persecutory ideas. However, many delusions are not persecutory and some persecutory ideas are not delusions.

The Paranoid Spectrum

To clarify this distinction and to include the entire array of paranoid conditions encountered in couple therapy, following Cameron (1974), the concept of a *paranoid spectrum* is used here. At one extreme is suspiciousness without delusions. The other extreme consists of disorders in which a panoply of persecutory and other delusions are found together with fragmentation of thinking and mood disturbances. Lorr (1964) proposed six stages in the progressive development of paranoid disorders: (1) hostile attitude toward the world; (2) open expression of hostility; (3) feelings of resentment toward others; (4) blaming others for their misfortune; (5) believing that others are conspiring against them; and (6) believing that thoughts, emotions, and actions are being controlled by external forces. Stage 5 signals a disorder of delusional intensity. Romney (1987) later confirmed Lorr's model from interviews with psychotic inpatients. As the disorder progresses, each stage is succeeded and incorporated by the next. Whether paranoia advances depends on aggravating and mitigating influences including life events and treatment.

The spectrum model of paranoia has important implications for the practice of couple therapy. Evaluation for paranoia should be considered even among clients showing simple hostility, resentment, and a propensity to blame others for their own misfortune—all of which are seen in most couples early in treatment. Paranoid delusions may already be present or may develop at a later time. Delusions signal the presence of a severe disorder requiring comprehensive evaluation by a psychiatrist.

Delusions and Overvalued Ideas

Delusions are, first and foremost, beliefs. For purposes of this chapter, a delusion is "a reality judgment which cannot be accepted by people of the same class, education, race and period of life . . . and which cannot be changed by logical argument or evidence against it" (Anderson & Trethowan, 1973). For a belief to be considered a delusion, evidence must be present from the interview or reports of reliable others that the holder is totally convinced of the belief. Ideas which appear to be firmly held, but are given up or doubted by the holder when challenged by appeals to logic, common sense, the laws of nature, or observation, are overvalued ideas. Beliefs held in common with others from a similar sociocultural group, especially religious beliefs, are not delusions.

Types of Delusions

Although suspicion of others is the most common type of delusion, the couple therapist may also encounter any of the five types delusions:

1. *Persecutory* delusions are unsupported convictions that someone (usually the holder of the belief) has been targeted for harm by others. Persecutory delusions are commonly associated with intense, negative emotions and with impulses to act against others (Appelbaum, Robbins, & Roth, 1999). They are typical of schizophrenia and bipolar disorder, but are also very common in Alzheimer's disease and other dementing disorders, including early and mild cases. Because persecutory delusions are extremely disturbing, they often give rise to actions that bring the client to the attention of others, including physically aggressive behavior and suicide attempts.

2. *Jealous* delusions are unsupported beliefs that one's sexual partner is being unfaithful. Sometimes referred to as the *Othello syndrome*, these phenomena are incompletely distinguished in the literature from morbid, pathological, or obsessional jealousy, which are generally understood as nondelusional preoccupations with sexual infidelity of a love

partner. Jealous delusions are frequently present without other delusions and without other psychiatric symptoms and, although persisting over many years, are associated with less functional disability than other delusions (Crowe, Clarkson, Tsai, & Wilson, 1988). Nevertheless, hostility, verbal threats, family murder, and family murder with suicide are seen with delusional jealousy (Leong et al., 1994). Treatments commonly found effective for obsessive–compulsive disorder (OCD), including the selective serotonin reuptake inhibitors (Stein, Hollander, & Josephson, 1994), and behavioral psychotherapy (Cobb & Marks, 1979), are effective in treating jealous delusions, suggesting that they represent an atypical form of OCD. Jealous delusions are also seen in various cerebral pathologies. As many as one-sixth of individuals with dementia have jealous delusions, making organic brain disease the most common underlying associated pathology (Soyka, Naber, & Volcker, 1991).

3. *Grandiose* delusions are unsupported beliefs that one is famous, rich, or powerful. Religious themes are very often prominent. Typical in bipolar disorder, grandiose delusions are also observed in schizophrenia and delusional disorder.

4. *Erotomanic* delusions are unsupported beliefs of being secretly loved by another person, usually a wealthy, prominent person. Initial elation and hope soon turn to disappointment and anger toward the presumed lover and action that leads quickly to police attention may follow. The grandiosity of these delusions suggests that erotomania is a variant of bipolar disorder (Signer & Swinson, 1987).

5. *Somatic* delusions are unsupported beliefs that one's health or appearance is abnormal. These clients commonly seek out primary care physicians and medical specialists for a wide array of symptoms for which no physical basis can be found and about which the client remains deeply preoccupied despite repeated reassurance.

Single and Multiple Delusions

Individuals with a paranoid disorder may hold delusions of one or several types simultaneously. Those presenting with any single type of delusion are more likely to have an underlying medical illness than those presenting with multiple delusions (Malloy & Richardson, 1994).

Bizarre Delusions

Many delusions embody beliefs that are plausible even if very unlikely. By contrast, *bizarre* delusions are patently absurd and grossly violate the laws of nature. For example, Russell Weston, Jr., the man who murdered two security guards in the U.S. Capitol in 1998, revealed in subsequent psychiatric examination the bizarre delusions that the government was spying on him through his neighbor's satellite television antenna, that people who are killed are not really dead, and that he possessed the ability to reverse time (Verrengia, 1998). Individuals presenting with bizarre delusions are invariably found to have schizophrenia, schizoaffective disorder, or bipolar disorder and require psychiatric attention.

Delusions, Awareness of Illness, and Referral Pathways

Individuals with delusions usually do not recognize that they have an illness and show an irrational skepticism about the efficacy of mental health treatments. Because they are convinced that something is wrong outside of themselves, paranoid individuals do not gravitate toward clinicians. They are more inclined to seek out lawyers or the police (if feeling persecuted), primary care physicians and nonpsychiatric medical specialists (for somatic delusions), stockbrokers and real estate agents (if grandiose delusions predominate), or (in the event of erotomanic and jealous delusions) their targets (Manschrek, 1996). Most commonly, someone else insists on mental health referral. A partner, because of relationship distress associated with paranoia, may seek couple therapy, and paranoid individuals may agree to couple therapy while refusing other types of mental health referral.

Physical and Mental Conditions Associated with Delusions

Physical Illness

When delusions are present, a number of physical, substance abuse, and mental conditions need to be considered. Physical illnesses should be considered first because they often lead to progressive functional impairment if untreated. Delusions may be the first manifestation of dementia, seizure disorder, or a wide range of systemic diseases in previously healthy adults, and may occur after a delay of weeks to years in individuals who have sustained traumatic brain injury. Evaluation includes a medical history, physical examination, and laboratory testing. Once an underlying physical condition is treated, delusions may subside or completely disappear.

Substance Abuse

Alcohol and substance abuse is considered next in the evaluation of clients presenting with delusions because untreated substance abuse will undermine the efficacy of all other treatments offered. Delusions have been observed in acute and chronic abuse and dependence, and in withdrawal syndromes associated with most drugs of abuse. For a variety of reasons, substance abuse may be denied or minimized by both partners seen in couple therapy.

Mental Disorders

The most common mental disorders associated with delusions are schizophrenia, schizoaffective disorder, bipolar disorder with psychotic features, major depression with psychotic features, and delusional disorder. Among delusional individuals referred for couple therapy, schizophrenia and schizoaffective disorder are in the minority because marriage rates in individuals with these disorders are low (Jonsson, 1991). Schizophrenia and schizoaffective disorder are severe psychotic disorders characterized by bizarre and nonbizarre delusions together with varying degrees of illogical thinking and disorganized speech. Associated functional impairments limit opportunities for work and marriage in most cases. Long-term treatment with antipsychotic medications, especially the newer so-called "atypical" antipsychotics (olanzapine, risperidone, quetiapine, ziprasidone, aripiprazole, and clozapine), substantially reduces symptoms and partially restores functioning in most individuals.

Individuals with bipolar disorder marry at rates similar to the general population but are more frequently embroiled in serious marital conflict (Levkovitz, Fennig, Horesh, Barak, & Treves, 2000). Although depression, elation, and irritability usually predominate, psychotic symptoms are just as frequently a source of relationship strain. Long-term treatment with mood stabilizers (lithium, divalproex, carbamazepine, lamotrigine, and others) in combination with antipsychotics is necessary for the control of mood symptoms and delusions.

Delusional disorder (paranoia in the older literature) is an uncommon condition characterized by *nonbizarre* delusions, few other psychiatric symptoms, and preserved functioning. Delusional disorder is associated with a later age of onset, fewer episodes of hospitalization, and better response to antipsychotic treatment than schizophrenia (Munro & Mok, 1995). Although there are no data on marriage rates of individuals with delusional disorder, both marriage and marital distress are likely.

Paranoid personality disorder is also seen in clients referred for couple therapy because of behaviors (demanding, arrogant, mistrustful, driven, unromantic, moralistic, and acutely vigilant toward the external environment) that are a source of relationship discord (Akhtar, 1990). The psychotic disorders described above should be considered in clients presenting with a habit of suspiciousness even when delusions are not obvious. Some clients will reveal delusions on careful evaluation, and can benefit from specific treatment.

Comorbid Disorders and Associated Phenomena

In addition to physical, substance abuse, and mental disorders, clients with delusions frequently present with other conditions that become a focus of clinical attention. Comorbid disorders complicate the primary condition, intensify symptoms, increase functional disability, interfere with response to treatment, and aggravate the relational discord that leads to referral for couple therapy. Some common comorbid disorders are reviewed here.

Domestic Violence

Although there is a modest association between mental illness and violence against the general population, there is no clear association between delusions and domestic violence (Else, Wonderlich, Beatty, Christie, & Staton, 1993). Domestic violence is frequent in *nonparanoid* personality disorders including borderline, antisocial, and narcissistic conditions (Cramer, 1999), and there are a number of case reports of delusions in domestic violence offenders. However, delusions do not predict violence in prospective studies (Appelbaum, Robbins, & Monahan, 2000.

Shared (Induced) Psychotic Disorder

The syndrome of *folie à deux* is now referred to as shared or induced psychotic disorder. This is a rarely observed phenomenon in which a delusional individual living in a close and socially isolated dyad influences the other, usually more impressionable member to adopt the same delusion (Sacks, 1988). Because one-third of published cases involved married couples (Silveira & Seeman, 1995), induced psychotic disorder should be considered if a socially isolated couple is referred for treatment, especially in association with a history of psychiatric hospitalization in one partner. There is a risk of serious violence in this disorder (Kraya & Patrick, 1997). It has been reported in individuals with mental retardation, dementia, and cocaine abuse, but it is also seen in schizophrenia.

Noncompliance with Treatment

Refusal to take medications as prescribed and refusal to follow other treatment recommendations are common sources of functional impairment, family burden, and family discord in mentally ill adults (Lindstrom & Bingefors, 2000). Therapists treating couples in which one partner is receiving medication for a paranoid disorder need to screen for couple interactions that support or disrupt medication compliance. Although clients usually admit medication noncompliance when asked directly (George, Peveler, Heiliger, & Thompson, 2000), assessment of compliance is more effective when the inquiry occurs in the presence of a partner.

Personality Disorders

Individuals with major psychiatric disorders, including paranoid disorders, commonly present with concurrent personality disorder (Carpenter, Clarkin, Glick, & Wilner, 1995). These conditions may aggravate relationship conflict and become a focus of clinical attention in couple therapy along with a paranoid disorder.

Life Events

As with other conditions, paranoid symptoms may be aggravated by ordinary events in the life of the family. Retterstol and Opjordsmoen (1991) reported onset of delusional disorder in a number of men and women at the birth of a child. Referral to couple therapy commonly occurs following life events because of this association.

Assortative Mating

Assortative mating—the tendency for married individuals to be more similar on certain traits than would be expected by chance alone—occurs in association with similarities in age, educational, religious and vocational backgrounds, and lifestyle preferences. Assortative mating has been reported in individuals with a variety of mental disorders. Although there are no reports on assortative mating in paranoid disorders, the prevalence of the phenomenon in related disorders suggests that couple therapists should consider psychiatric illness in the partners of paranoid individuals referred for couple therapy.

CLINICAL CONSIDERATIONS

To summarize the literature bearing directly and indirectly on paranoia in couples, individuals with paranoid conditions marry often, are subject to high rates of relationship discord, are likely to have partners with emotional problems, are often unaware of having a mental disorder, and are skeptical of the value of mental health services. Although they may avoid mental health clinicians, they may accept referral to a couple therapist. Many such individuals, especially those with good overall psychosocial functioning, respond well to specific treatment.

Although couple therapy has been found to be effective in the treatment of many mental disorders, it has not been studied systematically in the paranoid disorders. Im, Wilner, and Breit (1983) reported a series of interventions found useful in managing jealousy in couple therapy. De Silva (1997) described a comprehensive methodology for assessing jealousy in couple therapy and reviewed related treatment strategies. Few other reports, and virtually no systematic empirical work, have been published on paranoid disorders in couple therapy. Nonetheless, there are certain principles useful in treatment of couples with a paranoid partner (referred to here as "paranoid couples").

Alliance Formation

Svensson and Hansson (1999) found that talking to "someone who understands" is very important to individuals with serious mental illness. Meissner (1976) went further, stating that the therapeutic alliance is the most critical phase in treatment of individuals with paranoid disorders.

Before starting therapy with a paranoid couple, I remind myself that individuals with paranoid disorders are at a disadvantage when it comes to trusting other people. More often than not, revealing their ideas has been met with negative, judgmental, or dismissive reactions, reinforcing a belief that understanding and acceptance are unlikely. The expectation of similar responses from the therapist, or from the nonparanoid partner, hangs over couple therapy from the outset.

Therapists can complicate matters because listening with a neutral stance to each partner's version of relationship troubles in a conjoint session is very likely to bring out any existing delusions. It is easy to be drawn into challenging delusions exposed at the beginning of treatment. I have often found myself thinking, "This is preposterous!" Then I have to remind myself that trust is the basis for getting at truth. Although grappling with delusions may eventually be necessary, it is never useful until the paranoid partner feels heard and understood.

Things can also get out of hand if the nonparanoid partner reacts judgmentally to delusions. This may occur due to shock (if the delusions have not been apparent at home) or exasperation (if they have been a frequent topic), but also due to embarrassment. There is something peculiarly distressing about seeing one's husband or wife sharing bizarre ideas with an outsider. Nonparanoid partners may need to distance themselves from such ideas to attest to their own sanity.

Whatever the motivation, critical reactions to delusions need to be contained promptly, lest treatment collapse in the assessment phase. I accomplish this by promptly moving to protect and reestablish the usual framework of neutral listening needed for couple assessment. After listening just long enough to be sure that the nonparanoid partner is attacking a delusion, I stop the interruption, usually by saying, "I'm going to ask you to hold off on giving your side of this until I get a good understanding of your [husband's or wife's] experience here." Sometimes, facial expression or tone of voice signals that the nonparanoid partner is in distress or the interruption continues. Then I acknowledge the distress while reemphasizing the need to listen, saying something like, "Look, I can see this is upsetting you, but I really need to hear your partner out on this. Then I do want to come back to you to hear about your experience." I may expand on this by underscoring that couple therapy has to begin with a thorough understanding of each partner's experience of their troubles, which requires listening without interruption and without debate.

Individual versus Conjoint Assessment

Because there are no empirical data to guide us, experienced therapists argue for and against use of parallel individual sessions in assessment of couples. Those in favor underscore the need to provide a setting in which sensitive information (e.g., abuse and ruminations about harming others; past affairs) can be disclosed. I favor using only conjoint sessions to assess paranoid couples in light of the particular sensitivity about collusion among others seen in clients with paranoid disorders. Very infrequently, however, a nonparanoid partner has such a strong reaction to hearing delusions being made explicit that brief individual meetings may be needed to reestablish the treatment framework. If one gets to this point, it is useful to remember that assessment necessarily highlights dysfunction before strengths get revealed. Looking back and forth between husband to wife, the therapist can say, "Look, this is obviously so upsetting that I am going to ask each of you to meet with me separately . . ." (not "privately" which would convey an expectation of confidentiality), ". . . just for a few minutes. Then I would like to bring you back together and try again. Does that sound like a plan?" The therapist wants to keep explanation to a minimum here. So, only if the paranoid partner objects would one go on to say, "Well, for this to be helpful, your [wife or husband] needs to be able to listen while you and I talk . . . and I need to work with [him or her] so that can happen. Is that OK with you?" Here, one makes the nonparanoid partner's distress and intrusiveness the problem (a balancing intervention) and temporarily cedes control to the paranoid partner to offset the implicit concern about being overpowered by collusion.

If the paranoid partner cannot consent, I can let them know, again, that couple therapy requires a fair amount of listening without debating, and then ask them both to accept or reject this. Regretfully, this may result in the end of the treatment. However, if the paranoid member cannot bear some separation and their nonparanoid partner cannot tolerate some conjoint neutral listening, the prospects for couple treatment are not bright.

More often than not, one will elicit an agreement to proceed. Beginning with the nonparanoid member, I address only the distress about delusions while conveying the need to share what is said with their paranoid partner. "Now, can you tell me what is so upsetting that you can't listen to what your [husband or wife] is saying?" If the person is at a loss to explain, I go on with, "Is it embarrassing? . . . Is she or he leaving something out? . . . Are you afraid she or he is going to hurt you? . . . Or someone else? . . . Do you think she or he is getting sick? . . . Are we not getting to other things that you think are more important?" thereby alluding progressively to all the usual sources of distress while not taking sides. When the source of distress has been expressed, I continue with a series of awareness interventions: "Well, the problem is, I need to hear [him or her] out on this, . . . and your reactions are gonna stop that. . . . You know, for me to work with the two of you, . . . everything has to take place in the open, with both of you present all the time."

If I still don't get an agreement to work within this framework, I add, "Can you do this?" to give the nonparanoid partner a way out if couple therapy is proving to be overwhelming. I have never had anyone walk out on that question. Rather, it serves to clinch a particularly distressed partner's agreement to work within the established framework of couple therapy. Finally, I prepare to return to the conjoint meeting with, "Now, I need to tell [him or her] about this, you know . . . in order to get us back on track." In the separate meeting with the paranoid member, I convey the nature of their partner's distress and report that she or he has agreed to continue conjointly. I look for indications of an awareness that the ideas being expressed are "over the top," but inquiry concerning this is continued conjointly.

Assessment

Once the framework for neutral conjoint listening has been established, the focus shifts to the joint crafting of a statement of the couple's difficulties that includes the paranoid experience and associated behavior, as well as all the usual sources of relationship difficulties. De Silva's (1997) approach to assessment of marital jealousy can be extended into a general methodology for assessing all kinds of paranoia:

The Paranoid Experience and Associated Behavior

The therapist should listen and question in as neutral a way as possible. I develop a detailed picture of the paranoid experiences and behavior, looking in particular for how these beliefs shape the day-to-day life of the paranoid partner and for any awareness of the ideas being symptoms of illness. I ask for details, stopping only when I become aware of distress in any of the three of us. Here is an example. Suppose a husband reports that his wife has told him that someone has been coming in at night, moving furniture around and, once, changing colors in paintings hung in their living room. I turn to the wife immediately for confirmation, asking, "Is this so, what your husband is saying?" I turn to the wife because to continue asking the husband about her symptom would be treating her as an object; I ask for confirmation because she may or may not acknowledge it. If she confirms the husband's report, I might ask, "What did you notice?" . . . "Starting how long ago?" . . . "Is anything missing?" . . . "Were there any signs of a break-in?" . . . "Is there anyone you suspect of doing this?" . . . "Why would someone do this to you?" Eventually I would ask, "How has this affected your life?" and, as a part of the same inquiry, "Doesn't this frighten you?" because it ought to, and fear of harm is the core experience implicit in persecutory delusions. I could also ask, "Besides your husband, who else have you told?" and "How did they react?" which brings me a step closer to the next part of the assessment while giving me a chance to assess the wife's openness to commonsense reactions and the level of awareness that the belief is a sign of something wrong within.

The Nonparanoid Partner's Responses

By now, the nonparanoid partner has had a chance to hear about the paranoid belief in a lot of detail, probably more detail than ever. Turning to the husband in this example, I might ask, "Is there anything more that your wife hasn't mentioned?" to search for more strange beliefs and changes in behavior left out of the wife's report, and then, "What are your concerns about these experiences?" This is where many partners will suggest that they are living with a crazy person. Although that may be so, I clarify my role in relation to these reports by saying, "Well, I am not qualified to give an opinion about that. You came to me because of some difficulties you are having with each other and perhaps this is one of the things you are having difficulty with. But then, what we ought to be addressing here is the distress you have each experienced and how this has forced a change in your lives with each other. That's what a couple therapist ought to be doing something about. . . . So my question to you is, how has what your wife is reporting been affecting your life?" Only then will I have the husband telling his wife and me how this has turned his life upside down and he's scared for her, for their children, and for their life together. Only then might I find out that he doesn't sleep well anymore and doesn't want their friends around anymore out of fear that they will find out what his wife is thinking about and that this will be the end of their friendships.

The Impact on Functioning

Every type of paranoia has its own unique impact on the ability of both partners to carry out their primary roles of breadwinner, lover, and parent. One needs to survey the activities of each partner, looking for areas of impaired functioning but also looking for areas where functioning has not been affected and where strength is to be found in spite of paranoia.

The Couple's Shared Emotional Burden

Now the therapist is in a position to have each partner go over in more detail the emotional impact of delusions. In this part of the assessment, one tries to build up a picture of how one partner's strange ideas have brought fear and other disagreeable feelings to both, and how each partner's sense of well-being is being threatened. One wants to emphasize, here, that each is carrying an emotional burden related to the symptom.

Violence, Verbal Aggression, and Intimidation

Although paranoia does not predict violence, the therapist needs to look for other predictors of violence in paranoid couples because of the intense emotions arising in couple interactions that surround paranoia. Violence occurring at other times, not associated with paranoid symptoms, is a predictor of violence in these couples. Jealous delusions are commonly associated with verbal aggression and intimidation related to the fear of abandonment or betrayal. If there is a history of violence or intimidation, one needs to make an assessment of the need for immediate containment or partner training on how to access help in emergencies.

Comorbid Mental Disorders

Paranoia is frequently accompanied by other mental disorders, especially by substance abuse and affective disorders. Couples therapists need to search for evidence of these other disorders in the paranoid partner, with particular reference to conditions requiring psychiatric referral and treatment. One also needs to look for mental disorders in the nonparanoid partner in light of the phenomenon of assortative mating. As a rule, specific treatment of any comorbid mental disorder will improve the outcomes achieved in couple therapy.

Coordination of Care

Many couples with a paranoid member are referred to couple therapy during or immediately after an episode of inpatient treatment or crisis intervention. The referral may be part of a comprehensive treatment requiring involvement of several clinicians and agencies. Referrals may be made simultaneously to a psychiatrist for medication, to a case manager for supervision and advocacy, and to an individual therapist. Day hospital treatment or vocational rehabilitation services may be included. Public agencies including the police, courts, social service, and disability determinations may also be involved.

There are no data bearing on the impact of coordination of care on the outcome of couple therapy for paranoid disorders. However, there is a wealth of data and experience in related conditions all pointing to two conclusions. First, addressing all problems, through multimodal treatment plans, is associated with better long-term outcomes in many serious and persistent mental disorders. Second, coordination of treatment planning among multiple clinicians is vital to achieving the full potential of multimodal treatment plans.

A typical concern for all clinicians working with paranoid clients is how to achieve coordination of care without triggering fears of collusion. When a couple therapist is called on to work as part of a team, the client and his or her partner have usually already agreed to the multimodal treatment plan. Nevertheless, the couple therapist needs to reaffirm their consent whenever joint meetings are being planned. It may help to spell out what is usually reported to other clinicians and what does not get reported. I might say, for example, "Let's go over how your treatment team conferences work. You have agreed to my talking to your psychiatrist and your case manager, right? . . . OK, good. Now, usually all they want to know from me is that you are still coming and working hard on making your marriage better, understood? I don't have any interest in going beyond that . . . *except* that if I ever thought that one of you was about to do some *harm*, then I would let someone know about that. Is that understood?" If I cannot get an endorsement of that kind of basic safety arrangement, with or without the involvement of other clinicians or agencies, I withdraw from being that couple's therapist.

Often, the best way to engage in coordination activities with paranoid couples is to schedule conference calls to take place during conjoint sessions. Alternatively, one can go over what is going to be reported to others with the couple before each joint planning conference and then tell the couple what was discussed at the next conjoint session. I find that, either way, it is a good idea to ask both partners, "Now before the conference, do either of you have any concerns about what might get shared? Anything at all?" By making the possibility of a concern explicit, the couple therapist helps clients who fear collusion to learn to use and trust collaboration among their clinicians.

Psychopharmacology

At the outset of work with paranoid clients and their partners, one needs to consider the role that medication will play in a comprehensive treatment plan. I consider all newly referred clients showing paranoid symptoms as potential responders to drug treatment and inform the couple, as soon as the treatment alliance permits, that drug treatment may substantially alleviate some of the distress and problems in functioning associated with paranoid symptoms and improve the outcome of couple therapy. Because many clients with paranoid symptoms have avoided medication, one may have to make this recommendation several times before it is accepted, and some clients never accept it despite repeated evidence of distress and dysfunction.

Psychoeducation

Information about psychiatric illness and its treatment has been offered to family members with increasing frequency and candor in the last 30 years. For example, partners of bipolar couples have shown enhanced awareness of illness after receiving such information (van Gent & Zwart, 1991). Similarly, family psychoeducation is a preferred treatment in schizophrenia where specific outcomes can be identified as treatment goals (Dixon, Adams, & Lucksted, 2000). Worthington and Drinkard (2000) have proposed use of psychoeducation in promoting reconciliation in estranged couples.

I have found that explaining paranoia often promotes empathy in the nonparanoid individual and awareness in their paranoid partner. It can increase the commitment of both persons to specific treatments

such as medication therapy, and prepare the couple to engage in behavioral contracts aimed at limiting the impact of paranoid behavior on
the couple's interactions. I may say to paranoid couples, "You need to
know that this is happening to you because a tiny clump of cells in your
brain, about the size of your smallest fingernail, has gotten overactive
and is sending unusually strong messages to other parts of your brain.
The medication you are taking will restore that area of your brain back
to its usual level of activity and then your brain will function more normally overall." Because individuals with paranoia are often exceptional-
ly sensitive to bodily changes brought about by medications, I always
give special emphasis to side effects, describing what they are, and making a solemn commitment to do everything I can to minimize their impact. Finally, I say, "Look, I am recommending that you take this medication and I honestly believe it will relieve your paranoia, but I can't
make you take it and so it is up to you to take it or not."

As a couple therapist, one can challenge clients with paranoia to
ask for this kind of explanation. When the couple reports improved
functioning, their therapist can ask the paranoid partner to consider
whether it is related to use of medication. One can ask about side effects and encourage frank discussion of side effects with the prescribing
psychiatrist. And the couple therapist can mediate on behalf of the
paranoid individual when their nonparanoid partner is pushing too
hard about medication. In the latter circumstance, the nonparanoid
member may need to be informed that most people who don't like to
take medications or who are having bad side effects almost always try to
find out what they can get away with by going off the medications and
seeing what happens.

Behavioral Couple Therapy

Much has been written about treatment focused on behavior change in
couple therapy and this approach is elaborated elsewhere is this volume. Paranoid behavior is often an expression of underlying pathology
that is only partially responsive to specific treatment and that may wors-
en or ameliorate without warning. As a result, one needs to anticipate
that paranoid behavior will fluctuate throughout couple therapy. Precisely for this reason, couple therapy is of particular benefit in the treatment of paranoid behavior when combined with appropriate specific
treatment and with psychoeducation tailored to underlying conditions.
Teaching couples to think of paranoid behaviors as symptoms which,
like asthma attacks and headaches, may be triggered by events and interactions, can prepare couples to respond differently and earlier with
future relapses and, by doing so, to contain their effects on the couple's

and family's functioning. I have found that many nonparanoid partners can learn to process increasing paranoid behavior as responses to stressful events in the family or at work. Once that learning is established, it becomes possible for the nonparanoid member to deal with their paranoid partner as "a stressed out mate" rather than as "a crazy person." Examples of this kind of altered interaction are illustrated in the case description that follows.

CASE ILLUSTRATION

Alice and Marvin were referred to me in the late 1970s following Alice's first and only psychiatric hospitalization. Couple treatment continued, with declining frequency of contact, over the next 22 years.

Alice and Marvin emigrated to the United States when Alice was 20 years old for reasons related to Marvin's professional career. At the time of referral Alice was 42 and was occupied principally as a homemaker and mother of three children ranging in age from 14 to 22. Her only other activity of significance was sculpting, which she had taken up as a solitary pastime and would later incorporate into her delusional system. She had received individual outpatient psychotherapy for depression off and on for 6 years and, following that, a short and unsuccessful course of couple therapy.

For several months prior to hospitalization Alice was showing more persecutory thinking but refused to return to her psychiatrist. A visit to her home country that was planned as a rest went badly. She became very distraught and frankly delusional, telling her family that signals were being sent among conspirators as part of a plot against her, eventually including the bizarre belief that planes were flying overhead to signal her location. She was seen by a psychiatrist, returned to the United States, refused to see her own psychiatrist due to a belief that he was part of the plot, worsened, took an overdose of diazepam, filled her bathtub with water and tried to drown herself. Discovered by her husband, she was hospitalized for 2 months. The hospital diagnosis was paranoid schizophrenia, because some of Alice's delusions were bizarre and no contributory medical or substance abuse problems were identified then or at any later time. She received individual, group, marital, and multiple family group treatments and was started on imipramine for depression, fluphenazine for delusions, and benztropine for neuromuscular side effects of fluphenazine.

In addition to treatment of her paranoia, marital problems addressed in treatment included emotional distance associated with Marvin's long work hours and remote, stoic interpersonal style, and Alice's indecisiveness in household matters. To these problems was added Alice's increasing isolation, which she attributed to the children no longer needing her. Had she been in her home country, she would have involved herself socially with other women in the family as the children grew. In the United States, away from her family and having avoided social contacts outside the family, her interests turned toward theater and traveling. However, Marvin enjoyed neither of these activities and, due to mounting college expenses, felt that they could not enter into either of Alice's interests to the extent she desired.

The referral to a psychiatrist who would address both paranoia and marital discord flowed from the hospital assessment in which both concerns were seen to be prominent and interacting. At the time, I was one of the few psychiatrists in my area accepting referrals for marital and family therapy. Couple treatment focused extensively on restructuring their relationship into a more contemporary working partnership adapted to Alice's persistent discomfort in social contact with peers. During treatment, Marvin underwent a major "second career" shift, leaving his professional work behind and opening a home goods store. As the children left for college, Alice went to work in this business, interacting tentatively at first, and later more extensively with the public at the front counter and designing and arranging the store's presentation of goods.

Conjoint Assessment and Treatment

Because most of my clinical work in the 1970s was family therapy, I arranged to see the couple jointly in the intake appointment. The entire treatment was conducted conjointly with a handful of exceptions—individual sessions with Alice at times when she was in acute distress and when Marvin was unavailable due to demands of his job. In the initial 2-hour interview, all six aspects of De Silva's (1997) conjoint assessment for paranoia were addressed. As Alice told the story of her mounting distress, suicide attempt, and hospitalization, Marvin cut in to highlight delusions, which she was overlooking in her telling of the story. This became the opportunity to set ground rules about listening and interrupting. There was consensus that neither wanted a recurrence of the situation leading to Alice's suicide attempt.

Pharmacotherapy

The next session was focused almost entirely on drug treatment. Although fully compliant with medication in the hospital and in the immediate posthospital period, Alice began a campaign against medication in this session, coming back again and again to certain side effects and to her worry that the medications would cause permanent physical harm. In keeping with prevailing treatment standards and existing empirical reports on risks of discontinuing medications, I recommended continuation of both antidepressant and antipsychotic medications. In the course of this intervention I learned that Marvin was completely in favor of medications, which he saw as essential treatment of Alice's psychosis.

Psychoeducation

In light of Alice's persistent concerns about side effects, I launched directly into a detailed explanation of the purpose of her medications, how they worked, how they were to be taken, and the risks she would incur by discontinuing them. I began a process, which would unfold again and again over many years, of hearing out every one of Alice's concerns about side effects while challenging Marvin's repeated dismissals of side effects as inconsequential or exaggerated. The aim in this intervention was to underscore the validity of Alice's experience and the quality of life burden associated with having a chronic illness. I treated side effects that could be ameliorated and commiserated with her about others that she had to live with.

Behavioral Treatment of Paranoia

By the fourth session, 6 weeks into treatment, it was possible to put forward an interpersonal model of Alice's persecutory delusions. By this time, the alliance was sufficiently strong that she was able to tolerate Marvin reporting to me that, at home, she had been asking him if he noticed that some of her sculptures had been altered. Marvin's disclosure made it clear that Alice had a heretofore undisclosed belief that unknown individuals entered their home under cover of night and carved new lines to completed works that were displayed in their home. Assessment showed that Alice had held this belief firmly for some time. She had not disclosed it to any of her former clinicians. Moreover, disclosure was unlikely except in the context of conjoint treatment because she feared, as many paranoid individuals do, that disclosure would lead to rehospitalization.

Marvin insisted that this belief was evidence of paranoia plain and simple. Alice attributed it to being cut off from friends. Working from a family therapist's desire to acknowledge both sides of any story, I took the position that the important task was to figure out how their divergent explanations were linked. I suggested that Alice was particularly prone to becoming preoccupied about alteration of her works when she was isolated. Addressing Alice (and, of course, speaking at the same time indirectly to Marvin), I suggested that she learn to use her paranoid thinking as a barometer. When paranoid thinking got more intense, that would indicate that some part of their relationship needed healing. Turning to Marvin, I suggested that he learn to be more playful when she came out with paranoid statements at home, so as to set up a climate of curiosity and self-observation. Doing this would also, I thought, give him a way to interact with Alice about her paranoia, which, while acknowledging its existence, would help to get her redirected toward activities and involvement with people.

In sessions over the succeeding 6 weeks, Alice spontaneously revealed an interest in getting the house in shape to invite company over. Later there was much talk about getting out to the theater more often, and some action on that front. Still later, the business started by Marvin became a social outlet for Alice. As she continued to sculpt, concerns about her work being altered receded, and her obvious artistic talents were put to use in arranging the store window for each season.

Although the couple treatment went on to address their other marital problems, persecutory ideas took center stage from time to time, usually at times of major family stress. She was paranoid again when her brother visited for the first time, and during the long period of her mother's final illness and the return trip to their home country for the funeral, and still later, to dispose of her mother's estate. Each resurgence of paranoia served as an opportunity to reinforce the paradigm that paranoia was a signal of stress and that the stress needed the couple's attention.

Addressing Noncompliance

Compliance with medication almost invariably falls off in individuals who have had a single psychotic episode. In fact, virtually all such clients who I have followed for any period of time eventually try to do without medication. Many are so relentless that their physicians cut doses until eventually the dose is too small to prevent a relapse. Those individuals whose physicians refuse to reduce medications find another physician or go off the medication on their own. Sometimes, family members support this covert noncompliance.

With this couple, both things happened. Alice complained relentlessly about side effects, so I halved the dose every 3 months (the customary interval for dose decreases). However, at the time of the last decrease, Alice stopped medications altogether, concealing her noncompliance from Marvin and me. Within 3 weeks, Marvin was reporting in a couple session that he thought that she was unduly suspicious again. Within a week, he was on the phone between sessions (a necessary deviation from conjoint proceedings when relapses are suspected) to report that Alice had admitted to being off medications for 3 weeks. Over the phone, she agreed to resume fluphenazine at half the original discharge dose, but only with Marvin's insistent support for my recommendation. At the next conjoint session 4 days later, she revealed that she had been off medication for 5 weeks, not 3, and agreed to continue medications at the recommended dose despite continued complaints about side effects impacting the quality of her life.

Shifting to Maintenance Treatment

Eventually, Alice and Marvin showed evidence of an ability to manage paranoia more independently. Alice came to terms with the need for indefinite continuation of medication therapy. Marvin became adept at initiating the line of thinking that paranoia signaled the existence of some relationship issues that needed mending, and Alice more easily accepted his lead. At the same time, their problem solving improved enough so that, apart from the need for continued management of paranoia, couple therapy per se was no longer needed. Nevertheless, almost all contacts had been conjoint, and Marvin's contribution to their improved coping skills was considerable. In addition, they appeared to enjoy continuing to come in once in a while together. For all these reasons, follow-up sessions that focused mostly on medication management were held conjointly in the final years of my part of their treatment. When I eventually moved from their area, I recommended a continuation of that format to the psychiatrist who assumed responsibility for Alice's care.

CONCLUSIONS

Couple therapy often plays a central role in the treatment of paranoid conditions. Paranoid symptoms, including all kinds of delusions, usually point to the presence of serious physical or mental disorders that are often helped by specific treatments, including antipsychotic medications, but are not typically put into full remission. Symptoms come and go over the years. Sometimes changes in symptom severity are obviously connected to life events. Sometimes other illnesses are added to the mix or the client goes off medications or picks up street drugs or alcohol. Various kinds of therapy are usually needed in conjunction with medication to attain the best possible control of paranoia and to sustain the paranoid client's commitment to specific treatments.

For paranoid clients in a stable relationship, couple therapy should always be offered and is sometimes accepted as part of a comprehensive package of services aimed at multiple problems. A couple therapist should maintain a focus on the entire relationship and not just paranoid phenomena, but can play an important role in promoting understanding about paranoia on the part of both partners. The better the couple is able to function as a partnership, the better the paranoid individual will manage the symptoms of his or her underlying condition.

Because paranoid conditions usually do not go away but, instead, run a relapsing and remitting course over decades, the need for various therapies, including couple therapy, usually comes and goes. Couple therapy need not be a constant in the mix of services making up a comprehensive treatment plan. Rather, there is often a need for a "refresher" from time to time, usually at times when life events like births, deaths, children moving out, relocations, and the like contribute to a period of particular stress. As illustrated by the case of Alice and Marvin, it is especially helpful in times of stress to have access to a couple therapist who already knows the couple and is already trusted by them. Often, one or two meetings at times like these by a known and trusted person gets the couple out of a hole quickly. In the absence of this kind of continuity, other clinicians, including case managers, individual therapists, and psychiatrists can help fill in the gaps for a couple therapist who is new to the case. Opportunities for collaboration among several clinicians who, as a rule, are involved with these clients and their partners are needed and should be sought out whenever their presence is known.

Finally, paranoid conditions usually travel with one or more companions—other physical and mental disorders that have their own symptoms, course, and treatments. Clients presenting with paranoia very often have resorted to street drugs or alcohol, sometimes to treat symptoms, sometimes showing paranoia only after drugs are used. Manic and depressive episodes frequently are associated with persecutory, grandiose, and somatic delusions. These and other conditions alter the course of paranoia and need to be addressed as part of a comprehensive treatment plan. Especially in these complicated cases, multiple services provided in support of a couple's functioning greatly improve the odds of a favorable outcome.

REFERENCES

Akhtar, S. (1990). Paranoid personality disorder: A synthesis of developmental, dynamic, and descriptive features. *American Journal of Psychotherapy, 44*(1), 5–25.

Anderson, E. W., & Trethowan, W. H. (1973). *Psychiatry* (3rd ed.). London: Baillière, Tindall.

Appelbaum, P. S., Robbins, P. C., & Monahan, J. (2000). Violence and delusions: Data from the MacArthur Violence Risk Assessment Study. *American Journal of Psychiatry, 157*(4), 566–572.

Appelbaum, P. S., Robbins, P. C., & Roth, L. H. (1999). Dimensional approach to delusions: Comparison across types and diagnoses. *American Journal of Psychiatry, 156*(12), 1938–1943.

Birtchnell, J. (1986). Psychiatric disorders in marriage. *British Journal of Hospital Medicine, 35*(6), 409–412.

Cameron, N. A. (1974). Paranoid conditions and paranoia. In S. Arieti (Ed.), *American handbook of psychiatry* (2nd ed., pp. 676–693). New York: Basic Books.

Carpenter, D., Clarkin, J. F., Glick, I. D., & Wilner, P. (1995). Personality pathology among married adults with bipolar disorder. *Journal of Affective Disorders, 34*(4), 269–274.

Cobb, J. P., & Marks, I. M. (1979). Morbid jealousy featuring as obsessive–compulsive neurosis: Treatment by behavioral psychotherapy. *British Journal of Psychiatry, 134,* 301–305.

Cramer, P. (1999). Personality, personality disorders, and defense mechanisms. *Journal of Personality, 67*(3), 535–554.

Crowe, R. R., Clarkson, C., Tsai, M., Wilson, R. (1988). Delusional disorder: Jealous and nonjealous types. *European Archives of Psychiatry and Neurological Sciences, 237*(3), 179–183.

De Silva, P. (1997). Jealousy in couple relationships: nature, assessment and therapy. *Behaviour Research and Therapy, 35*(11), 973–985.

Dixon, L., Adams, C., & Lucksted, A. (2000). Update on family psychoeducation for schizophrenia. *Schizophrenia Bulletin, 26*(1), 5–20.

Else, L. T., Wonderlich, S. A., Beatty, W. W., Christie, D. W., & Staton, R. D. (1993). Personality characteristics of men who physically abuse women. *Hospital and Community Psychiatry, 44*(1), 54–58.

George, C. F., Peveler, R. C., Heiliger, S., & Thompson, C. (2000). Compliance with tricyclic antidepressants: The value of four different methods of assessment. *British Journal of Clinical Pharmacology, 50*(2), 166–171.

Im, W. G., Wilner, R. S., & Breit, M. (1983). Jealousy: Interventions in couples therapy. *Family Process, 22*(2), 211–219.

Jonsson, S. A. (1991). Marriage rate and fertility in cycloid psychosis: Comparison with affective disorder, schizophrenia and the general population. *European Archives of Psychiatry and Clinical Neuroscience, 241*(2), 119–125.

Kraya, N. A., & Patrick, C. (1997). Folie à deux in forensic setting. *Australian and New Zealand Journal of Psychiatry, 31*(6), 883–888.

Leong, G. B., Silva, J. A., Garza-Trevino, E. S., Oliva, D. Jr., Ferrari, M. M., Komanduri, R. V., & Caldwell, J. C. (1994). The dangerousness of persons with the Othello syndrome. *Journal of Forensic Sciences, 39*(6), 1445–1454.

Levkovitz, V., Fennig, S., Horesh, N., Barak, V., & Treves, I. (2000). Perception of ill spouse and dyadic relationship in couples with affective disorder and those without. *Journal of Affective Disorders, 58*(3), 237–240.

Lindstrom, E., & Bingefors, K. (2000). Patient compliance with drug therapy in schizophrenia. Economic and clinical issues. *Pharmacoeconomics, 18*(2), 106–124.

Lorr, M. R. (1964). A simplex of paranoid projection. *Journal of Consulting Psychology, 28,* 378–380.

Malloy, P. F., & Richardson, E. D. (1994). The frontal lobes and content-specific delusions. *Journal of Neuropsychiatry and Clinical Neurosciences, 6*(4), 455–466.

Manschreck, T. C. (1996). Delusional disorder: The recognition and management of paranoia. *Journal of Clinical Psychiatry, 57*(Suppl. 3), 32–38.

Meissner, W. W. (1976). Psychotherapeutic schema based on the paranoid process. *International Journal of Psychoanalysis and Psychotherapy, 5,* 87–114.

Munro, A., & Mok, H. (1995). An overview of treatment in paranoia/delusional disorder. *Canadian Journal of Psychiatry, 40*(10), 616–622.

Retterstol, N., & Opjordsmoen, S. (1991). Fatherhood, impending or newly established, precipitating delusional disorders. Long-term course and outcome. *Psychopathology, 24*(4), 232–237.

Romney, D. M. (1987). A simplex model of the paranoid process: Implications for diagnosis and prognosis. *Acta Psychiatrica Scandinavica, 75*(6), 651–655.

Sacks, M. H. (1988). Folie à deux. *Comprehensive Psychiatry, 29*(3), 270–277.

Signer, S. F., & Swinson, R. P. (1987). Two cases of erotomania (de Clerambault's syndrome) in bipolar affective disorder. *British Journal of Psychiatry, 151,* 853–855.

Silveira, J. M., & Seeman, M. V. (1995). Shared psychotic disorder: A critical review of the literature. *Canadian Journal of Psychiatry, 40*(7), 389–395.

Soyka, M., Naber, G., & Volcker, A. (1991). Prevalence of delusional jealousy in different psychiatric disorders. An analysis of 93 cases. *British Journal of Psychiatry, 158,* 549–553.

Stein, D. J., Hollander, E., & Josephson, S. C. (1994). Serotonin reuptake blockers for the treatment of obsessional jealousy. *Journal of Clinical Psychiatry, 55*(1), 30–33.

Svensson, B., & Hansson, L. (1999). Relationships among patient and therapist ratings of therapeutic alliance and patient assessments of therapeutic process: A study of cognitive therapy with long-term mentally ill patients. *Journal of Nervous and Mental Disease, 187*(9), 579–585.

van Gent, E. M., & Zwart, F. M. (1991). Psychoeducation of partners of bipolar–manic patients. *Journal of Affective Disorders, 21*(1), 15–18.

Verrengia, J. B. (1998, July 26). Father says Weston blasted 12 cats. *Associated Press.*

Worthington, E. L., & Drinkard, D. T. (2000). Promoting reconciliation through psychoeducational and therapeutic interventions. *Journal of Marital and Family Therapy, 26*(1), 93–101.

CHAPTER 12

Narcissistic Disorder

JILL SAVEGE SCHARFF
CARL BAGNINI

CONCEPTUALIZATION OF THE
NARCISSISTIC PERSONALITY

Narcissistic personality disorder is defined as "a pervasive pattern of grandiosity, need for admiration, and lack of empathy that begins by early adulthood and is present in a variety of contexts" (American Psychiatric Association, 1994, p. 658). The pattern is inflexible, persistent, maladaptive, disabling, and distressing. This diagnosis is estimated to affect 1% of the general population and is found in up to 16% of the clinical population. Half to three-quarters of the group diagnosed with narcissistic personality disorder are male. In our view, this percentage is tilted toward males because the greater emotional expressiveness of narcissistic women tends to generate diagnostic categorization in the borderline and histrionic groups.

Adolescents are narcissistic, being self-centered and impervious to their parents' needs, but normally they grow beyond it. Some narcissistic traits may appear in normal adults. Only when these traits are distressing and impairing is the diagnosis of narcissistic personality disorder made. In later years, narcissistic traits may emerge as a full-blown personality disorder when declining mental ability and physical competence puncture grandiosity and the required admiration is harder to attract.

Narcissistic individuals are self-important, boastful people who aggrandize themselves and belittle others. They are entitled, exploitative, and insensitive. They think that they are unique and should be appreciated as being special. They often prefer to associate with people whom they regard as brilliant, beautiful, or famous in order to emphasize their own superiority. Beneath this veneer of overinflation of self lies a weak self-esteem system. They waste time seeking praise and feel unduly hurt if it is not forthcoming. They are often described as having huge egos but in fact their egos are extremely fragile and need constant boosting. They appear to be self-sufficient but they are really hugely dependent on others for emotional supplies. They may be quite charming and seductive, but below the exterior they are cold and unresponsive. They are arrogant, haughty, selfish, disparaging, and envious.

In the world of work they may perform at a low level in order to avoid competition that could lead to defeat and humiliation. On the other hand they may perform at an outstanding level, pushed on by ambition. At some point they experience a downfall as they react badly to adversity, criticism, and unfavorable decisions. In social life they feel vulnerable to slights and rejections (real or imagined). They either withdraw in a state of hurt and shame or fight back with contempt and rage.

The Origins of Narcissistic Personality Features

Traumatized children who are not given words to encode their memories of the trauma and are not encouraged to express their reactions may develop a narcissistic cocoon to shield them from further trauma (Scharff & Scharff, 1994). Children raised as extensions of self-absorbed parents instead of feeling valued for their individuality become narcissistic. Whether the parent has overvalued or denigrated the child depends on how the parent has felt about the part of himself or herself that the child represented at any one moment. The child builds a narcissistic personality in identification with the parent, worshipped on the surface but beneath the bravado, denigrated. When the child's self is treated as a part of the parent, it cannot be autonomous and self-determining. The self creates a defensive, grandiose state of self-sufficiency and seeks admiration from others to confirm its worth. Narcissism is a result of the miscarriage of the normal process of identification (Modell, 1993).

Narcissistic Partners in Love and Marriage

Narcissistic personality disorder may be commoner in men than women, but many women have narcissistic features that cause them as much trouble in their work and social lives, even if other features skew the diagnostic picture. Narcissistic traits create a cocoon that protects from further hurt and prevents closeness (Modell, 1975). Narcissistic people are afraid that intimacy means fusion with another and loss of the self (Solomon, 1989). So, when the narcissistic person marries, the spouse chosen is up against a formidable challenge. He or she is likely to feel frustrated by the elusiveness of the perfect butterfly that is promised but never emerges. Narcissistic people have great difficulty in achieving intimate relationships, because they do not relate to their partners as people having needs and personality attributes. They behave in ways that allow them to regulate distance and appear powerful to avoid the humiliation that follows if their fragility is revealed (Lansky, 1985). Their sense of entitlement and superiority means that their partners must either kowtow to their narcissistic mate and accept a denigrated position or must aspire to ideals of perfection that keep threats to self-esteem at bay. Being afraid of not existing as an independent entity, the narcissistic individual seeks agreement and validation from the partner. There is no concept of mutual interaction and shared development.

Narcissism may be expressed in hypomanic behavior, overspending, drinking to excess and overeating to feed the hollow ego, verbally abusive scolding, physical abuse, having affairs, and pairing emotionally with a child to exclude and hurt the denigrated spouse. The narcissistic traits may be colored with histrionic features that dramatize the self and secure the attention of onlookers to ward off fears of being empty and uninteresting. Narcissistic traits may be associated with paranoid and antisocial features when withdrawal is the form of defense that is dominant. Narcissistic traits may be expressed as substance abuse in the form of drinking or snorting cocaine to get a physical feeling of needs being met. When narcissism reveals itself in the form of preoccupation with appearance it may lead to excessive exercise, anorexia, and purging as the perfect body is hatefully pursued inside the self rather than being sought and enjoyed in the body of the loved one.

In the average courtship, a state of narcissistic overvaluation happens normally. People fall in love and each thinks the other is wonderful. When one of the lovers is narcissistic, this state of finding the self and the other wonderful may be prolonged into the marriage to a ridiculous extent that does violence to the reality of the spouse or it may give way to profound disappointment when expectations are not met. For example, during courtship the narcissistic fiancé might ooze with charm and romantic appeal. Another woman might hate it, but his inhibited, unselfishly good fiancée finds in him an attribute that she cannot find in herself, and she cherishes it in him. Such hero worship is short lived because the other side of the narcissistic persona is abusive and demanding (Glickhauf-Hughes & Wells, 1995). After the marriage, he cannot remain charming and the wife no longer finds him to be everything that she is not. Then the partners have to accept each other as they really are, and that means accepting aspects of oneself too, which may prove impossible in a narcissistic state of nonawareness.

If there was an intense sexual courtship, an exciting attachment may last for a while, but only if the narcissist is viewed as the great lover. Should the other person require attention to detail, or express preferences not within the narcissistic partner's lovemaking repertoire, deep feelings of inadequacy may result, and take the form of complaints, withdrawal, or excuses. Disillusionment is painful for the narcissistic personality. Since only one lover is truly wonderful, the other must be bad.

What type of marital partner is suitable for the narcissistic individual, and what kind of marital pattern will result from the bonding of the two personalities? The other partner's personality may be narcissistic also, or it may be borderline (Lachkar, 1992; McCormack, 1989, 2000; Slipp, 1984), obsessional (Barnett, 1975), or masochistic (Glickhauf-Hughes & Wells, 1995). The borderline is loved for expressing emotionality that the narcissist is not capable of, but trouble comes when emotionality turns to rage and escalating bids for attention. The obsessional partner tries too hard to be perfect and feels driven by increasing demands from the narcissist who cannot be satisfied. The masochistic partner submits to the denigration that keeps the narcissist's self-esteem propped up by comparison. The narcissistic spouse succeeds in aggrandizing the narcissistic partner until their mutual envy tears the marriage apart.

To put it simply, the ideal partner for a narcissist is either a stunning knockout, or a devoted audience! But such a partner does not lead to growth. The narcissist's partner seeks an ideal love object in order to mend deficiencies in self-esteem and to meet unacknowledged infantile needs, not to grow through an appreciation of difference and a mutual, loving negotiation.

In every intimate relationship there is tension between the needs of the self and its strivings, and the needs of the loved one. Partners want to be together but they need to feel separate too. For marriage to work, the couple must find a way to transcend the tension of opposing forces between two different psyches (Colman, 1993). A person with a secure self brings substance to the couple relationship. He does not lose his individuality and yet he adapts to the personality of the woman he loves. A person with a narcissistic self is both insecure and apparently self-sufficient. This interferes with bonding and intimacy in marriage. When the couple then seeks therapy, the narcissistic state complicates the establishment of a therapeutic alliance.

THE NEED FOR AN INTENSIVE
PSYCHODYNAMIC APPROACH

Couples with a narcissistic partner (and there may well be narcissistic issues in both members of the couple) are hard to engage and difficult to treat. The therapist must take a long-term view of the case. A few sessions getting at the symptoms and the couple's complaints about each other may make a dent in the armor, but will only increase the need for better armor. We advise the therapist to take time to get to know the couple and to let the couple build trust. That means asking more about every sign of distrust and nonengagement in the opening sessions so that anxiety can be put into words and faced in relation to the therapist as assessment and therapy proceed. What helps the narcissistic person to emerge from the cocoon is a favorable environment in which past traumas can be remembered, unhooked from their present incarnation in the marriage, reworked in safety over time, and so detoxified. This calls for an intensive, long-term, psychodynamically oriented approach. Within that spectrum, we recommend object relations couple therapy for narcissistic issues in marriage.

THE OBJECT RELATIONS APPROACH TO COUPLES

Our approach to couple therapy is based on the Scharffs' (1991) integration of the individual object relations theories of Fairbairn (1952) and Klein (1946/1993) and the work of Bion (1970) on mother–infant interaction. In object relations theory, we think of the individual personality as a system of parts built up from experience with the mother and others in the family of origin. The infant is born as a whole self that is ready to engage with the mother and the family. In the course of infantile dependency, the child encounters both satisfaction and frustration of the drives to be autonomous and to be in a relationship. Satisfying experience is recorded in a conscious area of the self in the form of an accepted internal object. Infants deal with unsatisfying experience by taking the unmanageable aspects of frustration into the self where they are repressed as bad internal objects. The self divides into parts of the ego that relate to these objects and the frustrated, craving feelings that they elicit. We call these unconscious systems of ego, object, and affect *internal object relationships* and we find that they are constantly seeking to return to consciousness and be integrated into the self.

The state of being in love offers hope of acceptance of these hidden parts of the self. When two people fall in love, they do so in response to an attraction between these internal object relationships of

which they are unaware. The fit between these internal object relationships, and whether they are open to modification by learning from experience with the other person—new experience that is different from
that of infancy—determines the nature of the marriage and its long-
term quality.

We use the concept of projective identification to help us understand marital dynamics as an extension of processes that begin in infancy. For example, an infant may deal with anxiety attached to internal-
ized parts of the mother by projecting the anxiety and feelings that go
with it (such as rage) outside the self and inside the mother instead.
This projection becomes a way of communicating the infant's state of
mind, as the mother feels acutely the distress her infant cannot describe
to her. The empathic mother is able to contain the infant's distress and
respond in a way that renders it more manageable. By contrast, the unresponsive mother is not available to help the infant who may keep up a
barrage of crying to engage her or may withdraw into a self-protective,
narcissistic cocoon.

Projective identification is the basis of empathy and the means for
communicating distress in adult relationships, too (J. Scharff, 1992). Individuals use projective identification for communicating deeply with
the personality of their partner and for defending against anxiety by
getting rid of it into the other person without acknowledging it. To put
it another way, in marriage, unwanted parts of the self, such as unac-
ceptably needy or aggressive parts, are projected outside the self and re-
found in the spouse where they may be hated or cherished (Dicks,
1967). If hated, the spouse is attacked with all the force directed against
the bad objects that would otherwise remain internal to the self. On the
other hand, these projected parts of the self may be cherished. If cherished, the partner whose personality resonates with these attributes is
met with indulgence—perfect for the narcissist. With commitment,
love, and satisfying experience in marriage, the defensive aspects of
projective identification become less necessary and the communicative
aspects predominate so that the other person can experience and so
understand what one is feeling, and care about it. A capacity for concern is essential for mature relating.

We believe that for a marriage to be mutually satisfying, self-
centered aims have to be subordinated in favor of intimacy. Narcissistic
partners cannot do that. They remain self-involved. They have a rigid
outlook and they do not relate to each other as whole persons (Klein,
1946/1993). Instead, they overuse the mechanism of projective identification to get rid of painful aspects of themselves and project them into
their partner. Then the narcissistic husband deals with his wife as if she
has traits that need a cocoon around them, like he does, and he may

overwhelm her with his wish to be the same as her or frustrate her by keeping his distance.

For example, a narcissistic man who is always working rarely sees his wife except when they go out to entertain clients. She amuses herself by spending the extra money he earns on expensive clothes and personal grooming. He enjoys the way she looks as a trophy on his arm. He does not confront her on her overspending but secretly he holds her in contempt. In this way he fails to acknowledge his own greed and exploitativeness and attacks it in his wife.

Such deficits reduce the capacity for intimacy with partners and for working with therapists. The therapist needs to observe how the narcissistic wife uses her husband and the couple therapist to support her functioning, and how the narcissistic husband craves the unconditional support of his wife. Such couples come for therapy when the partners who previously fulfilled their projected needs fail to cope with the feelings that they have to bear in doing so. The projective identification system of the marriage breaks down. Then the couple therapist is needed to release the gridlock and help the couple to adapt and develop a more flexible system for defending themselves, communicating their anxieties, tempering their needs, and satisfying each other's longings for understanding, connection, and pleasure (Ruszczynski & Fisher, 1995).

It is not easy for a marriage—or a therapeutic relationship—to modify malignant narcissism. Instead of putting their selves into the healing mix of the loving marriage, narcissistic people require their partners to mirror and validate their uniqueness so that their shameful insecurities can remain underground. Their partner is called upon to admire sufficiency and to overlook the narcissistic person's inherent selfishness and entitlement based in neediness. Hidden are longings, dependencies, and deficiencies, but beneath the surface lies tremendous shame about selfishness and neediness. These longings and fears are uncovered when the narcissist is faced with possible loss of the other, for instance when infidelity or divorce threatens.

The narcissist is prone to deny any and all disturbing attributes. Fantasy rules. Feelings make perceptions about self and other real; projections are experienced as realities. The constant need for affirmation precludes carefully appraising the reality of the other person. Dealing with the differences that should enrich the marriage is particularly difficult.

THE CHALLENGE TO THE THERAPIST

As we have said, narcissistic people have difficulty engaging in treatment. They want, and they feel they deserve, only the "best" therapist.

Anything less is an insult to their self-evaluation. Yet, they are terrified of depending on the therapist, even if they do convince themselves they have found the best therapist. They want us to feel impressed by them. They want us to want them as patients and to dedicate ourselves to their every need, to gratify their requests for special treatment, and to provide them with phenomenally intuitive understanding. We may find their expectations daunting. We may feel flattered. We may feel unbelievably appreciated for our work as their therapists, but more often we feel bored and irritated because they are unable to take in our interpretations. Loaded with honor, we may then be sunk without trace. We feel frustrated when we are unable to reach them or help them see beyond their own narrative. Any intervention can be felt as an assault, destructive to the ego and its peculiar wrappings and sensitivities to slights. We have to tread softly when we tread on this particular psychopathology and we have to be alert to the ever-present likelihood that our sincere efforts at understanding will lead instead to a degree of shame that threatens the continuity of the treatment.

THE TASKS OF COUPLE ASSESSMENT FOR THE NARCISSISTIC PERSONALITY

Setting the Frame

We establish the arrangements for meeting, the length of the session, and the fee. Then we note how the couple responds to the frame. How they deal with the boundaries of the professional relationship reflects the way they deal with each other, with significant members of their families of origin, and with authorities in their community. Any couple may ask to be seen in the evening or to have a reduced fee, but the narcissistic couple may expect it and be overly hurt or furious if special consideration is not offered.

Creating Psychological Space

We want to hear about whatever is on their minds. We do not take sides. We do not lead the session with many questions on standard inventories. We ask occasional questions for clarification as need arises, and other questions to link history to current experience in this marriage and this couple therapy. We do not pounce with astute observations, clever interpretations, or behavioral recommendations. By letting them take the lead in determining how to use the session, and by listening attentively and responding to the thoughts and feelings of both partners approximately equally, we ensure that the session becomes a space for thinking psychologically about their issues. The narcissistic couple may seem to dismiss the therapist's efforts but that is only because they cannot admit how much they need a secure, dependable environment in which to unwind their cocoon.

Listening to the Unconscious

We listen in a relaxed yet attentive way to the words, of course, but we also follow the back story, the unspoken conflict behind the narrative, by attending to silences, pauses, hesitations, and gestures. We listen for the associative flow between the paragraphs of their speech to detect the underlying theme. The narcissistic couple may have trouble communicating because they block feeling.

Following the Affect

We assess the feeling tone of each communication and the atmosphere of the session. Rare moments of affect in the here-and-now give us access to earlier moments of heightened tension in the families of origin. For example, newly married Mrs. A nags Mr. A to get rid of years of accumulated papers, childhood possessions, and mementoes of his bachelor life to which he is attached and for which he has plenty of storage space. He claims that she is piling on the pressure and it is driving him crazy. Suddenly she gets very agitated. The therapist asks whether her husband reminds her of anyone she had to deal with before. Now she says that her mother is a pack rat, a schizophrenic who refuses treatment, and who is unable to have relationships. Mrs. A gets rid of everything she doesn't need so as not to be like her mother. Mrs. A owns her own anxiety instead of projecting it onto Mr. A's similar but different behavior. Mr. A keeps everything to be like his mother and to hold onto his memories of her. For our way of working, allowing this to emerge is a more effective way of learning about the relevance of family history than taking a genogram or a formal family history inventory.

Transference and Countertransference

We connect with the couple in the depth of our personalities. We notice how we feel in their presence (Scharff & Scharff, 1991). Our personal reaction gives us a mirror image of their joint marital personality (Dicks, 1967). We can then interpret their repetitive, behavioral patterns and their impact on each other from inside our own experience. To continue with the above example, Mrs. A recites long lists of things to be got rid of. The therapist notes that the domestic problems she asks for help with represent a conflict over intimacy and old attachments. But Mrs. A doesn't leave any room for comment. At first, the therapist cannot find the space to make this interpretation, but if she does not succeed in doing so they will not get much from their session. She interrupts to say that like Mr. A she found the long list overwhelming now as it is in real life and that like Mrs. A she had great difficulty in finding space for herself. Then she says that Mrs. A is trying to find a way to express her feelings about her husband not making room for her and his new marriage, and Mr. A is reacting against the fear that she will leave no room for him. This intervention moves the discussion forward.

To work in this way, we need to prepare ourselves as a finely tuned, therapeutic instrument by having our own analysis or therapy, subjecting our interactions to process and review, and engaging in supervision, peer supervision, and consultation (Scharff & Scharff, 2000).

Interpreting Defense

These patterns of behaving, communicating, thinking, and feeling defend the couple from deep anxieties, the most primitive of which are the possible death of the couple and the negation of the hope of creating a family.

Confronting Basic Anxiety

Once we recognize the defenses we can figure out what anxieties they protect the couple from facing. Once the anxieties are named, the couple can connect them to their histories, disconnect them from their interactions with each other, and then develop strategies and solutions together for moving on securely to the next developmental phase of the couple's life.

COUPLE ASSESSMENT ILLUSTRATION: USING COUNTERTRANSFERENCE TO UNDERSTAND PROJECTIVE IDENTIFICATION

I (JSS) set the frame by agreeing to a 1-hour consultation. Because this was a consultative service to the low-fee clinic, there would be no fee. I began to create a psychological space by asking the couple to tell me about themselves and the problem they were working on, and then I waited to hear from them.

Cissy and Patrick told me that they had been married for only a short time. They came for couple therapy because conflict over Patrick's passion for his hobby and Cissy's longing for intimacy that had troubled them during their courtship had not been resolved by being married. Patrick denigrated marriage but he valued highly the commitment of being together exclusively.

I waited to hear more. I noted that Patrick looked at me apparently defiantly and Cissy looked at Patrick with a resigned look of frustration. Here I was attending to a nonverbal communication that expressed their dynamic before their words put it together for me. I learned that they had met at a prestigious university where they felt superior to the other students. They thought of themselves as gifted in a highly complex area of study. When I heard that neither of them now had full-time work in their field, I began to suspect narcissistic dynamics. They said that they had enjoyed getting together to laugh at everyone else. Now I felt sure of it. Cissy and Patrick began trying to tell me about Patrick's devotion to an idealistic organization and how Cissy felt about it, which should have been simple, but they used language that was so general and highly intellectual that I had no idea what they were actually talking about. I sensed that Cissy wanted a close relationship with Patrick and that Patrick wanted to be free to follow his own path.

Using my countertransference I noted that I felt excluded. I also felt like an idiot, too inferior to comprehend their discourse. I had experienced the way that Cissy and Patrick were defending themselves by locating feelings of inadequacy not in themselves, or even projecting them into each other, but locating them in other people, finding them to be inferior, and excluding them from their circle. Examining my feelings, I deduced that what they were defending against were probably anxieties about self-worth. What I said was that their highly intelligent way of talking left me feeling confused and excluded from their tight circle, and then I couldn't understand their pain. They were pleased to have their intellect admired, and I think that is what let them listen to the problem I was addressing of my being excluded from a position in which I could develop empathy.

Cissy and Patrick responded by telling me about a specific marital problem of lack of empathy. Extremely hesitantly, Cissy explained that Patrick was thoughtless, neglectful, and dismissive of her feelings. I thought that she was holding back a tremendous amount of rage at her attachment needs not being met by him, and which probably had not been met in her family of origin. She said he was constantly late, not minutes late, but hours late. Patrick said that he couldn't understand why Cissy worried if he was late, why she expected him to call her if he was detained, and why she felt neglected and depressed. She thought he didn't care about being together or making her happy. He thought that she didn't care about letting him do his work and do things his own way and so making him happy. For instance, he complained that she insisted that he buy a good suit to get married in without regard to the fact that buying clothes from arrogant salespeople and dressing up made him extremely uncomfortable. He concluded that she was not thoughtful about his concerns either but that he was the most thoughtless. He seemed proud of his accomplishment in being the worst.

Cissy was masochistic and depressed. Only Patrick qualified as having a narcissistic personality disorder. However, Cissy and Patrick as a couple had a shared narcissistic defense in which they bonded against the helpless, inadequate people in their world and held them in contempt. Patrick attempted to escape the bond by staying out late. When Cissy expressed longing to be with him or the wish to be considered when he couldn't be with her, Patrick felt that Cissy was trying to control him. Neither one felt cared about. Each of them thought less about the other's needs, fears, and wishes than they did about their own. I began to wonder about how neglected or dismissed they felt in their families of origin, but waited to see if the information would emerge spontaneously.

Cissy volunteered that she hated herself for being resigned to Patrick's behavior as her mother had been resigned to the callousness of her father. Her own marriage was conforming to the destructive image of her parents' marriage. This led to a discussion of Cissy's pain as a child who was responsible for keeping her parents together and who was the only reason that they went on living, but still she could not make them happy. Patrick illustrated the pain of his childhood with an example of being punished viciously when his behavior outside the home had upset the prominent neighbor that his parents admired. He said that his parents always cared more about their standing in society than about his physical and mental health. Now I could understand that Cissy was glad to have a husband whose ideals gave him more to live for than just herself, and Patrick was glad to have a wife who did not insist that he conform to her standards. Patrick and Cissy's narcissistic defenses were identifications with and against the parents they were dependent on but about whom they were ambivalent.

OBJECT RELATIONS COUPLE THERAPY TECHNIQUE

In therapy the aspects used in assessment to establish a basis for working with the couple continue to apply. Over time, the therapist's capacity for holding and containment become the main ingredients of a successful treatment.

Holding

Holding refers to the therapist's task of providing a safe psychological space over time in which the couple can feel accepted, not judged or blamed, and in which each member will be viewed as equally important and held equally accountable for the state of the marriage. We listen without intervening at first. We follow the affect and use it as a guide to the core issues of the relationship and their connection to early individual experience. We notice defensive patterns that repeat and, when the time is right, we point them out and ask the couple to think about what purpose they serve. This leads us gradually to a discussion of deeper issues, once the couple trusts our capacity to hold their anxieties and help them to put them into words. We call this our holding capacity.

The therapist's self is our most useful tool. We train ourselves in personal analysis or psychotherapy, in supervision, in discussion with peers, and in constant personal process and review of the clinical situation to be receptive to the manner in which the couple uses us as their therapist. As we experience, think about, and react emotionally at a deep level to the personality structures of the couple, we respond by reflecting back what we have noticed, relate it to the historical context, and interpret in the here and now (Joseph, 1985). We attend to their responses to separation at vacation time and between regularly scheduled sessions to learn how the couple deals with loss and separation anxiety. We work with a partner's dream, listening for associations by the dreamer and by the other partner. We regard the individual's dream as a communication from the couple to us.

The narcissist wants to be loved unconditionally, but the therapist offers only acceptance. We form an alliance on the basis of a nonjudgmental attitude, good reality checking, an appreciation of the separateness of minds, and the value of differentiated thinking, thoughtfulness, and concern. One person will often want the partner's narcissism confronted. We will do that, but we will also look out for narcissistic traits in both of them. We will always find that the person who is not diagnosed as narcissistic does have some narcissistic issues too that are buried in the more obvious problems of the narcissistic spouse. Perhaps they are not as crippling, but they are there contributing silently to problems of inaccessibility and entitlement. In fact, we find that more subtle forms of narcissism lie at the root of many couple problems.

How do we deal with a narcissistic wife who appears overly concerned for the health of her husband and yet she does not really sense what he is feeling at all? We think about what she is avoiding in herself. Perhaps she focuses on improving his comfort so as to avoid experiencing his pain, examining her role in causing his pain, and acknowledging her own pain. Perhaps she does not allow suffering since the relationship may be threatened if responsibility is sought for actual hurts or slights. As therapists we cannot afford to collude with this. We have to hold onto our own separate view of them individually and as a couple and to face pain where there is pain. Having attended to our own individuality, we are in a better position to help the couple move out of their state of complementary narcissism and face the reality of their separateness and their need for mutuality (Strean, 1985). We help them toward a state of individuation with improving capacities for empathic attention to losses, rage, sadness, and grief, and eventually to mature relating.

Containing

The term "containing" refers to the therapist's task of tolerating the couple's anxieties over time and allowing them to resonate at the deepest levels of the therapist's psyche so as to understand the couple from inside her own experience. She is then able to respond in words that give shape to nameless fears. As she creates with the couple a narrative of their marriage and of their childhood experiences, she shows them how to process their experience and meet the developmental challenges at the present stage of their marriage. As the couple works with her, the partners learn to do this for themselves. They identify with her containing function.

To work in this way with such couples, therapists must study their own reactions, their countertransference to the couple's transference. As therapy proceeds, the therapist may unwittingly play a role in recreating the couple's defensive patterns to avoid underlying anxieties. He may experience feelings, thoughts, fantasies, or sensory experiences such as visual or olfactory images that give a clue to the underlying dynamics of the couple. The therapist's analysis of how he feels helps him to understand what is being projected from one partner to another and from the couple to him. His observations of contradictions between a woman's supposedly benign motives and the actual effects of her behavior on her partner and on the therapist supply the basis for reality-based mirroring and interpretation. In a real sense the provision of a space for thinking anew is the single most powerful tool in working with primitive abandonment anxieties, the narcissist's deepest dread.

COUPLE THERAPY ILLUSTRATION: HOLDING, CONTAINMENT, AND INTERPRETATION

We will now present an example of holding and containment and the interpretation of mutual projective identifications in object relations couple therapy. We will emphasize the therapist's internal thought process as he worked to understand the couple.

Background

Paul and Anne had been married for 1 year before Paul arranged for couple therapy in which he hoped I (CB) would cure his wife. Paul was 40, Anne 45. This was a first marriage for both of them. Paul and Anne had the same goals and wishes: a marriage, children, achievements, physical health, and the acceptance of each spouse's family, but the real draw was tremendous physical appeal and instant sexual chemistry. They looked like Pierce Brosnan and Sharon Stone. Anne became hurt and enraged when Paul noticed how attractive the "real" Sharon Stone was, even though it was Anne who liked to imagine that Sharon Stone would find Paul attractive. Then Anne became convinced that Paul was no longer faithful to her. Paul referred to Anne as "my wife" rather than by name, which suggested to me that he thought of her as a possession that was no longer under his control.

First Session

Anne vehemently accused Paul of having an affair, of removing his underwear from the home, and comparing himself to young movie stars. Paul expressed fury that she was raging irrationally and threatening to divorce him because of things that meant nothing. Paul said that his spiritual advisor/therapist advised him that his wife's behavior was bizarre and needed therapy and medication if he was to get back his marriage. Paul insisted that Anne was the sick one and the cause of their problems. Anne said she had requested marital therapy 6 months ago and Paul had refused. He had little idea of a collaborative approach to them as a couple. Each partner's mirroring of the other as an exciting, idealized, romantic object was severely tested by shared attraction to an enviably admired look-alike. This diminished both partners' self-esteem and led to fears of competition and loss.

I asked for more details about their first year of marriage. They told me that Paul's father had died of cancer, Anne's mother had fallen ill, and her male companion had died suddenly; Paul had lost his boss and his new boss had tried to force him out. All through this they had been supportive, sympathetic, and available to each other. The marriage had not fallen apart then. Anne and Paul had clung to each other desperately in the face of attack by stressors outside the marriage. Now their bond was threatened by attraction to a competitor. Recovery from earlier trauma could not be complete because they did not know how to mourn.

Anne demanded that Paul own up to his selfish and flagrant betrayal, or get out. Paul demanded that Anne get treatment for her crazy ideas about him. Neither spouse took responsibility for any of the charges being hurled about. Paul viewed himself as the helpless victim of what he called his wife's "incipient psychiatric breakdown." Anne viewed herself as the victim of a distancing, self absorbed, betraying spouse. Paul looked to me for constant validation. Anne wanted me to confirm her perception of herself as the victim and justify her experience of rage and terror.

Using a technique of empathic mirroring, I commented that it was no wonder they were struggling after the trauma they had been through in their first year of marriage. They paused briefly and looked at each other, but they could not take in what I said. Neither of them could connect empathically to any process that led to this derailment of the marital relationship. Emotions continued to run high. Complaints and counteraccusations escalated. They wanted me to be like Solomon, wise in judgment of their case, but I viewed myself like a dormouse, stunned by the craziness of the Mad Hatter's tea party. I felt besieged by their demands that I take sides with no regard to my own separate thoughts or personality. I found it difficult to provide good psychological holding or to think coherently about them, but I did attempt to tune in to each of them.

My feeling of ineptness and incoherence stemmed from a countertransference response to narcissism. I reminded myself that the narcissistic person who seems psychically removed from the human environment, encased in a cocoon of grandiosity, omnipotence, and in Paul's case, pathological certainty, is not able to provide flexible and robust psychological holding for his fragile self. The narcissistic man is terribly fearful of compliance with the wishes of the woman he loves because it threatens his independence. However, he is also in desperate need of nourishment and he fears losing her as the person he really depends on. Love relations require comfort with mutual dependence, and so do sexual relations. Because of dependency conflicts in the narcissistic personality, love and sexuality in marriage threaten the integrity of the self.

Paul's demands that I comply with his point of view were charged with aggression. His demands on me were a defense against my detecting the narcissistic vulnerabilities that he wished to deny (Modell,

1975). Underneath his aggression lay a secret helplessness in response to the threat of complete loss of the woman I was expected to transform for his use.

Narcissistic people do not listen well and so the therapist must often repeat interpretations and comments. I said again that there had been too much trauma for such a young marriage to handle, and I guessed that the family had been under strain as well and less able to support the young couple. I said that they were upset with each other because their emotional bond had been under attack from too much fall-out to bear and that I believed that their rage and terror spoke for a powerful helplessness that could not be verbalized—at which Anne sobbed, and Paul went numb. This offered me a moment of emotional connection before Paul retreated to his imperious style and threatened divorce if Anne did not get the help I must give her. And Anne said he'd have to admit to the affair if she were to forgive him.

I felt some anger at their stubborn refusals to accommodate. I felt most anger at Paul's intrusive and demanding attempts to manipulate the couple therapy contract and continually try to get me to see Anne as sick. I balanced this reaction by feeling empathy for him being in such a panic, unable to convince his wife that he was faithful. Narcissistic people like Paul want a spouse (and a therapist) who is in complete agreement with them. An independent position produces abandonment anxiety and rage.

Second Session

In the next session, I said that Paul could not reduce his wife's threats to end the marriage if he did not own up to having an affair. He said he was not having an affair. He confessed to getting rid of his underwear and explained that it was because he had a slight leakage sometimes. Indignant, he complained that he was being blamed for taking six pairs of underwear outside the home as if he was seeing another woman!

Anne had interpreted the leakage as sexual infidelity and Paul had hidden his insecurity by trying to throw it away. Each of them was threatened by the other's excessive projection of disavowed bad parts of the self—Anne with being excluded, betrayed, unreasonably jealous, and sick, and Paul with being irresponsible, imperious, self-centered, and abandoning. They held onto this projective identification system stubbornly rather than recognizing their shared sense of threat, their shared helplessness in the face of trauma, and their fears of abandonment. They did not want to admit their dependency on each other for security and regulation of self-esteem. I wrestled with questions as I pondered the gridlock. What was the intolerable threat to Anne? Was there something beyond infidelity that terrified Anne so much that she had to threaten divorce from Paul? Was this panic perhaps a manifestation of a narcissistic object choice leading to escalating disappointment as each partner's performance in the marital task failed to serve grandiose motives?

I asked Anne to tell me more about the threat. She said that she could not help feeling that Paul was up to no good. He was bringing home magazines of men and comparing himself to them. He was always telling her how handsome he was, like the models in the magazines. She used to think he was self-centered, but not that much. And, they had not had sex in 4 months.

I asked them what they thought that meant. Paul said that they used to play a game of imagining they could be movie stars since they were so attractive. Paul justified his use of the magazines as just another game like that. I asked if this game with fantasies had fostered better sexual relations. They looked at each other as though they had been found out doing something illicit. But they cautiously went ahead to explore their memories of imagining love scenes between movie stars and how that had increased their mutual sexual desire.

I made little comment so as to allow them the space to begin their work and to enjoy the improved feeling that was now entering our work space. Capitalizing on the improved tone of the relationship, I asked Anne and Paul to hold off on their threats of divorce because these added more trauma to a situation that was already full of trauma, and the constant threat would prevent working with the marriage and sorting things out. Anne explained that she threatened divorce when she felt violent, or feared that Paul would divorce her, as his therapist seemed to be encouraging. Now it became clear that both members of the couple were using the threat of divorce in a desperate attempt to modify the other's use of them.

I asked Anne and Paul to tell me more about their sexual relationship now and in the early days. They described a tenuous beginning. Intense passions were kept inside, with desires and even affection strictly limited in family surroundings. Playful affection and kissing were minimal in their love life. The sexual bond was purely functional, they said. Sex consisted of manual touching of genitals toward orgasm. Intercourse was infrequent and short, just sufficient for Paul to achieve ejaculation. Anne was satisfied with the pleasure that she gave him.

The mood during this discussion was serious and halting. These facts were told with shame, as though I were a religious authority figure who might be looking for ways to censure them. I did not ask much, letting them add or subtract to each other's statements. Nor did I comment. It was becoming painful for me to hear of so much insecurity, anxiety, and adolescent uncertainty. The couple's lack of emotion and lack of playful intent made me sad.

The more I heard, the more I had to tolerate a dysphoric state in myself. The mourning process for their losses and traumatic experiences had become frozen. Mourning had to begin in me before they could become capable of it themselves. Once they could feel sadness and grief, initially through their therapist and then in themselves, they would be able to experience feelings of love. As this session progressed, Paul and Anne continued discussing their lack of sexual relations. As we ended, Paul shook my hand as they left the office. I think he was thanking me for my silent acceptance.

As a young couple Anne and Paul had been confronted with the impermanence of bonds. This had disrupted their confidence in the longevity of marriage. They had not developed a secure sexual relationship to maintain their marital bond and to provide pleasure and relief from stress. The threat to Anne of losing Paul to an affair and the threat to Paul of divorce from Anne provoked major anxieties and a sense of crisis that eventually filled the therapy space week after week. This was an expression of their despair and their resistance to sharing the therapy space for the good of the couple. They had to test their therapist with threats of divorce and termination before they could trust in his ability to work with them at the deepest levels of their anxiety and for as long as they needed. Subsequent sessions continued to focus on resolving Anne's paranoid anxieties about Paul's betrayal and his delusion that Anne was mentally ill before progressing to more fundamental anxieties about loss, damage, and lack of generativity.

CONCURRENT THERAPIES

During the course of assessing Anne and Paul, their therapist did not detect a level of anxiety or depression that would warrant medication. Behavioral sex therapy might become relevant to help them sustain vaginal intercourse more reliably, but not before Paul's fears of needing Anne while feeling persecuted by her accusations, and Anne's inhibition and envious projection of desire into other women, had been fully addressed in couple therapy. The question of alternative psychotherapy approaches was considered, especially in the face of the couple's deep resistance to sharing the therapeutic space for exploring how each contributed to impede their marital satisfaction. Individual therapy might seem a much easier choice for each of them. However, when an individual therapist supports a one-sided point of view that one spouse is the victim of the marriage, as Paul's advisor did, this creates in the patient an infantile attachment to the therapist and a nonselective identification based on adhering to the therapist's biased view. This is a major impediment to establishing couple therapy (Fisher, 1995). Individual therapy can often proceed concurrent with couple therapy if the couple therapist and the individual therapists trust and respect each other's work. It is possible to integrate to good effect what has been learned in the partners' individual therapies into conjoint couple sessions.

THE GOALS OF OBJECT RELATIONS COUPLE THERAPY

We do not aim for symptom removal. We aim for fundamental character change. We are not teaching the narcissistic person to avoid expressing those traits. We are working toward their being unnecessary in the context of a loving marriage. On the other hand we do not privilege marriage over divorce. Our role is to help the couple appraise their marriage, explore what can be done to bring satisfaction to each partner, and arrive at a commitment to marriage or divorce. Divorce is not necessarily a failure of couple therapy. For instance, in the case of Paul and Anne, their therapist had to be prepared for the possibility that couple therapy might lead to divorce, given the degree of the narcissistic pathology, the resistance, the short duration of the marriage before trouble hit, and the tenacity of Paul's defensive strategy of scapegoating Anne. Only if couple therapists can face the possibility of failure of the marriage, can they deal with the anxieties that compromise the couple's relationship.

IMPLICATIONS FOR RELATED
THERAPEUTIC APPROACHES

We believe that object relations theory of narcissistic personalities and their marital interaction can be useful to extend understanding in other psychodynamic couple therapy models where personality change and adaptability are the goals. Even if the treatment goals are for cognitive mastery or behavioral restructuring, our way of thinking and working can enhance the establishment of the alliance. We have emphasized that the defensive, fragile nature of narcissistic personalities and their marriages requires special attention to the holding environment, sensitive pacing of interventions, and the careful creation of the therapeutic alliance. Systems and strategic therapy models that do not take account of this are prone to stalemate. Then the therapist may feel bored, flooded, or unable to remain impartial and detached. Therapeutic interventions under these conditions reflect an anxious response to being ignored or deprecated. The therapist tries too hard to think up things to do so as to feel effective, rather than experience the deadening feelings of being with a narcissistic person or couple. It is more beneficial to the couple for the therapist to tolerate the feelings of boredom and worthlessness and use the experience to understand and talk about the couple's affect. Couples may have highly charged emotional reactions or may leave treatment because of therapist-directed action-oriented interventions that do not take account of narcissistic resistance and vulnerability. Of course, negative therapeutic reactions may occur at any time and within any treatment, but techniques that ignore resistance and vulnerability will surely fail.

We advise trying to maintain a state of mind that follows the aims of the narcissistic individual and their impact on the partner. We recommend looking out for the other person's hidden investment in the narcissistic partner's narcissistic equilibrium. We track the affect, monitor frustrations, and detect the aims of various behaviors. We pay particular attention to the infantile origins of the current mode of relating in the marriage.

With narcissistic personalities, the holding and containment deficits in the relationship and the individual's past derivatives present a regressed and pain-driven situation. Our theory and clinical experience guide us to tread softly and gradually with these patients. We attend to the developmental deficits, transferences between the partners, and their projections onto the therapist. Most importantly, we work with the couple's conflict over longing for intimacy and fearing intimacy, wanting to give love but needing to protect the self from imagined attack and depletion. This powerful ambivalence presents the greatest challenge to the holding and containing function of all types of therapies. Without a secure alliance, no treatment can occur, whichever school of therapy is at work.

CONCLUSION

The study and treatment of narcissism in couples requires careful, lengthy assessment of developmental, interpersonal, and intrapsychic dimensions. Because couple therapy is extremely difficult with this narcissism-dominated population, therapists have tended to conclude that individual therapy of the self-psychology school is the treatment of choice. On the contrary, individual therapy may collude with the narcissistic problem. We find that object relations couple therapy provides a perspective on the inner world of narcissistic relating that is useful for an in-depth understanding of marriages that present this pathology. The intrapsychic lens enlarges our view of the interpersonal world of the couple and vice versa. Our knowledge of the marital joint personality translates into techniques in which we provide a psychological holding space in which the couple can express their narcissistic defenses, explore, and then modify them. Couples on the brink may be unable to share in couple therapy no matter how receptive the therapist is to their narcissistic issues. Nevertheless, receptivity and knowledge of early object relations maximize the couple therapist's effectiveness in engaging and sustaining therapy with the couple threatened by unhealthy narcissism.

REFERENCES

American Psychiatric Association. (1994). *Diagnostic and statistical manual of mental disorders* (4th ed.). Washington, DC: Author.

Barnett, J. (1975). Narcissism and dependency in the obsessional–hysteric marriage. *Family Process, 11,* 75–83.

Bion, W. (1970). *Attention and interpretation.* London: Tavistock.

Colman, W. (1993). Marriage as a psychological container. In S. Ruszczynski (Ed.), *Psychotherapy with couples* (pp. 70–96). London: Karnac.

Dicks, H. V. (1967). *Marital tensions: Clinical studies towards a psychoanalytic theory of interaction.* London: Routledge & Kegan Paul.

Fairbairn, W. R. D. (1952). *Psychoanalytic studies of the personality.* London: Routledge.

Fisher, J. (1995). Identity and intimacy in the couple: Three kinds of identification. In S. Ruszczynski & J. Fisher (Eds.), *Intrusiveness and intimacy in the couple* (pp. 74–104). London: Karnac.

Glickhauf-Hughes, C., & Wells, M. (1995). *Treatment of the masochistic personality.* Northvale, NJ: Jason Aronson,

Joseph, B. (1985). Transference: The total situation. In E. Bott Spillius & M. Feldman (Eds.), *Psychic equilibrium and psychic change: Selected papers of Betty Joseph* (pp. 156–167). London: Routledge, 1989.

Klein, M. (1993). Notes on some schizoid mechanisms. In *The writings of Melanie Klein* (Vol. 3, pp. 1–24). London: Karnac. (Original work published 1946)

Lachkar, J. (1992). *The narcissistic/borderline couple: A psychoanalytic perspective on marital treatment.* New York: Brunner/Mazel.

Lansky, M. R. (Ed.). (1985). Masks of the narcissistically vulnerable marriage. In M. R. Lansky (Ed.), *Family approaches to major psychiatric disorders* (pp. 2–12). Washington, DC: American Psychiatric Press.

McCormack, C. (1989). The borderline/schizoid marriage: The holding environment as an essential treatment construct. *Journal of Marital and Family Therapy, 15,* 299–309.

McCormack, C. (2000). *Treating borderline states in marriage.* Northvale, NJ: Jason Aronson.

Modell, A. (1975). A narcissistic defense against affects and the illusion of self-sufficiency. *International Journal of Psycho-Analysis, 56,* 275–282.

Modell, A. (1993). The narcissistic character and disturbances in the holding environment. In G. H. Pollock & S. Greenspan (Eds.), *The course of life* (Vol. 6, pp. 501–517). Madison CT: International Universities Press.

Ruszczynski, S., & Fisher, J. (Eds.). (1995). *Intrusiveness and intimacy in the couple.* London: Karnac.

Scharff, D., & Scharff, J. (1991). *Object relations couple therapy.* Northvale, NJ: Jason Aronson.

Scharff, J. (1992). *Projective and introjective identification and the use of the therapist's self.* Northvale NJ: Jason Aronson.

Scharff, J., & Scharff, D. (1994). *Object relations therapy of physical and sexual trauma.* Northvale, NJ: Jason Aronson.

Scharff, J., & Scharff, D. (2000). *Tuning the therapeutic instrument.* Northvale, NJ: Jason Aronson.

Slipp, S. (1984). *Object relations: A dynamic bridge between individual and family treatment.* New York: Jason Aronson.

Solomon, M. F. (1989). *Narcissism and intimacy: Love and marriage in an age of confusion.* New York: Norton.

Strean, H. (1985). *Resolving marital conflicts: A psychodynamic perspective.* New York: Wiley.

CHAPTER 13

Posttraumatic Stress

SUSAN M. JOHNSON
JUDY MAKINEN

Posttraumatic stress disorder (PTSD) and depression are the two mental health problems that most often accompany significant relationship distress (Whisman, 1999). An anxiety disorder such as PTSD certainly tends to interfere with the formation and maintenance of satisfying close relationships. It is also clear that the lack of such relationships, at the very least, impedes coping mechanisms and prevents healing and growth, and at worst, exacerbates and perpetuates anxiety and depression. Just how crucial the quality of significant relationships is when it comes to dealing with traumatic stress is, however, only now being fully recognized. As McFarlane and van der Kolk note (1996, p. 24), emotional attachment to significant others is the "primary protection against feelings of helplessness and meaninglessness." The impact of traumatic experience is most often best predicted, not by trauma history, but by whether survivors can seek comfort in the arms of another (van der Kolk, Perry, & Herman, 1991)—that is, whether they have a bond that offers them a safe haven and a secure base. The promise of couple therapy is just this, that the creation of a more stable, loving relationship can offer such a haven, as well as a secure base on which to stand and learn to deal effectively with the echoes of traumatic experience.

THE EFFECTS OF TRAUMATIC STRESS

Perhaps the most significant criticism of the DSM-IV description of PTSD is that this problem is described as rare or unusual. Whereas many people succeed in bearing the scars of trauma in ways that allow for relatively fulfilling lives, there is increasing evidence that PTSD, first formulated to reflect the problems of war veterans, is not that rare at all, particularly in people who seek out a therapist. In a large national sample in the United States, 12.3% of women reported having PTSD at some time in their life, and 4.6% were experiencing PTSD at the time of the study (Resnick, Kilpatrick, Dansky, Saunders, & Best, 1993). In a separate study, over 9% of people in an urban suburb were suffering from PTSD (Breslau, Davis, Andreski, & Peterson, 1990). This is the same rate of prevalence generally found for major depression. Feminist writers also stress that traumatic events are not "uncommon" as suggested in the DSM, especially for women and children (Root, 1992; Waites, 1993) and that even relatively low magnitude stressor events can result in significant PTSD symptomatology in vulnerable populations (Litz & Weathers, 1994). As Foa and Rothbaum (1998) point out, PTSD poses a serious health problem in North America, especially for women. Given such statistics and the long-term negative impact of PTSD symptoms on survivors and their relationships, it is clear that couple therapists are likely to see a significant number of trauma survivors from a variety of traumatic events in their practices.

It is also important to note that victims of trauma, whether this trauma is a one-time event such as rape, or a longer term event such as engagement in combat or childhood physical and sexual abuse (CSA), develop a range of disorders such as depression, substance abuse, eating disorders, or general anxiety disorders, as well as full blown or partial symptoms of PTSD. Additional diagnostic categories that further differentiate the effects of trauma have also been suggested. Specifically, complex PTSD or disorders of extreme stress, not otherwise specified (DESNOS), have been suggested as ways of recognizing the effects of CSA, where individuals experience a basic "violation of human connection" (Herman, 1992, p. 154) at a young and vulnerable age. This violation is perpetrated by those they depend on the most, and impacts the development of personality, the victim's sense of self, and how he or she makes sense of the world. Such survivors are particularly likely to be self-denigrating and to inflict harm on themselves. This may reflect the fact that one of the only ways a victim can understand such abuse at such a tender age, and maintain the needed bond with an abusing parent, is by believing that he or she deserved or invited it. The very self of the victim is then viewed as contaminated or bad and deserving of punishment. These survivors are likely to be diagnosed with such personality disorders as borderline or hysterical personality disorder and often use extreme strategies such as self-mutilation or starvation to regulate their distress. These strategies then, in the long term, tend to maintain their distress and negative sense of self.

PTSD was recognized as a formal diagnosis by the American Psychiatric Association in 1980. The essence of PTSD reflects the essential nature of helplessness in the face of inescapable terror. Such terror is fundamentally disorganizing and creates inner and outer chaos. By its very nature trauma overwhelms attempts to regulate and integrate experience. The most essential feature of traumatic experience and its aftermath is an inability to regulate one's emotional life (van der Kolk, McFarlane, & Weisaeth, 1996). One of the first trauma theorists, Henry Krystal (1978), noted that trauma results in a "de-differentiation of affect" that results in the loss of the ability to identify specific emotions and to use emotions as guides to the significance of environmental cues or as guides to appropriate action. The "speechless terror" of trauma (van der Kolk, 1996, p. 193) is then often expressed by bodily symptoms and somatization. Given that the regulation of emotion and the sending of emotional signals are essential organizing elements, if not the defining features of the dance between intimates (Johnson, 1998), it is not difficult to understand that traumatic stress creates chaos in close relationships. The primary symptoms of PTSD are:

1. *Intrusive reexperiencing.* Dreams, intrusive thoughts, and emotional reactions to internal or external trauma cues are included in intrusive reexperiencing. Such reexperiencing skews the survivor's experience of and engagement in the present moment. For the partners of such survivors, these responses often make the survivor seem like an unpredictable stranger who lives in a different world and speaks a different language; as a client once described it, this world is "full of ghosts and demons."

2. *Numbing and avoidance.* Attempts to restrict exposure to inner and outer trauma cues by numbing and avoidance also constrain and restrict the survivor's engagement with life in general. Most CSA survivors, for example, have considerable problems engaging in sexual intimacy with their partners, and a restricted range of affect that they can comfortably express. There is evidence that, although grouped together in the DSM, these two symptoms are best viewed separately (Foa & Rothbaum, 1998). Numbing, or the shutting down of affect, may be a reaction to the other intrusive symptoms of PTSD. This symptom appears more difficult to treat than others, does not seem to respond to traditional individual and group treatments, and predicts distress in survivors' relationships (Riggs, Byrne, Weathers, & Litz, 1998). In a recent study (Foa, Hearst-Ikeda, & Perry, 1995) numbing symptoms best distinguished victims with PTSD from those without PTSD. Irritability also clustered with the numbing factor in this study, suggesting that anger may serve to protect from continuous anxiety when avoidance fails to do so.

3. *Hyperarousal symptoms.* The most common hyperarousal symptoms seem to be general hypervigilance and irritability. For a survivor, the whole world is dangerous. Not only this, but his or her internal warning system has gone awry and is "now a problem rather than a solution" (Waites, 1993, p. 22). The modulation of anger and irritability is a very frequent problem that survivors and their partners bring to couple therapy. As a client stated, "I am so thin skinned, she looks at me wrong and I bleed."

All these symptoms, as well as "solutions" to these symptoms that in themselves become toxic, such as cutting one's body to exit states of numbness and dissociation, interact with each other and can become a "trap" (Shalev, 1993). In this trap, one level of impairment (or one set of symptoms and way of dealing with those symptoms) blocks self-regulatory healing processes from occurring on other levels. It is easy to see why trauma survivors tend to be overrepresented among those who seek out the help of therapists.

THE TREATMENT OF TRAUMA

The traditional treatment of trauma has involved individual therapy, with a particular focus on the therapeutic nature of the alliance with the therapist (McCann & Pearlman, 1990), augmented by group therapy to address interpersonal symptoms and medication. Cognitive-behavioral approaches, particularly those that focus on prolonged exposure, as well as dynamic and experiential approaches have been found to be effective in relieving symptoms such as flashbacks (Brom, Kleber, & Defares, 1989; Foa & Rothbaum, 1998; Paivio & Nieuwenhuis, 2001). However, the general consensus in the field appears to be that the impact of trauma, particularly complex PTSD, is multileveled and multifaceted. Effective treatment therefore requires a set of specific interventions and different treatment modalities aimed at specific issues and problems.

Until very recently, couple interventions were not seen as part of this treatment package. This is now beginning to change. This may be because, first, there is increasing recognition of the extent of complex PTSD, particularly PTSD arising from childhood physical and sexual abuse. There is also more awareness of how such trauma impairs personal relationships and how this impairment then exacerbates an individual's problems and prevents healing. If a survivor is unable to trust others, for example, then the isolation he or she experiences will tend to maintain or exacerbate symptomatology. Second, there is a recognition that the interpersonal symptoms of trauma, such as avoidance and numbing, may be at the heart of PTSD (Foa & Rothbaum, 1998) and that these symptoms are more difficult to treat. In fact, there is growing evidence that group therapy approaches do not, as previously assumed, significantly impact these difficulties (Saxe & Johnson, 1999). The need for other kinds of interventions that address these symptoms has then become pressing. Third, couple therapy is emerging from the shadows of family therapy and becoming a sophisticated modality in its own right (Johnson & Lebow, 2000) with substantial evidence as to its effectiveness (Baucom, Shoham, Mueser, Daiuto, & Stickle, 1998). There is also increasing evidence that viewing people in the context of their interpersonal relationships allows for the effective treatment of problems, such as depression, that have traditionally been addressed in individual therapy (Leff et al., 2000). Fourth, and perhaps most significantly, the role of what Bowlby (1969) called a safe haven and a secure base—that is, a soothing and reliable relationship with a significant other—in coping with and healing from trauma is being recognized, not just by professionals, but by traumatized individuals and their partners who are seeking out couple therapy. As we recognize the fact that "a secure bond is the primary defense against trauma-induced psychopathology" (Finkelhor & Browne, 1984, p. 36), the relevance of couple interventions for traumatic stress becomes clear. For CSA survivors such interventions may be crucial and may be the only ones that offer a real antidote to the violation of human connection that these survivors have experienced.

Given the nature of trauma and its impact, what kind of couple therapy might be most appropriate? Both empirically validated approaches to couple interventions, cognitive-behavioral and emotionally focused approaches, have been applied to couples dealing with trauma (Follette, 1994; Johnson & Williams-Keeler, 1998; Johnson, in press, 2002). This chapter focuses on the use of emotionally focused couple therapy (EFT) with traumatized couples. It is useful to think of the couple, rather than the individual, as traumatized because in many cases a survivor's spouse has been secondarily traumatized as a result of living with the survivor (Barnes, 1998; Nelson & Wampler, 2000). EFT appears to be particularly well suited to addressing the needs of traumatized couples in that it focuses upon affect, and PTSD is essentially a problem of affect regulation, processing, and integration. EFT is also particularly suited to working with trauma survivors because it focuses specifically on attachment and the building of secure bonds (Johnson, 2003). As an experiential humanistic approach, it is also explicitly collaborative and focuses on validating and affirming clients. This is essential in a client population where self-blame has been found to mediate adjustment (Coffey, Leitenberg, Henning, & Turner, 1996). Feminist writers in particular have stressed the need to depathologize the effects of trauma and the constricted ways of coping that survivors often develop (Root, 1992).

Recent research (Johnson, Hunsley, Greenberg, & Schindler, 1999) also suggests that the results for EFT are better and more stable than those found for other models. A meta-analytic study of treatment outcomes found that 90% of distressed couples improved and 70–73% of couples recovered from relationship distress after EFT interventions (10–12 sessions). A study on the process of change (Johnson & Talitman, 1997) found that these results were not as heavily influenced by initial distress levels as behavioral models were. This is important in relation to traumatized couples because they tend to be more severely distressed than other couples facing relationship problems. As yet, there are only descriptive data on outcomes with EFT and trauma survivors. Over a decade, in a hospital clinic and in a university center, these clients have taught us how to adapt the EFT model to their needs.

THE EFT MODEL

The EFT model integrates a constructivist experiential approach (reflecting the work of Rogers, 1951) with a systemic approach (reflecting the work of Minuchin & Fishman, 1981). The EFT therapist focuses on how each partner continuously constructs his or her experience and does so in a way that both reflects and creates the interactional patterns that define the couple relationship. The therapist considers self and system and how they both define each other. So the EFT therapist would help a traumatized client, who had been diagnosed with borderline personality disorder, articulate and share with her partner how she longs for closeness and fears being alone but how, when she reaches for closeness, she is suddenly flooded with traumatic fears and images of violation. So she reaches, but then angrily pulls back, and her partner withdraws in confusion and despair. The therapist then would help these clients see such patterns and how they defined the relationship between them, as well as slowly helping each of them to take new steps and create a dance where she can ask for comfort and he can stay emotionally engaged. The three stages of EFT—the deescalation of negative cycles and stabilization, the creation of new stances and patterns of interaction that foster open responsiveness and more secure bonding, and lastly, consolidation and integration—are very similar to the steps in the change process suggested by individual trauma therapists such as Mc-

Cann and Pearlman (1990). Throughout EFT the emotional experience of self in relation to other is articulated and expanded and the impact of traumatic experience on each partner's sense of self and ability to engage the other is clarified.

EFT interventions fit very well with recent research on the nature of relationship distress as elaborated in the work of Gottman and colleagues (Gottman, 1994; Gottman, Coan, Carrere, & Swanson, 1998) and Pasch and Bradbury (1998). This research stresses the power of emotional cues, such as facial expression, to define close relationships and the centrality of emotional engagement in predicting the course of such relationships. This research also delineates the same patterns of negative interaction as are outlined in the EFT literature, such as critical pursuit followed by defensive withdrawal, and stresses the need for a reorganization of interactional patterns such as these on a systemic level, rather than a focus on finding solutions to pragmatic issues and problems. This research also parallels the theoretical and research findings on attachment theory (Bowlby, 1969; Cassidy & Shaver, 1999), which is the theory of relatedness on which the EFT model is based (Johnson & Whiffen, 1999). For example, both attachment theory and the research mentioned above emphasize the role of soothing, comforting interactions in relationship definition. Research on secure attachment has found that, in general, such attachment is associated with more open, flexible communication and responsiveness to relationship cues.

DIFFERENTIAL ASSESSMENT AND TREATMENT PLANNING

First, it is important to note that traumatized couples face particular difficulties that other couples who come for therapy, who face the wounds of loss and abandonment or betrayal and the pain of isolation and rejection, do not. In traumatized couples, all these hurts are exacerbated by traumatic stress and the need to cope with such stress. Most often, couples come to therapy when the individual survivor has articulated and explored his or her trauma in individual therapy and now wishes to deal with the ways in which the echoes of traumatic experience negatively impact his or her key relationship. Individual therapists also refer survivors and their partners for couple therapy, often because the process of recovery is blocked by the difficulties in the survivor's main attachment relationship. However, occasionally a survivor will enter couple therapy with traumatic experience that is untouched and even unnamed. This person will then need the therapist's help in articulating this experience and support in seeking out individual therapy. Even when survivors have been through a course of individual treatment, there are still special considerations during the first few sessions to which the couple therapist needs to attend.

First, these couples are often severely distressed and responses such as aggressive blaming or defensive distancing tend to be more extreme. Also, the therapist has to be particularly careful to assess the possibility of violence and substance abuse in the relationship. The question is: If the survivor cannot use his or her intimate relationship to regulate traumatic stress and tame fear—for example, to deal with flashbacks as they occur—how then does he or she deal with this stressor? The therapist needs to be aware of any tendency to self-injury or uncontained rage against others and set up contingency plans to contain such behaviors. In the beginning of therapy, the therapist also needs to educate partners about the impact of trauma on close relationships. For example, most survivors of childhood abuse do not feel entitled to comfort and care and are too ashamed to speak of their needs even to their partner. The survivor's partner may also need support to understand the nature of trauma and how it impacts his or her partner's ability to respond to relationship cues. In our experience, confiding about the specific nature of a trauma has often been quite limited, even in long-term relationships. The therapist has to then include education about traumatic stress in the beginning stages of therapy and explicate how the symptoms of PTSD impact the relationship and render experiences that partners usually find rewarding, such as lovemaking, problematic.

In setting the goals of therapy the therapist has to be careful to allow for the "indelible imprint" of trauma (van der Kolk, 1996). A survivor of childhood sexual abuse may need to shape very specific and more limited goals around sexuality and confiding than partners who have not been so traumatized. The therapist needs to consult with other therapists who may be involved with a traumatized partner and integrate the goals and process of couple therapy with the process of change in these other therapies. Finally, and most importantly, the alliance with the therapist tends to be more fragile and has to be constantly monitored. In the beginning of therapy, it is crucial to emphasize the collaborative nature of the alliance and maximize the safety and predictability of the therapy process. It is important that the therapist be as genuine and transparent as possible so that the sessions can quickly become a safe haven and secure base for both clients, even when they are facing their most overwhelming fears.

EFT FOR SURVIVORS AND THEIR PARTNERS:
THE PROCESS OF CHANGE

EFT, being experiential and collaborative in form, does not include a formal period of assessment. In experiential models, assessment is ongoing and treatment begins with the first encounter with the therapist. The therapist constantly focuses on how each partner constructs his or her emotional experience and how this construction guides the process of interaction.

However, the therapist usually has individual sessions with each partner at the beginning of therapy to assess issues such as levels of commitment and possible contraindicators for couple therapy, such as violence in the relationship. With traumatized couples the level of traumatization and coping mechanisms can be formally assessed with questionnaires (see Johnson, 2002; Wilson & Keane, 1997). However, our experience has been that focused interviews that outline interactional patterns and help each partner articulate a clear account of how the echoes of trauma impact emotional engagement and bonding in the couple relationship are more useful. The therapist might ask: Can the survivor ever step out of numbness or irritability and ask to be held and reassured? Can the partner ever see past these behaviors and offer caring in spite of the survivor's defensiveness? Can partners conceive of a relationship characterized by accessibility and responsiveness where they could create a safe haven in which the effects of trauma could be confronted and healed?

The most important factors seem not to be how distressed a couple is when the partners enter therapy (this does not appear to be a particularly good predictor of outcome in EFT in any case; Johnson & Talitman, 1997), but instead the level of commitment to the relationship and the process of therapy, and the nature of the trauma. Complex PTSD (Herman, 1992), where individuals have experienced violation by attachment figures, usually requires that the change process proceed slowly and in small steps, with routine minor relapses. Couples have taught us that the natural tendency to turn to an attachment figure at times of danger and to protect those we love from danger is a powerful ally in the treatment process if the therapist can use this frame. In particular, male partners can find it rewarding to know that they are able to protect and comfort their wounded partner in a special way that facilitates healing. If a survivor copes with traumatic stress by becoming abusive then the general guidelines for working with abusive couples apply (Bograd & Mederos, 1999). For example, the survivor must take responsibility for his or her abusiveness and comply with rules to contain this behavior.

In the beginning deescalation stage of therapy, the therapist helps traumatized partners articulate the interactional cycles that sabotage positive emotional engagement, and specify how the echoes of trauma and attempts to cope with such echoes play a part in these cycles. Nontraumatized partners may discount or minimize such echoes, and this is often wounding to the survivor and tends to maintain relationship distress. The therapist may have to support these partners to understand how the echoes of trauma can distort relationship experiences. For example, a partner may need help to be able to hear that his wife dissociates at a certain point during lovemaking and that this experience has never been what he assumed it was—that is, a positive experience of connection. Partners may need help to formulate specific boundaries or ways to foster a sense of safety and begin to share their underlying emotional realities with each other. For the first time, nontraumatized partners may be able to share their fear of the survivor's rage, their despair at his or her sudden distance, or their confusion at his or her acute sensitivity to any kind of rejection or criticism. For the first time, survivors may begin to share the images of violation that arise and call out to them, compelling them to push their partner away just as intimate contact becomes a reality. As one partner remarked, "I am starting to understand. Her first concern, her obsession, is with danger. She is listening for warnings of doom. She doesn't hear the love in my voice." His partner was then able to tell him how he could help her hear the love in his voice and how this music could in fact, when she could really hear it, soothe her and offer her the safety she longed for. The couple began to be able to view the negative cycle and the echoes of trauma as robbing them of the connection they needed and to have confidence in their ability to face such echoes and improve their relationship. The relationship became more stable and less distressing and the couple was then ready to move into stage 2 of therapy. At this point they could begin to create new and more intimate dances that offered new ways to cope with PTSD and depression and new corrective emotional experiences that acted as antidotes to the effects of trauma.

In the second stage of therapy, key change events are gradually constructed that offer each partner a corrective emotional experience of engagement and connection. This involves not only numerous small steps in risking and trusting but the exploration of key emotional responses, attachment issues, and the model of self that emerges at key points in partners' interactions (Johnson 1998, 2002). For example, a survivor will, with much support from the therapist, begin to be able to tell her partner about her fears and terror and her longing for his support. However, when he then offers this support, she will pull back and reject it. The therapist will then help this client regulate and organize her emotions and explicitly formulate her sense of self as unworthy, contaminated, and unlovable and therefore better hidden and disowned, that blocks her acceptance of love and caring. The therapist also supports the other partner to remain accessible and responsive.

Let us look at the above process in a little more detail. The EFT therapist constantly helps clients piece together their emotional experience in a manner that lends itself to the construction of new kinds of interactions with partners. For example, the therapist will reflect and validate a survivor's helplessness when she awakes from nightmares and feels unable to call on her partner for comfort. The therapist will use evocative questions, conjectures, and concrete images to give a survivor's experience form, shape, and color. So a survivor might say, "I see his back. He doesn't want to hear my crazy nonsense. I should be able to handle this after all these years." The therapist will validate how terrifying the nightmares are and how the survivor always has to deal with them alone. He or she will then explore the label "crazy" and how the survivor's self-doubts and shame cue her withdrawal from her partner. This kind of exploration of key emotional experiences, where the therapist walks through the experience with the client and helps the client organize and expand this experience, bringing unclear or marginalized elements to the fore, is then used to create new enactments. For example, in the above scenario, the therapist might help the client crystallize her formulation of the above experience, namely that if she wakes her partner and asks for comfort, she "knows" that she will hear what her abusing father always told her, that she is pathetic and defective. She will then be overwhelmed by her sense of abandonment and lose the fragile sense of connection she has with her partner. The therapist explicitly helps her share this with her partner with as full a sense of emotional engagement as possible. Her partner, supported by the therapist, then is able to respond reassuringly. He is also able to express his fears that he will not "do it right" and will then further injure his partner. This opens up new levels of dialogue that can become microfocused (as when she tells him specifically how to hold her so as to soothe her) or macrofocused (as when they talk of their attachment needs and how both of them need reassurance from the other as to their value and significance in the other's life).

After more secure emotional engagement can be achieved, partners can be more open about their trauma symptoms and how these symptoms impact them, and can replace dysfunctional coping mechanisms, such as self-mutilation, with strategies such as confiding and asking for physical comfort. Such strategies then strengthen the survivor's sense of agency and the bond between the spouses.

In the final stage of therapy, these strategies are consolidated and a new sense of identity, new ways of experiencing and dealing with emotions and attachment needs, and new validating frameworks for understanding trauma and relationship distress are integrated into oneself and one's attachment system. There is evidence that EFT is able to create stable change in distressed relationships (Johnson et al., 1999). Nevertheless, the process of change is longer and includes more blocks and impasses than with nontraumatized couples. The therapist also has to be more meticulous about the process of consolidation. Relationship partners are supported to create a coherent narrative of their relationship problems, including how the trauma connects to these problems, and how they have resolved them and can continue to strengthen their bond. Negative patterns do still occur, but the couple is able to disengage from these patterns and does not allow these lapses to define their relationship. We also encourage couples to create simple rituals to maintain the safety and connection in their relationship. These can be simple greeting and leaving rituals or set times and formats for interaction. For example, one couple agreed to have breakfast together, and if the day had contained "snares and snakes" to share these with each other before going to sleep at night. Another couple agreed to a bedtime ritual with two kinds of hugs. It was agreed that the survivor initiated hugs at this time. One kind of hug signaled that limited contact was best and the other kind of hug signaled that the survivor was able to be physically and emotionally close. One of the positives in dealing with traumatized couples is perhaps that, when facing any kind of demon, if a partner stands close and faces the demon with the survivor, the connection with that partner tends to become particularly tangible and resilient.

CASE ILLUSTRATION: LAND MINES AND HURRICANES

Mike and Cathy, a young couple in their mid-30s, had been married for about 10 years when they entered therapy for relationship problems that had escalated over the past few years. Cathy, an administrative assistant, was referred for couple therapy by her individual therapist, who was treating her for nightmares. A consultation with her therapist revealed that she also had reexperiencing, avoidance, and hyperarousal symptoms and had since received a diagnosis for PTSD. In addition, she was very reactive and often dissociated. For example, during arguments with her coworkers or her husband, she often had no recollection of what transpired between them. Mike, a successful lawyer, had received individual therapy for clinical depression and assertiveness training. He was no longer in therapy but reported that he still felt depressed.

Although both partners appeared committed to their relationship and the raising of their 5-year-old daughter, they indicated that their primary concern was a lack of trust and safety in their relationship. Each understood the problem in terms of the other partner's short-comings. Their pattern of interaction was attack–distance, with Cathy critically attacking and Mike distancing himself and sometimes shutting down for days. On the Relationship Questionnaire (Bartholomew & Horowitz, 1991), they both endorsed a fearful–avoidant attachment pattern indicating that they both desperately needed and at the same time feared closeness. They both scored 75 on the Dyadic Adjustment Scale (DAS; Spanier, 1976), which indicated that they were severely distressed (a score of 70 is typical of divorcing couples). Given that they were both symptomatic and dealing with the echoes of being violated by past attachment figures and both had developed insecure strategies in this relationship, the therapist expected the process of therapy to be arduous.

The attack–distance cycle became very apparent in the first session. Cathy was extremely verbally abusive and denigrating, contemptuously labeling Mike as incompetent, pathetic, and a loser. Mike remained passive and quietly pointed out that he hoped therapy would eventually "fix" Cathy. Further exploration of their families of origin revealed a long history of maternal physical abuse for both partners. Mike described his family as a matriarchy and recalled his father as passive or absent from the home. He recounted how his mother would physically abuse Mike and his siblings and how he learned to acquiesce as a means of avoiding abuse. Cathy's mother was extremely physically and verbally abusive and would also deliberately withhold affection. When her mother went on a "rampage," Cathy would lock herself in her room or flee through her bedroom window when it became unbearable.

Their traumatic histories often were played out in their own relationship. When Mike sensed any tension or potential danger he would "run and bunker" himself against the "storm" and would recoil from physical touch from Cathy. Feeling rebuffed and worthless, she would then panic and "freeze." Her only line of defense was to "sling verbal assaults." Although Mike prided himself for remaining physically present, the constant attacks on his character resulted in him shutting down completely. The couple had little or no intimacy and their sexual relationship was nonexistent. Given their abusive backgrounds and the level of their distress, it was reassuring to the therapist (JM) that, in both couple and individual assessment sessions, they reported that there had been no physical abuse between them.

Being fully aware that trust was a key issue, the individual sessions were used to foster a working alliance with each partner. In the individual session with Mike, he commented that Cathy did not trust him, had never trusted anyone, and had no reason to trust a therapist. The therapist, however, did not have difficulty creating an alliance with either partner. The therapist made a point of validating and legitimizing each partner's experience and their positions in the relationship, and also being as transparent as possible and working collaboratively with them.

In the next few sessions, the intensity of the couple's negative interactions began to deescalate. They were encouraged to talk about their underlying feelings (e.g., fear, hurt, shame, and disgust). As they talked about their experience of the relationship, the therapist helped both partners to relate their sensitivities, learned in their past traumas with attachment figures, to specific cues in their present interactions. They were able to see how they became caught in negative cycles that then confirmed both partners' fears. Cathy was also confronted about her angry outbursts, and the impact they had on Mike and on the relationship was made explicit. A firm agreement was made that she would refrain from directing her anger toward Mike in this manner and alternatives were given (e.g., tell him she is upset, take a time out, take several deep breaths and count to five). As she began to talk about underlying feelings, specifically her panic and fear of being abandoned and alone, he began to emerge a little from his "protective armor." The negative cycle became slower and gentler, positive interactions increased and the couple became more hopeful.

The ongoing difficulty with this couple was that they were both extremely insecure and fearful, which created a paradox. As Mike became more accessible and emotionally engaged and the therapist supported this change, Cathy would get caught up in a new fear and would respond with, "I don't trust you" or "I'm not sure I want closeness now." Mike interpreted her apprehension as rejection, and would then begin to slip back into a withdrawn position.

The following excerpt gives a flavor of how the trauma was reflected in the cycle and shows a more permanent shift from a withdrawn position to reengagement on Mike's part and the beginnings of a more trusting stance on Cathy's part. This time, Mike asserted himself by setting limits and Cathy did not get so caught up in her fear.

MIKE: There are so many triggers, and I never know when something will happen or when Cathy will get upset.

CATHY: That's right . . . it's always like that. Even when I go to a movie with Mike I'm still tense—I can't just be there for me and be comfortable. I'm worrying that we're making too much noise, if Mike's head is too big, you know, you know I'm always outside of myself.

THERAPIST: You're watching for danger and worrying. (*Cathy nods vigorously.*) Sounds like it's really hard to be in contact with Mike when you are always out there scanning for danger. You get preoccupied with danger, it grabs all your attention?

CATHY: It's so true! (*Laughs*) I mean I can't, you know, just on the weekend I started for the first time in a long time to be able to concentrate—I actually had a sense of the movie.

THERAPIST: You're so vigilant and cannot relax and enjoy the moment, any moment.

CATHY: Exactly, yeah. I rarely get to the point of calm and peace. I don't feel safe because I know something will happen.

THERAPIST: To relax and be yourself is hard—because you don't feel safe?

CATHY: That's right, yeah, umm, it's almost like, like I know we are going to run into a problem. And then somebody does something, or Mike says something that sets me off, and everything goes from calm to chaos in an instant. It gets so confusing, like a battle. Yep, that's it, nothing is stable . . . and I'm alone and I panic.

THERAPIST: You feel totally alone, you panic, chaos comes in a moment—it is always a battle—

CATHY: Yeah, absolutely. And that's where it gets confusing, right at that moment, because I lash out at him (*looking at Mike*).

MIKE: Yeah, just like the other day when we went out to eat and something triggered Cathy. I was busy eating, I didn't even notice until she got angry.

THERAPIST: (*to Mike*) But then you were very much aware of her anger. (*Mike begins to weep.*) What was happening for you?

MIKE: Oh (*sniffs*), I was terrified because I knew there was nothing I could do. It's too late already. It's hopeless. So, I just wait until the storm, or rather the hurricane, passes. When she is angry, she attacks me, insults me, and I don't even know why. I give up, shut down, go back inside my armor.

CATHY: (*to therapist*) Wait a minute. What I see are two very different scenarios. One where Mike does something specific to annoy me and at other times he doesn't have to do anything, but somehow he still poses a threat. So. . . .

THERAPIST: Either way the threat is still there. Is it that you feel alone and can't connect with him?

CATHY: Yeah, and something snaps in me, like, like all of a sudden there's danger, like I stepped on a landmine. (*Therapist nods and re-*

flects.) All of a sudden, it's full battle. It just comes. It's like I'm whacked (*weeps*). The war is over but the landmines still exist.

THERAPIST: Even when he is physically there, you sense that suddenly you are alone in a dangerous world and that sets panic and fear off inside you. My sense is that you have felt shut out and unable to connect with him and that sparks off all your helplessness—the helplessness you felt when you were little.

CATHY: Yeah (*weeps*), because I still can't let go of the fact that I can't trust Mike. He is not really there for me.

THERAPIST: So you stand on this landmine called "I'm alone" and it sets off a whole visceral response, right? The panic sets in and the panic is that he has deserted you?

CATHY: (*Nods and tears.*) And when I look at him, I get scared. To me his expression is strange. He looks flat. He looks evil.

THERAPIST: Somehow Mike becomes the enemy.

CATHY: Yeah, he is not there for me. He is not Mike.

THERAPIST: Suddenly he seems so dangerous, you can't trust him.

CATHY: Yes, but it is the filter, it is how I see the world when I step on these landmines. I cannot trust anyone, my whole world is not safe.

MIKE: (*to therapist*) Is this like the Vietnam War vets who hit the ground when a car backfires?

THERAPIST: Exactly, and what I hear is that both of you have come from traumatic backgrounds. And everyday situations, though they may look quite innocent and innocuous, are about life and death and survival. For you Mike, I kind of get the sense that when you feel you are in danger you bunker yourself to protect yourself from danger. Cathy then goes into a state of panic. She is back in that dangerous place where she has to take care of herself and everybody around her becomes a potential enemy.

MIKE: Yes, that's it (*weeps*), it's tough, so hard. . . .

THERAPIST: But Mike, you are much stronger and are more present than before. I have seen you here in the session be a source of support for Cathy when these landmines go off. Maybe you can help ground her by reassuring her that you are not the enemy?

MIKE: Yes, I think now I can. But to come out I have to know that it is safe. I have to set limits. Like she cannot verbally attack me like that. When Cathy gets angry and smacks me with insults that imply I'm not OK, I feel completely rejected. When I feel rejected, I shrink back and she only gets my outer shell.

THERAPIST: What you are saying is that when you're hurt, you protect yourself by shutting down emotionally.

MIKE: Yeah, that's it. And when I come forward it is very gradual and very tenuous, but it takes almost nothing to put me back there. Her attacks have the power to destroy me. They permeate my very being. So when she insults me at 8 o'clock, she cannot expect me to be warm, affectionate, and sexy at 10 o'clock. I can't do it, I can't.

THERAPIST: So, staying fully present is very risky.

MIKE: Yes, I am willing to try, but no more attacks. I am not the enemy.

THERAPIST: You want to be there for her? (*Mike nods.*) Can you tell her that?

MIKE: (*Leans forward.*) I want to be there. I'm tired of hiding. It makes me feel small. I want to hold you when you're scared, but I won't be yelled at. I need to feel accepted and valued too.

THERAPIST: Can you hear him, Cathy?

CATHY: Yes, I'm starting to, yesterday when I began to go into a panic, he stayed with me and said "You are my Cathy." Those words really really helped. (*cries and Mike tentatively puts his hand on her arm.*)

This process continued for several more sessions. The task then was to help Cathy begin to confront her fears and to risk asking for comfort and caring from Mike. Several times he would begin to take a risk by being more present and responsive to her needs. In these moments a protective voice in her head would begin to scream, "Don't, you're beginning to let your guard down, don't, don't trust." When he met her resistance, he would withdraw for a moment. The therapist would reflect the process and access underlying feelings. The more engaged and assertive Mike became, the less panicked Cathy felt and the relapses into the negative cycle decreased substantially. Eventually, Cathy was able to differentiate moments when her fear would simply arise, without any clear cue from Mike, and she would tell him, "I'm sorry I snapped at you, it's not about you, it's about me." At other times when she felt abandoned by him, Cathy was able to check with him.

CATHY: (*to therapist*) The other day I came home from a stressful day of work and touched his arm and he flinched, and then had that look, like he was so far away. I was afraid because he seemed so distant. But this time, instead of panicking and yelling at him, I asked if he had gone away again or was he just preoccupied. And, he said he was just tired and I had caught him by surprise. We talked and it was better. I needed to know he was there, to be heard, to lean on him.

THERAPIST: Tell him please, can you?

CATHY: I like it when I can connect with you, when you're attentive. I need to know that I can lean on you, and that you care.

MIKE: I am here for you, but sometimes I'm tired or preoccupied and don't always feel like talking, but I'm still very much here.

THERAPIST: You're here right now.

MIKE: That's right, but sometimes I'm tired or just plain upset. I need to put my feelings on the table and not be judged.

CATHY: (*to Mike*) I like that, I mean, I need to know when you are upset. I prefer to know how you feel rather than have you just disappear. I cannot bear that anymore. I have to know I can reach and find you.

THERAPIST: Can you reach right now? Can you ask for his reassurance?

CATHY: (*Beams at Mike and silently mouths, "Hug?"*)

MIKE: (*Smiles back and stands up and pulls Cathy to him into an embrace.*)

By the end of 28 sessions of couple therapy, this couple had made momentous gains. Cathy scored 100 and Mike scored 102 on the DAS (a score of 100 usually signifies a nondistressed relationship). They had moved from a preoccupation with self-protection and constantly coping with fears triggered by a vast number of cues, to identifying their underlying feelings and expressing their needs. Their trauma histories that had once dominated the relationship and perpetuated the negative cycle became more peripheral. Although the old cycle occasionally reemerged, they were more adept at negotiating their way through these times and were able to discuss what they needed. For instance, when either partner stepped on a "landmine," they recognized each other's need for temporary distance as a way to "diffuse the impact of the blast," but would reconnect when they were able to listen effectively and comfort each other. In the consolidation phase of therapy, the couple were able to construct a coherent narrative about their relationship and how each person's wounds and fears from traumatic incidents in the past sparked their negative interactions, as well as how they were now able to reassure and support each other and help each other heal some of those wounds. They were able to create islands of connection and comfort together in their everyday life that made the world a generally less dangerous place. Cathy agreed that she would also benefit from further work on her sensitivities and symptoms related to her history of abuse and began to work more intensively with her individual therapist. It is our experience that if the couple can establish a safe base in their relationship, this then potentiates the survivor's growth in individual therapy. The specific reactions of close family members are also the most powerful variables in the maintenance or loss of treatment benefits in anxiety disorders (Craske & Zoellner, 1995).

A SAFER COUPLE RELATIONSHIP: THE NATURAL ARENA FOR HEALING FROM TRAUMA

It is easily argued that the most important goal in the treatment of PTSD is the reduction of fear (Foa, Hearst-Ikeda, & Perry, 1995). It is also easily argued that, as Bowlby (1973) put it, being alone makes cowards of us all. If the trauma that has poisoned an individual's life is essentially a violation of human connection, a safe and comforting human connection, not just with a therapist but with an attachment figure, also offers the perfect antidote to that poison. More specifically, the process of emotionally focused couple therapy directly addresses the seven elements of recovery from traumatization outlined by Harvey (1996). These are, first, authority over remembering and second, the integration of affect with such remembering. These are fostered by a secure base where remembering can be tolerated and dealt with. The third element is the creation of affect tolerance and the lessening of both undue alarm and numbing. This then fosters the next element of recovery, symptom mastery, and healthy coping. The fifth element is the enhancement of self-esteem and cohesion. Secure attachment is associated with a more positive, articulated, and cohesive sense of self (Mikulincer, 1995). The sixth element is the creation of new meaning that transforms traumatic experience; for example, the compassion of one's partner can transform one's self-blame and inability to grieve. The last element is the creation of the ability to trust others. As a client so eloquently stated, "Really getting that he loves me, and that I can rest in his love—that's made all the difference. That's like water in the desert."

REFERENCES

Barnes, M. F. (1998). Understanding the secondary traumatic stress of parents. In C. R. Figley (Ed.), *Burnout in families: The systemic costs of caring* (pp. 75–89). Boca Raton, FL.: CRC Press.

Bartholomew, K., & Horowitz, L. M. (1991). Attachment styles among young adults: A test of a four-category model. *Journal of Personality and Social Psychology, 61,* 226–244.

Baucom, D., Shoham, V., Mueser, K., Daiuto, A., & Stickle, T. (1998). Empirically supported couple and family interventions for marital distress and adult mental health problems. *Journal of Consulting and Clinical Psychology,* *66,* 53–88.

Bograd, M., & Mederos, F. (1999). Battering and couples therapy: Universal screening and selection of treatment modality. *Journal of Marital and Family Therapy, 25,* 291–312.

Bowlby, J. (1969). *Attachment and loss: Vol I. Attachment.* New York: Basic Books.

Bowlby, J. (1973). *Attachment and loss: Vol II. Separation.* New York: Basic Books.

Breslau, N., Davis, G. C. D., Andreski, P., & Peterson, E. (1991). Traumatic events and posttraumatic stress disorder in an urban population of young adults. *Archives of General Psychiatry, 48,* 218–222.

Brom, D., & Kleber, R. J., & Defares, S. (1989). Brief psychotherapy for post traumatic stress disorders. *Journal of Consulting and Clinical Psychology, 57,* 607–612.

Cassidy, J., & Shaver, P. (Eds.). (1999). *Handbook of attachment: Theory, research, and clinical applications.* New York: Guilford Press.

Coffey, P., Leitenberg, H., Henning, K., & Turner, T. (1996). Mediators of the long term impact of child sexual abuse: Perceived stigma, betrayal, power-lessness and self-blame. *Child Abuse and Neglect, 20,* 447–455.

Craske, M. G., & Zoellner, L.A. (1995). Anxiety disorders: The role of marital therapy. In N. S. Jacobson & A. S. Gurman (Eds.), *Clinical handbook of couple therapy* (2nd ed., pp. 394–410). New York: Guilford Press.

Finkelhor, D., & Browne, A., (1984). The traumatic impact of child sexual abuse: A conceptualization. *American Journal of Orthopsychiatry, 55,* 530–541.

Foa, E. B., Hearst-Ikeda, D. & Perry, K. L. (1995). Evaluation of a brief cognitive behavioral program for the prevention of chronic PTSD in recent assault victims. *Journal of Consulting and Clinical Psychology, 63,* 948–955.

Foa, E. B., Riggs, D. S., & Gershuny, B. S. (1995). Arousal, numbing and intrusion: Symptom structure of PTSD following assault. *American Journal of Psychiatry, 152,* 116–120.

Foa, E. B., & Rothbaum, B. O. (1998). *Treating the trauma of rape: Cognitive behavioral therapy for PTSD.* New York: Guilford Press.

Follette, V. (1994). Survivors of child sexual abuse: Treatment using a contextual analysis. In S. C. Hayes, N. S. Jacobson, V. M. Follette, & M. J. Dougher (Eds.), *Acceptance and change: Content and context in psychotherapy* (pp. 255–272). Reno, NV: Context Press.

Gottman, J. (1994). *What predicts divorce?* Hillsdale, NJ: Erlbaum.

Gottman, J., Coan, J., Carrere, S., & Swanson, C. (1998). Predicting marital happiness and stability from newly wed interactions. *Journal of Marriage and the Family, 60,* 5–22.

Harvey, M. (1996). An ecological view of psychological trauma and trauma recovery. *Journal of Traumatic Stress, 9,* 3–23.

Herman, J. L. (1992). *Trauma and recovery.* New York: Basic Books.

Johnson, S. M. (1998). Listening to the music: Emotion as a natural part of systems theory. *Journal of Systemic Therapies* [Special issue], *17,* 1–17.

Johnson, S. M. (2002). *Emotionally focused couple therapy with trauma survivors: Strengthening attachment bonds.* New York: Guilford Press.

Johnson, S. M. (2003). Introduction to attachment: A therapist's guide to primary relationships and their renewal. In S. M. Johnson & V. E. Whiffen (Eds.), *Attachment processes in couple and family therapy* (pp. 3–17). New York: Guilford Press.

Johnson, S. M. (in press). An antidote to post-traumatic stress disorder: The creation of secure attachment in couples therapy. In L. S. Atkinson (Ed.), *Attachment and psychopathology* (Vol 2.). Cambridge, UK: Cambridge University Press.

Johnson, S. M., Hunsley, J., Greenberg, L., & Schlindler, D. (1999). Emotionally focused couples therapy: Status and challenges. *Clinical Psychology; Science and Practice, 6,* 67–79.

Johnson, S. M., & Lebow, J. (2000). The coming of age of couple therapy: A decade review. *Journal of Marital and Family Therapy, 26,* 23–38.

Johnson, S. M., & Talitman, E. (1997). Predictors of success in emotionally focused marital therapy. *Journal of Marital and Family Therapy, 23,* 135–152.

Johnson, S. M., & Whiffen, V. E. (1999). Made to measure: Adapting emotionally focused couples therapy to couples attachment styles. *Clinical Psychology: Science and Practice, 6,* 366–381.

Johnson, S. M., & Williams-Keeler, L. (1998). Creating healing relationships for couples dealing with trauma: The use of emotionally focused therapy. *Journal of Marital and Family Therapy, 24,* 25–40.

Krystal, H. (1978). Trauma and effects. *Psychoanalytic Study of the Child, 33,* 81–116.

Leff, J., Vearnals, S., Brewin, C. R., Wolff, G., Alexanders, B., Asen, E. Dayson, D., Jones, E., Chisholm, D., & Everitt, B. (2000). The London Depression Intervention Trial. Randomized controlled trial of antidepressants v. couple therapy in treatment and maintenance of people with depression living with a partner: Clinical outcome and costs. *British Journal of Psychiatry, 177,* 95–1000.

Litz, B.T., & Weathers, F. W. (1994). The diagnosis and assessment of post-traumatic stress disorder on adults. In M. B. Williams & J. F. Sommer (Eds.), *Handbook of post-traumatic therapy* (pp. 19–37). Westport, CT: Greenwood Press.

McCann, I. L., & Pearlman, L. A. (1990). *Psychological trauma and the adult survivor.* New York: Brunner/Mazel.

McFarlane, A., & van der Kolk, B. (1996). Trauma and its challenge to society. In B. A. van der Kolk, A. C. McFarlane, & L. Weisaeth (Eds.), *Traumatic stress* (pp. 24–45). New York: Guilford Press.

Mikulincer, M. (1995). Attachment style and the mental representation of the self, *Journal of Personality and Social Psychology, 69,* 1203–1215.

Minuchin, S., & Fishman, H.C. (1981). *Family therapy techniques.* Cambridge, MA.: Harvard University Press.

Nelson, B. S., & Wampler, K. S. (2000). Systemic effects of trauma in clinic couples: An exploratory study of secondary trauma resulting from childhood abuse. *Journal of Marital and Family Therapy, 26,* 171–183.

Paivio, S., & Nieuwenhuis, J. A. (2001). Efficacy of emotion focused therapy for adult survivors of child abuse: A preliminary study. *Journal of Traumatic Stress, 14,* 109–127.

Pasch, L. A., & Bradbury, T. N. (1998). Social support, conflict and the development of marital discord. *Journal of Consulting and Clinical Psychology, 66,* 219–230.

Resnick, H. S., Kilpatrick, D. G., Dansky, B. S., Saunders, B. E., & Best, C. L. (1993). Prevalence of civilian trauma and posttraumatic stress disorder in a representative national sample of women. *Journal of Consulting and Clinical Psychology, 61,* 984–991.

Riggs, D., Byrne, C., Weathers, F., & Litz, B. (1998). The quality of intimate relationships of male Vietnam veterans: Problems associated with posttraumatic stress disorder. *Journal of Traumatic Stress, 11,* 87–101.

Rogers, C. (1951). *Client-centered therapy.* Boston: Houghton-Mifflin.

Root, M. P. (1992). Reconstructing the impact of trauma on personality. In L. S. Brown & M. Ballou (Eds.), *Personality and psychopathology: Feminist reappraisals* (pp. 229–265). New York: Guilford Press.

Saxe, B. J., & Johnson, S. M. (1999). An empirical investigation of group treatment for a clinical population of adult female incest survivors. *Journal of Child Sexual Abuse, 8,* 67–88.

Shalev, A. Y. (1993). Stress versus traumatic stress: From acute homeostatic reactions to chronic psychopathology. In B. A. van der Kolk, A. C. McFarlane, & L. Weisaeth (Eds.), *Traumatic stress* (pp. 77–101). New York: Guilford Press.

Spanier, G. (1976). Measuring dyadic adjustment. *Journal of Marriage and the Family, 38,* 15–28.

van der Kolk, B. A. (1996). The complexity of adaptation to trauma. In B. A. van der Kolk, A. C. McFarlane, & L. Weisaeth (Eds.), *Traumatic stress* (pp. 182–213). New York: Guilford Press.

van der Kolk, B., McFarlane, A. C., & Weisaeth, L. (1996). *Traumatic stress.* New York: Guilford Press.

van der Kolk, B., Perry, C., & Herman, J. L. (1991). Childhood origins of self-destructive behavior. *American Journal of Psychiatry, 148,* 1665–1671.

Waites, E. A. (1993). *Trauma and survival: Post-traumatic and dissociative disorders in women.* New York: Norton.

Whisman, M. A. (1999). Marital dissatisfaction and psychiatric disorders: Results from the National Comorbidity Survey. *Journal of Abnormal Psychology, 108,* 701–706.

Wilson, J. P., & Keane, T. M. (Eds.). (1997). *Assessing psychological trauma and PTSD.* New York: Guilford Press.

CHAPTER 14

Childhood Sexual Trauma

BARRY W. McCARTHY
MIA SYPECK

Child sexual abuse, especially incest, has been widely discussed in the professional and popular literature. There are vastly different conceptual and treatment models for understanding and intervening with adults who have a history of childhood sexual victimization. The predominant model is based on concepts from the self-help book *The Courage to Heal* (Bass & Davis, 1988) that emphasizes the critical importance of identifying feelings (including repressed memories), receiving validation for the courage to disclose personal stories of victimization, using self-help and other resources to assert autonomy, and the importance of confronting the perpetrator. Trauma concepts and interventions are as much influenced by the self-help movement (e.g., Incest Survivors Anonymous) as any other factor.

This chapter focuses on couples where one or both partners report a history of childhood sexual abuse and trauma. The authors discuss conceptualizing, assessing, and treating this complex issue in couple therapy. Clinical paradigms are in conflict, especially whether to focus on child abuse issues and resolving these before addressing couple issues of intimacy and sexuality. An alternative paradigm is to focus on couple sex therapy (McCarthy, 1995) with an emphasis on the individual as a "partner in healing" (Maltz, 2001). In this model, vulnerabilities caused by child sexual abuse are carefully assessed and integrated into couple treatment. This chapter is based on that model and cognitive-behavioral therapeutic strategies and techniques. These strategies can be and are used by a range of clinicians and integrated into other theoretical systems (Follette & Pistorello, 1995; Maddock & Larson, 1995; Trepper & Barrett, 1986).

The therapist is challenged to use a number of skills, including individual assessment and therapy, couple assessment and therapy, assessment and treatment of trauma, and assessment and treatment of sexual dysfunction. The model espoused emphasizes (1) promoting individual and couple awareness and empowerment; (2) assuming personal responsibility; (3) understanding that present behavior is multicausal, multidimensional, and not controlled by past trauma; (4) respecting individual and couple differences; (5) problem solving; (6) underscoring being a survivor; and (7) integrating intimacy and sexuality into the couple's relationship. The core therapeutic cognition is "living well is the best revenge."

It is crucial for clinicians to be aware that conceptualizations and interventions can be iatrogenic rather than therapeutic. The risk of iatrogenic outcomes is greater in treating sexual trauma than in any other area of mental health (McCarthy, 1997). A key concept in the therapeutic management of childhood sexual trauma is to explore the adult's memory of events in a respectful, empathic, nonblaming manner (Courtois, 2000). The appropriate format for this exploration is an individual developmental history session rather than a couple session. The clinician helps the client to explore (1) cognitions, feelings, and behavior involving the abusive incidents; (2) cognitions, feelings, and behavior in dealing with the trauma; and most importantly, (3) present cognitions, feelings, and behavior regarding the trauma, intimacy, and sexuality. By exploring these areas, the person can make the crucial distinction of honoring the importance of sexual abuse, while not allowing it to control individual sexuality or couple intimacy.

Although there is a plethora of treatment models, books, and case reports about the effects of child sexual abuse, unfortunately a dearth of empirical data remains regarding assessing effects and successful treatments (Rind, Tromovitch, & Bauserman, 1998). There is a vast clinical literature on treatment of children who have been abused, but little empirical validation of treatment models (Saywitz, Mannarino, Berliner, & Cohen, 2000).

There is a great deal of public and clinical discussion about the severe and continuing impact of sexual abuse on adult sexuality. However, there are no solid empirical data on frequency or types of dysfunction associated with child sexual abuse (Bartoi & Kinder, 1998). Nor are there any empirically validated treatments. Clinical data emphasize inhibited sexual desire (ISD), nonorgasmic response, and vaginismus for females. There are even fewer data for males with a history of sexual abuse, although erectile dysfunction, ISD, and ejaculatory inhibition are believed to occur at higher rates. Depending on type of trauma and gender factors, the person might have deficits in intimacy, sexuality, or in integrating intimacy and eroticism.

Many important conceptual and treatment questions remain, including:

1. Should the clinical focus be on recalling and reworking past abuse or being a survivor in the present?
2. Is the optimal therapeutic focus on damage from abusive experiences or resilience and pride in being a survivor?
3. Is the primary treatment modality individual, couple, or group?
4. What are the advantages and risks of long-term versus time-focused treatment?
5. Is the therapeutic strategy to heal the inner child or build confidence in the adult survivor?
6. How important is it to elicit memories of past abuse? Is there a danger of promoting false memories?

The area of sexual trauma generally, and treatment of adults who were sexually victimized as children specifically, is one of the most controversial in mental health. The most adversarial issue is the conflict over "recovered memories of abuse" (Knapp & Van De Creek, 2000). The politicization of the field and increased lawsuits and countersuits are particularly distressing. When the adult sues a parent, family member, teacher, or religious figure based on memories recovered years later during psychotherapy or focused memory recovery therapy, is this therapeutic or iatrogenic? Litigation changes the focus from a mental health issue with the emphasis on recovery to a legal issue based on monetary damages, "black and white" legal judgments, and use of coercive tactics and threats to force settlement. The legal process can become a quagmire, draining time and energy and straining the couple bond. The recovered memory controversies have decreased professional and public respect for the sexuality field.

Although estimates vary widely with divergent operational definitions and subject samples (Haugaard, 2000), the best estimate is that one in three female children and one in six male children have a significant sexual experience with an adult or with an adolescent who was at least 5 years older. This includes "hands off" incidents such as voyeurism, exhibitionism, obscene phone calls, and sexual harassment. "Hands on" incidents range from vaginal or anal intercourse to fondling the child's genitals to the child being coerced to give or receive manual or oral stimulation.

Two factors that increase the long-term negative impact of sexual abuse are use of force or violence and breaking a close trust bond (Mc-Carthy, 1990). The factor of violence (less than 15% of hands-on incidents) represents a different dimension and is better categorized as sexual assault. The combination of violence and sexuality can have a multiplicative effect, especially for middle-class children who have been sheltered from violence. The impact of breaking a trust bond (with a parent, stepparent, sibling, minister, teacher, or youth counselor) can be particularly impactful for trust issues in subsequent adult intimate relationships.

A helpful conceptualization for assessment and treatment of abuse is the "levels of victimization" model (McCarthy, 1986). The first level is the sexual abuse itself: what happened, with whom, duration, cognitions, behaviors, and feelings at the time. The second level is how the child dealt with the abuse: was anyone told or was it a "shameful secret." Was there police, counseling, or court involvement? Was this intervention helpful or did it further confuse or stigmatize the child? What the child wants is for the abuse to stop, to be able to understand what happened, not to feel blamed or stigmatized, for the adult to apologize, to have a nonabusive relationship with him, and to receive a positive sexuality education which helps put the abuse in perspective. Unfortunately, these needs are seldom met. The great majority of adult clients do not feel that sexual abuse issues were dealt with well at the time or afterward. The third level is the most important and is the focus of this chapter: the effects on adult psychological and sexual functioning. The core variable is whether the person views herself and acts as a victim or a survivor. Traditionally, she was a silent, passive victim; but now the trend is to be a vocal, angry victim. The essence of being a victim is that past trauma control present feelings and behavior, including intimacy and sexuality. The victim model emphasizes vulnerabilities and deficits that cast a huge shadow over the individual, emotional and sexual intimacy, and couple therapy.

In contrast, the conceptual models of Maltz (2001), Meichenbaum (1994), Compton and Follette (1998), and McCarthy and McCarthy (1993) emphasize confronting the victim role and building a healthy, secure sexuality. This therapeutic strategy focuses the individual and couple on the present and future rather than allowing them to be controlled by past trauma. For the individual who was abused, gaining personal control of sexuality, feeling she deserves sexual choice, having the partner honor her veto, and experiencing sexuality as voluntary, mutual, and pleasure oriented, are crucial learning experiences. When the person experiences desire, arousal, orgasm, and emotional satisfaction, she feels like a sexual survivor. The self-esteem of a survivor includes (1) acceptance of self, including integrating past abusive incidents; (2) realizing that the perpetrator, not self, is responsible for abuse; (3) living in the present, not stuck in shame, anger, or guilt about the past; (4) feeling she deserves psychological and sexual well-being; (5) viewing sexuality as voluntary, comfortable, intimate, and pleasurable; and (6) establishing an intimate, functional couple sexual style.

COUPLE THERAPY AND CHILD SEXUAL ABUSE

The major therapy decision is whether to use couple therapy as the primary modality rather than individual or group therapy with a focus on past sexual abuse. Each individual states their needs and wants as part of the clinical assessment. In the majority of cases, couple therapy is the treatment of choice. Couple therapy focusing on the one–two combination of personal responsibility, combined with being a member of an intimate team, is the optimal strategy for change as well as maintaining individual and couple gains. These cases challenge the clinician to use and integrate skills of individual therapy, couple therapy, trauma therapy, and sex therapy. This requires high levels of clinical judgment and sensitive sequencing of interventions. The assessment/intervention process allows treatment to be individualized rather than be dependent on a rigid formula or rule-governed therapy. There are three therapeutic focuses: (1) the couple's emotional relationship; (2) the couple's sexuality; and (3) integrating vulnerabilities and sensitivities from childhood sexual trauma into self-acceptance as a survivor and valuing intimate sexuality.

INDIVIDUAL AND COUPLE ASSESSMENT ISSUES

Assessment is not an isolated component, but an ongoing process dependent on feedback from therapy interventions and sexual exercises. The assessment phase involves an initial couple meeting, followed by individual history-taking sessions, and a couple feedback session. In addition, release of information forms are obtained to contact previous individual, trauma, or couple therapists. It is fascinating to hear the perceptions of past therapists, as these are often different from clients' own perceptions and experiences.

The initial meeting is scheduled as a couple session to reinforce the concept of sexuality being a couple issue. This session focuses on assessing the couple's readiness and motivations to address problems, past attempts to understand and change, determining what did not work in the past so that mistakes are not repeated, and identifying potential stresses or pitfalls. At least one individual session is crucial in assessing psychological and sexual issues (especially trauma) from the past and in the present. The therapist begins with an introduction to the goals of the session:

> "I want to understand your psychological and sexual development, attitudes, and experiences, both before meeting your partner and during your relationship. We will explore both problems and strengths. At the end, I will ask if there are sensitive issues or secrets that you do not want shared with your partner. These will not be discussed without your permission. But I need to understand these issues in order to be of help."

This session provides the clinician with critical information for treatment planning as well as helping the client to feel understood, respected, and valued.

In exploring childhood issues, the first question is how and where the person learned about sexuality. This facilitates exploration of family, religious, and educational background. Other questions include childhood sex play, feelings about self-exploration and masturbation, first orgasmic experience by self and with others, body image perceptions and feelings, as well as dating experiences. Was touching comfortable or problematic? How old was the person when he or she left home to live independently? After this chronological review, the client is asked, "As you look back on your childhood and adolescence, what was the most negative, confusing, traumatic, or guilt-inducing experience you had?" Approximately one in four people (especially males) will disclose an experience they had not previously reported. In addition to the major sources of trauma—childhood sexual abuse, incest, and rape—other negative experiences include contracting a sexually transmitted disease, an unwanted pregnancy, being sexually rejected or humiliated, guilt over masturbation or fantasies, a sexual dysfunction, unsuccessful first intercourse, being peeped on or exhibited to, receiving an obscene phone call, or being sexually harassed. A sad reality is that negative sexual experiences are an almost universal occurrence for both females and males.

In a sensitive, nonjudgmental manner, the clinician explores any negative incidents in three time frames. The first frame involves attitudes, behaviors, and emotions at the time of the incident. The second frame is who (if anyone) was told and how the incident was dealt with. Traditionally, abusive experiences were kept as shameful secrets. Incidents are now usually revealed but not dealt with well, leaving the child feeling confused and blamed. The third time frame is the present: Does she see herself as a survivor or a victim? Has she shared the traumatic experience with her partner fully, in a cursory manner, or is it still a secret? How does it affect the couple's sexual relationship and how does she want this dealt with in therapy?

At the end of the sexual history, the therapist should ask another open-ended question: "As you review your entire life, including this current relationship, what was the most confusing, negative, or traumatic experience you've had?" Again, approximately one in four clients will bring up an unreported experience. In reviewing negative or traumatic incidents, one should assess how well the person dealt with the incident at the time and its impact on self-esteem and sexuality. Is there a need for an additional session to explore this experience and make a determination of whether couple therapy is the best modality? Does the person need individual psychotherapy or specific trauma work, either individually or in a group?

The second issue is how much the partner knows and whether he is empathic. Is he capable of being a partner in healing or does he blame her or want revenge against the perpetrator? If the client has not shared her abuse history, why not? Is she willing to share it now? What does she want from her partner? How does she predict he will react? Does she hope to integrate past trauma in couple therapy, handle it separately, or postpone it until later? What if she wants it to remain secret? The therapist cannot decide this for her, but can share an assessment, clinical judgment, and recommendations.

Optimally, sharing the story of childhood sexual trauma is part of the feedback session. The feedback session is a core component in couple sex therapy (McCarthy, 2002). It can be quite impactful and highly motivating. In order to discuss issues fully, this is often scheduled as a double session. By integrating childhood sexual trauma into the feedback, the intention is to increase understanding and empathy. This enhances motivation to address individual, couple, and sexual problems. The goal remains the same: to develop a comfortable, functional, and satisfying couple sexual style. The nonabused partner has an integral role in the change process. Interestingly, a woman is typically open to assuming this role when the male has been victimized. By comparison, the male partner of an abused woman may be empathic about the past, but is often eager to be a problem solver and to move on with the couple's sexual relationship.

In history taking with the partner, it is crucial to assess attitudes, feelings, and a potential to be supportive in dealing with past trauma and building an intimate relationship. Especially important is to assess the likelihood that the partner will blame or coerce. Can he be an intimate, supportive partner? Will other personal or relationship problems dominate the partner's reactions? An example is the person who feels so angry or resentful that he has no empathy for the sexual trauma. Another example is a woman who has felt neglected or blamed, so that her view of her partner is so rigid that she cannot respond to his own sexual abuse disclosure.

The role of the nonabused partner is to be empathic and supportive, not to take on the problem him- or herself. It is not therapeutic for the nonabused person or their relationship to feel traumatized. Two reactions are particularly problematic: The first and most common is to be overly sympathetic and treat the partner as a "wounded person"; the second is to be judgmental and to blame the partner for being abused. Ideally, an individual encourages his or her partner to deal with past trauma and to grow psychologically, sexually, and relationally. The challenge for the abused partner is to be a survivor in the present, to take pride and satisfaction in developing a healthy relationship and couple sexuality.

What if both partners have a history of sexual trauma or another form of abuse (e.g., physical abuse, alcoholic family, neglect, extreme poverty, family chaos)? This is commonly reported, although there is a dearth of empirical data. Each person's trauma history has to be carefully explored, including the meaning of the trauma. Even if the category of abuse is the same (e.g., incest or sexual abuse by a teacher), the experience and meaning may be different for each. What are the vulnerabilities and strengths each person brings to their emotional and sexual relationship? Can they work as an intimate team in dealing with trauma issues, relationship issues, and the couple's sexuality?

TREATMENT ISSUES

The treatment of choice is typically to integrate sexual trauma therapy, couple therapy, and sex therapy in a contract with one therapist. However, this sometimes is not possible due to practical factors (one or both partners are already involved with individual, group, or trauma therapies) or because of client needs (a partner needs intensive therapy focused on past trauma or is not motivated for sex therapy). Couple therapy is more likely to result in significant individual, couple, and sexual changes (Maddock & Larson, 1995). Even more important, these changes are more likely to be maintained and incorporated into the person's individual life as well as the couple's sexuality (McCarthy, 1999).

Initially, the therapist takes an active role in providing structure, presenting an optimistic view of change, and encouraging motivation

and engagement in the therapeutic process, especially cognitive and behavioral exercises. As therapy progresses, the clinician is less active and
directive, encouraging the couple to take responsibility and develop
their unique relational and sexual style.

The clinician is respectful of individual differences in regard to
abuse issues while supporting and encouraging the person and couple
to adopt a survivor stance. Insights about childhood abuse serve as an
impetus to use healthy coping in the present. An example was the real-
ization for a woman that as a child she experienced fear of choking as
her 23-year-old brother-in-law forced his penis into her mouth. This insight clarified why, although initially aroused by kissing her husband's
penis, she subsequently became anxious and repulsed when he wanted
to continue fellatio. His empathy for her abuse made him aware that
she was struggling with complex psychological issues, rather than blaming her for being stubborn or sexually manipulative. The wife's realiza-
tion that she had sexual choices and a right to "veto" any activity that
she found aversive allowed her to experience sexuality as pleasure oriented and mutual. The husband's honoring her veto established him as
a trusting and intimate friend, not a demanding, blaming male. It was
hard for her to say "yes" to intimate sexuality if she did not feel free to
say "no" to aversive, intimidating sex.

Confronting the "ghosts" of childhood abuse is important but not
sufficient in establishing healthy adult sexuality. In moving toward this
goal, a therapeutic cognition is that life is meant to be lived in the present, not controlled by guilt or trauma from the past. A helpful cognition for the nonabused mate is "you are a partner in healing." This involves respecting the other's feelings and veto. Just as important is
responding to a partner's requests for intimacy, pleasuring, and eroticism—for example, valuing pleasure-oriented sexuality, rather than demanding sexual performance. Unlike the perpetrator, one puts the
other's emotional needs ahead of one's own sexual needs.

Healthy sexuality involves each partner being capable of experiencing desire (positive anticipation and feeling deserving of sexual
pleasure), arousal (receptivity and responsivity to pleasure and eroticism leading to subjective and objective arousal), orgasm (the voluntary, natural response to high arousal), and satisfaction (feeling bonded
and better about oneself and one's relationship after a sexual experience; McCarthy & McCarthy, 1998a).

Sexual dysfunction is treated as multicausal and multidimensional.
Trauma predisposes the person to develop a dysfunction but present
negative experiences, attitudes, feelings, and avoidance are important
in maintaining sexual dysfunction. In other words, what originally
caused the sexual problem is often different from what maintains sexu-

al dysfunction. This is a particularly important concept because most clients (and many clinicians) believe that once childhood causes are identified, sex will take care of itself. When that does not happen, the couple reverts to guilt and blame. Theoreticians argue about whether dealing with child abuse is necessary before dealing with adult sexual issues, but it is certainly not sufficient. The couple, not just the survivor, needs to learn a new style of sexual thinking, talking, feeling, and experiencing. The essence of abusive sexuality is that it involves coercion or force, meets the sexual needs of the perpetrator at the expense of the child's emotional needs, and is manipulative and secretive. In contrast, healthy sexuality is voluntary, intimate, mutual, pleasure-oriented, and an integrated component of the couple's intimacy.

The one–two combination of personal responsibility for sexuality (including dealing with childhood sexual abuse) and working as an intimate team is the core therapeutic strategy. The nonabused partner cannot rescue the survivor; the survivor has to develop his or her own adult sexual voice.

GENDER ISSUES

The clinician needs to be aware of gender issues and incorporate these into the treatment process. It is important to assess and individualize interventions carefully, and not to fall into the trap of gender stereotypes. The typical female trap is to treat sexual abuse as a shameful secret that controls her sexuality. The typical male trap is to deny or minimize the abuse, yet internally feel deficient and less of a man. Neither gender trap promotes being a survivor, nor does it promote healthy couple sexuality. Feeling like a passive victim is not healthy, but feeling and acting like an angry victim is even less functional. The passive victim can learn to assert sexual feelings and rights and move toward intimate, interactive sexuality. Anger interferes with sexual desire and eroticism, and negates an intimate relationship. The angry person has to reduce negative emotions and develop a trusting approach to rebuilding intimacy and sexuality.

In many ways, the male survivor has a more difficult transition to intimate sexuality (McCarthy & McCarthy, 1998b). The male performance myth emphasizes that men are not supposed to have sexual questions, doubts, anxieties, or inhibitions. This sexual standard is harmful in itself, but is particularly burdensome for the male who as a boy denied the sexual abuse because such experiences were not supposed to happen. The fact that the perpetrator was a male adds both stigma and self-doubt about why he was chosen to be victimized. What does that mean about his sexual identity? In truth, child sexual abuse is not about sexual orientation, but rather is about a deviant arousal pattern toward children.

It is difficult for the male (whether as a child or adult) to identify the sexual experience as abusive, realize that the responsibility lies with the adult, not blame himself, accept the reality of the abuse without either minimizing it nor making it the controlling aspect of his life, deal with it so he feels like a survivor, and be open to the partner as his intimate sexual friend. It is his responsibility to confront the abuse, not as a "Lone Ranger," but as a vulnerable human being who is committed to being a fully functioning person. His partner's role is to be empathic, supportive, and urge him to deal with intimacy issues and grow from the trauma, not to be an avoidant or angry victim. Her sympathy and restraint from sexual requests inadvertently reinforces his remaining in the passive, angry, or avoidant role. A key element in being a resilient survivor is being open to the partner's emotional and erotic needs. Her sexuality can enhance his comfort and invite erotic response. The trap for the female is to dampen her erotic response so as not to intimate him. The trap for the male is to push her to go at his pace rather than hers. In order to overcome child sexual abuse each person needs to communicate and implement the one–two combination of personal responsibility and being an intimate team.

CASE ILLUSTRATION

Alicia and Trevor presented for couple sex therapy as a last ditch effort to salvage their 3-year marriage. They had been a couple for 2 years before marrying and had been in therapy the entire time they had known each other. The referral came from Alicia's individual therapist who believed that this dysfunctional marriage was interfering with her individual therapy. Alicia either had to resolve the problem or leave the marriage. Trevor's individual therapist did not endorse couple sex therapy because he believed that sex was an unimportant symptom of individual psychopathology. Two previous couple therapists, two couple enhancement workshops, and involvement in a couple's self-help recovery program had not resulted in significant change. Both Alicia and Trevor were ambivalent about their marriage. Trevor's individual therapist worried that Trevor would deteriorate and become suicidal if the marriage ended.

In the initial couple session, the clinician's perception was that they were a confused, demoralized, ambivalent couple experiencing a great deal of psychological pain. The clinician suggested a four-session assessment contract before asking them to commit to treatment. The idea of jointly assessing their situation and making a treatment decision was appealing to them. Alicia and Trevor gave the clinician permission to consult with their individual therapists, past couple therapists, as well as the psychiatrist who was medicating each of them. Consultations were conducted by phone. A crucial piece of information was that Trevor's individual therapist would be happy to have Trevor see another therapist because he felt stymied, found Trevor a poor therapy patient, and was defensive because of fear of a catastrophic outcome and lawsuit. The psychiatrist did not share this view, but she agreed that Trevor was not making progress in individual therapy.

The individual session with Alicia focused on her sense of being stuck in life. At 31 years of age, her career was stalled because she could not move to another city, her marriage was unsatisfying, they had not been sexual in 4 years, and the hopes and dreams she had when they met were shattered. Alicia wanted their marriage to succeed, but was not optimistic.

Alicia's childhood sexual trauma involved an incestuous relationship with her first stepfather that occurred over a 4-year period, between ages 7 and 11. Alicia's parents separated before she was born; the marriage was a result of an unplanned pregnancy. Alicia never doubted that her mother wanted and loved her. She grew up in a caring extended family with grandparents, aunts, uncles, and cousins. She was her mother's only biological child, although there were stepsiblings from each of her mother's three subsequent marriages. A stepsister from the second stepfather was an important person in Alicia's life. Her mother's present husband was viewed as a decent man, but Alicia felt that her mother had "settled."

The focus of Alicia's individual therapy had been on her incestuous relationship and her growing up in a chaotic home. The incestuous behavior did not involve intercourse or physical force. Alicia no longer blamed herself or her mother. Alicia's anger was in perspective and she felt like a survivor. As an adolescent and young adult, Alicia had been sexually functional, but felt great ambivalence about sexuality. She felt best about sex in her first 6 months with Trevor, but was disillusioned and depressed by the nonsexual state of their relationship that began almost a year before marriage. Alicia argued with herself as to whether this was Trevor's or her fault, or if they simply had a bad marriage. She desperately wanted children, a strong motivator to resolve the problem. Alicia had no secrets about the past. She did have a present secret: she masturbated once a month while fantasizing about other men. On reflection, she agreed that this was normal, and left it to the clinician's judgment whether and how to share this information.

Trevor's history taking turned into three sessions. There were a number of sensitive and secret issues regarding the past and present, most of which he had not discussed with his individual therapist. The biggest secret from the past was that as an adolescent and young adult, more than 20 men had fellated Trevor to orgasm. For a significant number, the scenario involved Trevor spanking them with his hand or a paddle while being fellated. He received a substantial sum of money that was used for tuition and books. This was a shameful secret Trevor had shared with no one prior to this session even though he had previously seen five therapists and two psychiatrists. Trevor was not worried regarding his sexual orientation because he felt no emotional attraction toward men, nor did he desire physical contact other than being fellated. The legacy left was a strong feeling of shame and avoidance of oral sex with Alicia.

Another secret was that Trevor masturbated once or twice daily. Rather than having inhibited sexual desire, which was what Alicia complained about, Trevor was inhibited specifically about partner sex. He used video material with a focus on women orally stimulating men, and he experienced a special erotic charge from viewing the man standing before a kneeling woman and ejaculating on her face. A sensitive issue was that Trevor worried about his ability to ejaculate intravaginally and impregnate Alicia. He had never discussed this with her. Trevor had not heard of the term "ejaculatory inhibition"; he was given bibliotherapy on ejaculatory inhibition, healthy use of sexual fantasy, and oral sexuality (McCarthy & McCarthy, 1998b). In two subsequent individual sessions, the therapist explored Trevor's misuse of individual therapy, his reluctance to share secrets with Alicia, fear of her reactions, and most importantly how motivated he was to revitalize the couple's sexuality and have children.

The feedback session was scheduled as a double session. Alicia agreed to be the note taker. A major function of the feedback session was to construct a narrative that helped the couple to understand the problem in a new way and motivate them to view this as resolvable. The word "secret" was not used, but instead the therapist talked of "vulnerabilities" and "inhibitions." The format used in the feedback session was followed throughout treatment, speaking of the "distant past" before they met, "their past" and how sexual communication and functioning had deteriorated, and "the present" regarding what each needed to do individually and as a couple to confront sexual avoidance and develop a comfortable, functional couple sexual style.

A crucial issue in understanding the distant past was to acknowledge that their abusive experiences were quite different and that they had dealt with them quite differently. Alicia's ability to resolve the incestuous abuse was acknowledged; Alicia wanted Trevor to see her as a survivor. Trevor's experiences of being manipulated and used sexually (even though he was given money and had orgasms) were clearly abusive. This description was relieving for Trevor and increased Alicia's awareness of Trevor's vulnerabilities. She was an empathic, not blaming, partner. Understanding vulnerabilities from childhood abuse and how these were different for each person was the basis for therapeutic interventions.

Knowing that each masturbated and was sexually functional was a good prognostic sign. The challenge was to integrate sexuality into personal self-esteem and develop a healthy couple sexual style. Each person had to challenge a "trap." Trevor's was to isolate sexuality into a rigid, secret dimension and avoid intimate sexuality. Alicia's was to feel hopeless and to switch from self-blame to partner blame. After this feedback, they were given the choice of whether to engage in an initial sexual exercise. Alicia took the initiative and said yes. The first exercise was to discuss how to build trust and develop a "trust–vulnerability" position (McCarthy & McCarthy, 2002).

The format of therapy sessions was first to explore attitudes, behaviors, and feelings generated from the previous week's exercises, then integrate attitudes and experiences (including child sexual abuse) from the distant and couple past with present feelings and experiences, and most importantly discuss exercises and challenges during the next week. An example during the sixth treatment session involved processing an exercise where Trevor intermixed manual and oral stimulation of Alicia to orgasm. When she tried to pleasure him, Trevor became quite anxious. A therapeutic theme was to reinforce positive learning and experiences. Alicia noted how involved and erotic Trevor had been and her belief that they would succeed sexually. Alicia noted how different this was from abusive sexuality; she wanted pleasuring to be a mutual experience. Trevor was pleased with his successful confrontation of inhibitions about giving oral sex, but pessimistic about his ability to receive pleasure and to overcome ejaculatory inhibition. His masturbation had decreased to once or twice a week when feeling desirous, not as a compulsive behavior tied to anxiety reduction and mood control. Still, Trevor was feeling pushed beyond his capability to change.

A key therapeutic strategy was to urge Trevor to confront his challenge, but not to coerce him to do a specific behavior (the latter is what happens in abuse). Trevor was comfortable with Alicia's nongenital touch, but terrified that she would try to stimulate him orally. In designing an individualized exercise, a clear prohibition was put on Alicia giving oral sex. This restriction allowed Trevor to be receptive to her stimulation. The therapist suggested that Trevor use self-stimulation during couple exchanges, and Alicia agreed to this. Although he chose not to use this technique, Trevor's rigidity regarding compartmentalized sex was gradually reduced. For the first time ever, he was orgasmic with Alicia's manual stimulation. This was a major breakthrough. At the following session, Trevor shared his fear about ejaculatory inhibition during intercourse. In a highly emotional interchange, Alicia told him how much she wanted the marriage and to have his child. Trevor genuinely shared the goal of a successful marriage and children, but feared he could not perform sexually and that Alicia would abandon him. Trevor was not a crier, but there were tears in his eyes. Alicia felt a deep understanding of Trevor and a belief in them as a couple that was as strong as her belief that she deserved to be a survivor. The therapist raised the alternative of using insemination with Trevor's sperm for conception. Realizing that this was an option dramatically reduced Trevor's fears.

In subsequent exercises, Alicia initiated the transition to intercourse at high levels of arousal. They utilized multiple forms of stimulation during intercourse, which facilitated arousal and ejaculation. A dramatic breakthrough occurred when Trevor asked Alicia to kiss his penis. Emotionally and erotically he became receptive and responsive to giving and receiving stimulation, including oral sex.

CONSOLIDATING THERAPEUTIC GAINS AND RELAPSE PREVENTION

Relapse prevention is an integral component of couple sex therapy, especially for inhibited sexual desire (McCarthy, 1999). The most important technique for Alicia and Trevor was to maintain a regular rhythm of sexual contact and not revert to avoidance. Guidelines presented in Table 14.1 are given to a couple early in therapy, referenced throughout therapy, and serve as the basis of relapse prevention.

When one or both partners have a history of child sexual abuse, an active program of relapse prevention is crucial. The naive hope that the couple can treat sexuality with benign neglect is self-defeating. Relapse prevention is an active process of generalizing and reinforcing positive sexual attitudes, feelings, and experiences. Each partner becomes aware of vulnerabilities and "traps." They are committed to maintaining sexuality as a positive relationship resource. In a healthy relationship, sexuality is not allowed to be secretive, guilt inducing, coercive, a symbol of shame, or a performance. Each partner owns his or her sexuality, and sexuality enhances the couple's emotional intimacy. The clinician helps the couple to develop an individualized relapse prevention program.

TABLE 14.1. Guidelines for Revitalizing and Maintaining Sexual Desire

1. The essential keys to sexual desire are positive anticipation and believing that you deserve sexual pleasure.
2. Change involves a combination of personal responsibility and being an intimate team. Each person is responsible for his or her own sexual desire, with the couple functioning as an intimate team to nurture and enhance desire. Revitalizing desire is a couple task. Guilt, blame, and pressure subvert the change process.
3. Inhibited desire is the most common sexual dysfunction, affecting two in five couples. Sexual avoidance drains intimacy and vitality from the couple's bond.
4. One in five married couples has a nonsexual relationship (being sexual less than 10 times a year). One in three nonmarried couples who have been together longer than 2 years have a nonsexual relationship.
5. The average frequency of sexual intercourse is between 4 times a week to once every 2 weeks. For couples in their twenties, the average sexual frequency is 2 to 3 times a week; for couples in their 50s, once a week.
6. The initial romantic-love or passionate-sex type of desire lasts less than 2 years and usually less than 6 months. Desire is facilitated by an intimate, interactive relationship.
7. Contrary to the myth that "horniness" occurs after not being sexual for a long time, desire is facilitated by a regular rhythm of sexual activity. When sex occurs less than twice a month, couples become self-conscious and fall into a cycle of anticipatory anxiety, tense and unsatisfying sex, and avoidance.
8. A key strategy is to develop "her," "his," and "our" bridges to sexual desire. This involves ways of thinking, talking, anticipating, and feeling which invite sexual encounters.
9. The essence of sexuality is giving and receiving pleasure-oriented touching. The prescription to maintaining desire is integrating intimacy, pleasuring, and eroticism.
10. Touching should occur both inside and outside the bedroom and be valued for itself. Both partners should be comfortable initiating touch. Touching should not always lead to intercourse. Both partners should feel free to say "no" and to suggest an alternative way to connect and share pleasure.
11. Couples who maintain a vital sexual relationship can use the metaphor of touching involving "five gears." First gear is clothes on, affectionate touch (holding hands, kissing, hugging). Second gear is nongenital, sensual touch that can be clothed, semiclothed, or nude (body massage, cuddling on the couch, showering together, touching while going to sleep or upon awakening). Third gear is playful touch that intermixes genital and nongenital touching; this can be in bed, dancing, or on the couch—clothed or unclothed. Fourth gear is erotic touch (manual, oral, or rubbing) to high arousal and orgasm for one or both partners. Fifth gear integrates pleasurable and erotic touch that flows into intercourse.
12. Personal turn-ons facilitate sexual anticipation and desire. These include the use of fantasy and erotic scenarios, as well as sex associated with special celebrations or anniversaries, sex with the goal of conception, sex when feeling caring and close, or sex to sooth a personal disappointment.

(continued)

TABLE 14.1 *continued*

13. External turn-ons (R- or X-rated videos, music, candles, sexy clothing, visual feedback from mirrors, locations other than the bedroom, a weekend away without the kids) can elicit sexual desire.
14. Women with hormonal deficits may use testosterone injections, patches, or creams to enhance sexual desire, but only under medical supervision. Medical problems and side-effects of medication can interfere with sexual desire and function.
15. Sexuality has a number of positive functions—a shared pleasure, a means to reinforce and deepen intimacy, and a tension reducer to deal with the stresses of life and the couple's relationship.
16. "Intimate coercion" is not acceptable. Sexuality is neither a reward nor a punishment. Healthy sexuality is voluntary, mutual, and pleasure oriented.
17. Realistic expectations are crucial for maintaining a healthy sexual relationship. It is self-defeating to demand equal desire, arousal, orgasm and satisfaction each time. A positive, realistic expectation is that 40–50% of experiences are very good for both people; 20–25% are very good for one (usually the man) and fine for the other; 20–25% are acceptable but not remarkable. About 5–15% of sexual experiences are mediocre, dissatisfying, or failures. Couples who accept this without guilt or blaming and try again when they are receptive and responsive will have a vital, resilient sexual relationship. Satisfied couples use the guideline of "good enough" sex.
18. If the couple has gone 2 weeks without any sexual contact, the partner with higher desire should take the initiative to set up a planned or spontaneous sexual date. If that does not occur, the other partner should initiate a sensual or play date during the following week. If that does not occur and they have gone a month without sexual contact, they should schedule a "booster" therapy session.
19. Healthy sexual desire plays a positive, integral role in a relationship with the main function to energize the bond and generate special feelings. Paradoxically, bad or nonexistent sex plays a more powerful negative role in a relationship than the positive role of good sex.

VALUE AND PROBLEMS WITH SELF-HELP AND POPULAR PROGRAMS

There are a number of books, articles, talk shows, and self-help groups focused on recovery from child sexual abuse and trauma. The prime thrusts of these approaches are to increase awareness and confront the traumatic history. These approaches have value in confronting secrecy and shame, feeling support for sharing one's story, removing stigma, and realizing that one is not alone. Unfortunately, trauma programs do not focus on couple issues, especially not on sexual function and dysfunction.

McCarthy (1992) argued that "the pendulum has swung too far" from denial of child sexual abuse to treating it as the prime component of adult self-definition. In conceptualizing, assessing, and treating adults with a history of childhood sexual trauma, past experiences are addressed in an empathic, respectful manner. It is crucial that the person not feel revictimized or blamed by their partner or while in therapy. The central concept, psychologically and sexually, is to be a "survivor" with couple therapy promoting being "partners in healing." The person develops his or her own voice and experiences the relationship as respectful, trusting, and intimate, which facilitates psychological healing and growth. Once individuals are able to experience desire, arousal, orgasm, and emotional satisfaction, they have taken back responsibility for their sexuality. Sexuality is viewed as voluntary and mutual. In choosing people and resources (including self-help and therapeutic resources), the survivor should use those which promote healing and growth. This approach is individualized, dependent on the person and couple rather than a rigid formula.

Trauma-based therapies, whether conducted individually or in a group, can enhance awareness and decrease stigma and isolation. Unfortunately, for some people this is iatrogenic by reinforcing the "angry victim" role or focusing on the past at the expense of the couple's functioning. Discriminating what is therapeutic and what is iatrogenic is especially crucial for self-help approaches (McCarthy, 1997). The modal response to self-help readings and groups is increased awareness, expression of feelings, support, and increased acceptance about past abuse. However, the emphasis on the past and expressing negative feelings can be immobilizing. There is little focus on the present or experiencing positive emotions. Sexuality, building trust, and relationship intimacy are ignored. The victim advocacy approach is fatally flawed for couple therapy (Maddock, Larson, & Schnarch, 1998).

SUMMARY

Understanding, assessing, and treating couples where one or both partners has a history of childhood sexual abuse is challenging. There is not a widely accepted or empirically validated clinical protocol. There is a dearth of data, especially treatment outcome data. The primary question is whether to focus on the past sexual trauma or on the present relationship. The authors advocate focusing on the couple's emotional and sexual relationship, with the caveat of respecting individual differences. The second question is whether individual, group, or couple therapy is the treatment of choice. The authors advocate couple therapy with a focus on these concepts: "Be a survivor and not a victim," "Be partners in healing," and "Living well is the best revenge."

Understanding and confronting the sexual abuse history is motivated by a focus on empowering the person to think, act, and feel like a
survivor and experience sexuality in a manner which enhances one's individual life and intimate relationship. In confronting the past, the couple bonds of respect, trust, and intimacy grow in strength and security.
Sexuality is experienced as voluntary, pleasure-oriented, and mutual. If
one partner vetoes a specific sexual behavior, their partner honors this.
Rather than sexuality being the "shameful secret" of abuse, it is experienced as a positive, integral component of the couple's relationship.

REFERENCES

Bartoi, M., & Kinder, B. (1998). The effects of child and adult sexual abuse on
adult sexuality. *Journal of Sex and Marital Therapy, 24,* 75–90.

Bass, E., & Davis, L. (1988). *The courage to heal.* New York: Harper & Row.

Compton, J., & Follette, V. (1998). Couples surviving trauma. In V. Follette, J.
Ruzek, & F. Abueg (Eds.), *Cognitive-behavioral therapies for trauma* (pp.
321–352). New York: Guilford Press.

Courtois, C. (2000). The aftermath of child sexual abuse. In L. Szuchman & F.
Muscarella (Eds.), *Psychological perspectives on human sexuality* (pp. 549–572).
New York: Wiley.

Follette, V., & Pistorello, J. (1995). Couples therapy: When one partner has
been abused. In C. Classen (Ed.), *Treating women molested in childhood* (pp.
129–161). San Francisco: Jossey-Bass.

Haugaard, J. (2000). The challenge of defining child sexual abuse. *American Psychologist, 55,* 1036–1039.

Knapp, S., & Van De Creek, L. (2000). Recovered memories of childhood
abuse: Is there an underlying professional consensus? *Professional Psychology, 31,* 365–371.

Maddock, J., & Larson, N. (1995). *Incestuous families.* New York: Norton.

Maddock, J., Larson, N., & Schnarch, D. (1998). *Beyond victimhood.* Workshop
presented at the Family Therapy Networker conference, Washington, DC.

Maltz, W. (2001). *The sexual healing journey.* New York: Harper Collins.

McCarthy, B. (1986). A cognitive-behavioral approach to understanding and
treating sexual trauma. *Journal of Sex and Marital Therapy, 12,* 15–19.

McCarthy, B. (1990). Treating sexual dysfunction associated with prior sexual
trauma. *Journal of Sex and Marital Therapy, 16,* 142–146.

McCarthy, B. (1992). Sexual trauma. *Journal of Sex Education and Therapy, 18,*
1–10.

McCarthy, B. (1995). Sexual trauma and adult sexual desire. In R. R. Rosen & S.
C. Leiblum (Eds.), *Case studies in sex therapy* (pp. 148–160). New York: Guilford Press.

McCarthy, B. (1997). Therapeutic and iatrogenic interventions with adults who
were sexually abused as children. *Journal of Sex and Marital Therapy, 23,*
118–125.

McCarthy, B. (1999). Relapse prevention strategies and techniques for inhibited sexual desire. *Journal of Sex and Marital Therapy, 25,* 297–303.

McCarthy, B. (2002). Sexuality, sex therapy, and couple therapy. In A. S. Gurman & N. S. Jacobson (Eds.), *Clinical handbook of couple therapy* (3rd ed., pp. 629–652). New York: Guilford Press.

McCarthy, B., & McCarthy, E. (1993). *Confronting the victim role.* New York: Carroll & Graf.

McCarthy, B., & McCarthy, E. (1998a). *Couple sexual awareness.* New York: Carroll & Graf.

McCarthy, B., & McCarthy, E. (1998b). *Male sexual awareness.* New York: Carroll & Graf.

McCarthy, B., & McCarthy, E. (2002). *Sexual awareness.* New York: Carroll & Graf.

Meichenbaum, D. (1994). *A clinical handbook/practical therapist manual.* Waterloo, Canada: Institute Press.

Rind, B., Tromovitch, D, & Bauserman, R. (1998). A meta-analytic examination of assumed properties of child sexual abuse using college samples. *Psychological Bulletin, 124,* 22–53.

Saywitz, K., Mannarino, A., Berliner, L., & Cohen, J. (2000). Treatment for sexually abused children and adolescents. *American Psychologist, 55,* 1040–1049.

Trepper, T., & Barrett, M. (1986). *Treating incest.* New York: Haworth Press.

CHAPTER 15

Physical Illness

GAIL P. OSTERMAN
TAMARA G. SHER
GWEN HALES
W. JEFFREY CANAR
REEMA SINGLA
TRACY TILTON

Nick and Anita have been together for 10 years. They share three children ranging in age from 8 to 2. Nick is 42 years old and Anita is 45. Nick is the primary breadwinner. Upon the birth of their first child, they agreed that Anita would stay home to take care of the children and the house. This arrangement worked well for the couple although finances were always a stressor. Several weeks ago, Nick was diagnosed with severe viral cardiomyopathy following a few-week period of extreme fatigue. Within a 24-hour period, Nick went from believing that the symptoms were related to the flu to being placed in an intensive care unit (ICU) and awaiting a heart transplant. Both Nick and Anita understand that a transplant is Nick's only chance for survival and that people often die waiting for an available heart. They also understand that even if a heart were found and a transplant conducted, there could be numerous postsurgery complications that could prove fatal at any time.

The issues confronting Nick and Anita are numerous and affect many levels of their lives, their independence, and their relationship. For example, individually and as a couple they will need to decide if and when Anita should return to work and for what reasons (e.g., salary, benefits). Additionally, they will need to decide the best way for the two of them to make medical decisions for Nick. These decisions include deciding who will be present at doctors' appointments, what information is needed to make decisions, whose decision it is ultimately if the two of them disagree, and what plans they need to make legally (e.g., living will, advance directives, durable power of attorney). Nick and Anita may need assistance in figuring out logistics such as new childcare arrangements, or making their home accessible for a wheelchair. Finally, they may need somewhere to turn for what we think of as general psychological attention. Each or both could need help with concomitant depression, anxiety, or grief. As a couple, they will face old relationship issues never resolved that tend to resurface at times of stress as well as new relationship issues emerging as a result of the medical crisis. Finally, they may seek social support that perhaps they will not receive from their friends who have not yet experienced chronic illness—but will. Couple therapy in the face of an illness can address any or all of these concerns for the patient, his or her partner, or both.

Although the medical community often views illness in a patient as an individual issue, a couple approach to illness is gaining attention in both clinical and research settings. This couple-based approach assumes that an illness affects not just the patient but those in the patient's immediate environment as well. Although couples tend to respond to an event such as a chronic illness as an interpersonal unit rather than as individuals in isolation (Lavery & Clarke, 1999), there is little information available to help us predict how a patient, his or her partner, and the relationship will respond to an illness.

COUPLES AND ILLNESS

There are many factors affecting how a couple approaches, copes with, and survives a medical crisis. These issues are both illness related—such as the severity, type and chronicity of the illness—and patient related— such as the gender, ethnicity, and age of the patient. Although there is a growing literature concluding that there are health advantages to being in a committed relationship or marriage (see Kiecolt-Glaser & Newton, 2001, and Schmaling & Sher, 1997, for reviews), this topic is beyond the scope of this chapter. Instead, we take a clinical approach to working with couples in which one or both people are medically ill and the ramifications for the patient, the partner, and the relationship of such an approach.

First, illness-related concepts are discussed, such as issues that surround the diagnosis of a medical illness, its chronicity, and specific ways to assess and intervene with a couple around the illness, especially as they relate to communication. Second, working with individual differences both between and within couples is addressed. Third, role changes for both the patient and partner in light of the illness are discussed. We provide clinical examples illustrating these concepts from both the literature and our own work with couples and illness. Finally, we return to Nick and Anita for a discussion of their treatment in light of these issues.

ILLNESS-RELATED ISSUES AND CONCERNS

Diagnosis of an Acute or Chronic Medical Illness

Although the health-enhancing properties of personal relationships have been well documented (Kiecolt-Glaser & Newton, 2001), the toll that an illness takes on relationships is less well known. The first issue facing couples, and often unknown at the onset, is whether an illness is acute or will take on a chronic course. This information will affect the economic and social cost of the illness, and how a couple's resources are allocated around it. Although several studies have examined the role of chronic illness for patients and their partners, few studies thus far have detailed the effects of acute illness on couples. Acute illnesses are often accompanied by a psychological crisis in most patients, whereby "the usual patterns of coping are blocked or useless" (Powell & Lively, as cited in Hart, Reese, & Fearing, 1981, p. 341). The illness may be perceived as a threat to the individual's self-esteem or significant relationships, thereby generating feelings of anxiety and helplessness. There are several reports that wives tend to report higher incidences of stress during the initial stages of an illness than their husbands, even when the husband is the patient (e.g., Ptacek, Pierce, Ptacek, & Nogel, 1999). Other investigations have found that when dealing with an acute illness, communication style generally predicts recovery. For example, in a study investigating the relationship between the articulation of subjective impairment and the course of illness in patients with hepatitis A, results indicated that patients initially expressing depressed mood had a more favorable course of illness, in that they needed a significantly shorter period of time for recovery than patients not expressing complaints about their situation (Rose, Scholler, Jorres, Danzer, & Klapp, 2000). The authors contend that articulating a depressed mood is an indication that patients are accepting of the sick role and that they have the capacity to adjust to their new situation.

Conversely, couples facing a chronic illness often need to brace themselves and mobilize their resources for upheaval over the long course. It is these couples in particular that this chapter targets. It is for these couples that old patterns of relating, communicating, dividing roles, and associated behaviors will be called into question, reorganized, or found to be an additional stressor on an already overtaxed system. It is for these couples that a couple-based approach to illness is particularly suited and an often necessary component of their medical care.

Patients and Couples Facing Terminal Illness

Couples in which one member is diagnosed with a terminal illness present a unique set of challenges to the clinician. Dealing with the individual who has the terminal illness is not a new issue for therapists, and several books have been written on this topic. However, little has been written about dealing with this from a couple's perspective.

In addition to their illness, a patient who is dying must confront several relationship issues. Spencer et al. (1999) identified several concerns in a sample of breast cancer patients. The cost associated with treatment and the subsequent financial burden that is placed on the surviving partner can engender a sense of guilt in the dying patient. Similarly, couples enter into a relationship anticipating that they will be life partners. When one is diagnosed with a terminal illness, it can lead to a sense of loss and grief because of lost time with the partner. If there are children in the family, the sense of loss felt at not seeing the children grow up may need to be addressed.

Both patients and their partners can show high levels of emotional disturbance when one member is facing death. As many as half of such patients have either depression or anxiety (Stedeford, 1981a); the partners of patients with a terminal illness also have been found to demonstrate symptoms of depression, anxiety, or anger as well as physical symptoms (Willert, Beckwith, Holm, & Beckwith, 1995). In many cases, partners are also acting as the primary caregiver for the patient, and the level of caregiver burden is associated with depression and preloss traumatic grief (Beery et al., 1997). That is, other than issues associated with dying, comorbid psychopathology in the patient and partner should be addressed through conventional means because it can seriously complicate the clinical picture (Schoevers et al., 2000).

INTERVENTION AND COMMUNICATION

Couples with acute, chronic, or terminal illnesses are not of one type. Throughout our own research and work with couples, we have emphasized the importance of not assuming that all couples with illness want or need the same type of intervention. As is the case with many current therapies with couples (e.g., cognitive-behavioral couple therapy), our work emphasizes giving couples tools to help them figure out what they want and need from each other. Although some patients may want to talk about their worries, fears, or related feelings, others may opt not to engage in such discussions. Similarly, although some partners might want to be as involved as possible in the medical details of the illness, others would prefer to stay more removed. Unlike work with an individual patient, any intervention with a couple requires not just understanding intercouple differences, but intracouple differences as well.

As a result, the importance of communicating needs, desires, and expectations is emphasized early on in working with couples with illness. The importance of communication style has been well documented within the cardiac literature but can be used as an example for many types of couples facing different types of diseases, both acute and chronic. For example, it has been demonstrated that open communication between male heart attack patients and their nonpatient wives resulted in wives reporting less difficulty with empathizing, an increased sense of being part of a "team," and less anxiety about the responsibility of their husbands' care than wives who reported problems with empathizing because of their husbands' uncommunicativeness (Bramwell, 1986). Similarly, Coyne and Smith (1991) addressed the issue of wives' distress when coping with their husband's myocardial infarction (MI). They found that 6 months post-MI, partners were as psychologically distressed as patients, and the associations between this distress and the quality of the marriage and the nature of their contact with the medical system were strong. Interestingly, partners' protective buffering of patients had a positive relation with their own distress; that is, those partners providing more protection for the patients evidenced the most distress.

Conversely, a related study examined the role of overprotectiveness in couples coping with MI (Fiske, Coyne, & Smith, 1991). Couples were surveyed in the areas of spousal hostility, spousal overprotectiveness, patient and spousal psychological distress, patient self-efficacy, patient functional disability, partner burden, discussions about the heart attack, and changes in closeness. Overprotectiveness was related to the couples becoming closer post-MI, whereas hostility was related to the couples becoming more distant and having fewer useful discussions about coping post-MI.

In our own work with cardiac patients, we have had many discussions with couples about the role that protectiveness plays in their relationship once one of them has been diagnosed as a "heart patient."

Again, differences among and within couples emerged. For some patients, being taken care of was welcomed and appreciated. As one patient stated, "I have always been the one taking care of others. It feels good to be taken care of for a change." Others have the opposite reaction. One patient told us, "I am becoming very resentful of the amount of time my husband spends checking up on me. I feel like I have no independence anymore, and I feel like a child." The same partner behaviors were being described by these two patients, but with very different responses that perhaps could not have been anticipated or even understood by the partner without attention focused on it. Hence, teaching techniques such as interactive problem solving (see Epstein & Baucom, 2002, for a review) can help patients and partners specify the problem and chart a behavioral course for addressing it.

We have also worked with couples with heart disease where the partner was angry with the patient for the illness. Although typically not expressed at the time of diagnosis, over the course of therapy it was revealed that the partner blamed the patient for their disease. This often takes of the form of statements such as, "I have been telling you for years to lose weight (or exercise or stop smoking) and you haven't. You did this to us and I am furious with you because of it." The strength of this assertion and its accompanying emotion are often a surprise for both the patient and their partner. It is our experience that emotional expressiveness training (EET; see Epstein & Baucom, 2002, for a summary) helps both people uncover, understand, and respond to the feelings of the partner. Here, solving a particular problem is not the goal of the communication. Instead, having patients and partners learn to express their own and listen to the other's feelings is tantamount.

As with other categories of illness, communication is often an important issue to address with couples facing terminal illness. Studies have shown that partners and their terminally ill loved ones often show very poor communication, characterized by denial and silence. In one study, 80 caregivers, most of whom were partners, were asked about the communication between themselves and their partner during their terminal illness. Most reported never having discussed the inevitability of death or the conclusion of their relationship. Only one caregiver out of 80 reported that they and their partner had been fully able to discuss and deal with the patient's impending death (Beach, 1995). For both partners and patients, the desire for open communication conflicts with the wish to protect both themselves and their loved ones from pain (Stedeford, 1981b).

Additionally, it has been suggested that the therapist working with terminal illness issues needs to help the patient understand and accept his or her own mortality and work to maximize the patient's quality of life to the time of death—or "to die in a state of psychological well-being" (Richman, 1995). The therapist also needs to help the couple such that both the partner and patient can work together in meeting their own needs as well as the needs of the other. This might include using emotional expressiveness training to help both partners express their fears, concerns, and desires about the dying process and helping each to express how much or how little they would like to focus on life after death for the surviving partner.

Finally, the therapist can use problem-solving exercises to help the partner prepare for and adapt to the loss and subsequent role changes that result when their loved one dies. Some issues that may develop are more logistical, such as patient care needs if the partner is away, managing family finances to pay for patient care costs, and planning for changes in responsibility after the patient has died. Other issues can be considered more psychological such as depression, anxiety, anger, or grief for both patient and partner. These are not mutually exclusive, but interrelated. For example, a well partner who is depressed may not have the physical or emotional energy to participate in financial planning, even though the well partner's financial situation demands attention. Also as death nears, therapists can be very helpful in helping partners say goodbye (Counselman, 1997). Therefore, it is important to consider and structure interventions for the patient, partner, and couple, anticipating both premortem and postmortem needs.

ILLNESS AND INDIVIDUAL DIFFERENCES

Our approach to working with couples assumes that couples differ in what they need, what they want, and what resources they have with which to work. However, couples also differ in who they are and what they bring to their relationship. Some of these individual differences relate to personality and demographics.

There is a growing body of literature focusing on personality style as it relates to how much medical information is sought during an illness and ways to determine the style of any patient or partner. Information-seeking style refers to a person's willingness to seek out and process information. The information-seeking style can affect how satisfied an individual is with the information they receive regarding their health. Two separate types of information seekers have been identified: "monitors" and "blunters" (Miller, 1987). This distinction is based on the difference between vigilance in the monitors, and avoidance in the blunters with regard to potentially threatening information. Monitoring is characterized as a confrontive coping style. More specifically, individuals with a monitoring style characteristically look for threat-relevant information. The opposite is true of blunters, who typically avoid threat-relevant information. The Monitoring and Blunting Style Scale (Miller, 1987) has been developed as an empirically-validated measure of the construct. In addition, the Threatening Medical Situations Inventory was created as a dispositional monitoring–blunting inventory, which refers to threatening medical situations only (Van Zuuren & Hanewald, 1993).

In our own clinical work, we view the role of the therapist, in part, as that of a coach in helping the patient and their partner learn about and ask for what they want or need in terms of their relationship and how it interfaces with the medical community. For example, we have helped couples learn that a husband may not want a lot of detailed information from his doctor about his chronic heart disease. He may prefer that the doctor tell him what to do to take care of himself and then do it (blunter). On the other hand, his wife, more of an information seeker (monitor), may want a lot of detailed information about how and why her husband's symptoms were occurring and why certain therapies were preferred over others. As a result of this divergent style, the couple gets frustrated with each other: He resents her continual questions and she resents what she perceives as his "withholding of information" and general "lack of intelligence" regarding his disease. Therapy for a couple like this consists of learning about these styles and then developing a plan to ease the stress each partner feels. For a couple similar to the one described here, problem solving may be used to figure out who will attend doctors' appointments and make the logistical plans around the medical directives (e.g., buying the medications, making ancillary appointments, doing the paperwork for insurance, and so forth). Although formal assessment of monitoring style might not be conducted, emotional expressiveness training (Epstein & Baucom, 2002) can be used to help each partner understand the frustrations of the other and the preferences each has for his or her own approach and why.

Of course, there are many other patient, partner, or couple-related factors that can affect the response to an illness and its course. These include gender, cultural background, stage of life, and time since diagnosis, although research in these areas has historically been thin and equivocal. For example, it has been found that women tend to report greater distress and marital dissatisfaction following a diagnosis of an illness, regardless of whether they are the patient or the partner (Morse & Fife, 1998; Northouse, Mood, Templin, Mellon, & George, 2000). However, it has also been found in a study of cardiovascular disease, that women who are patients do not appear to change their lifestyle significantly in response to chronic cardiovascular disease (Badger, 1992). Although the sample size in this latter study was small, the results highlight the need for caution in interpreting gender-based differences in response to illness or specific gender-based interventions.

By comparison, research on differences among cultures is more robust. There are differences in how couples of diverse cultural backgrounds face illness, and therefore in what kinds of help these couples may find most useful. Clinicians need to be aware of the need for bilingual services, the importance that spirituality and faith play for certain cultures, and how culturally isolated some patients from minority cultures feel in hospital and hospice settings (Talamantes, Lawler, & Espino, 1995). Additionally, people's concept of health care, where it should be based (e.g., at home versus in a hospital), and by whom it should be delivered can influence a clinician's progress with a couple. For instance, Chinese patients often subscribe to a concept of family-based health care, where the family on behalf of the patient makes decisions, which is unfamiliar to Western clinicians (Tong & Spicer, 1994). With such couples, the openness and honesty that Western psychotherapists value may not be appropriate goals (Brotzman & Butler, 1991).

The couple's age and stage of life at time of diagnosis can play a role in how they cope with the illness as a couple. Younger patients tend to have greater difficulty adapting to diagnosis and the changing caretaking responsibilities (Payne, 1992), experience more stress due to the illness occurring "off-time" in the normative life cycle (Revenson, 1990), and become more dependent on extended family, interrupting their efforts at individuation and forging a family unit of their own (Sherman & Simonton, 1999). Younger couples also tend to become more isolated in their illnesses compared to older couples because they have trouble finding other couples in their same age range to share the experience (Rolland, 1994). If these couples have young children, child-related concerns add an additional burden to the coping process. On the other hand, couples in midlife facing illness face different issues. Partners whose energies have previously focused on parenting and family life may feel empowered by the additional duties required of having an ill partner. Similarly, it has been found that a partner previously devoted largely to career may feel open to the chance to spend more time in a nurturing family role when confronted with illness in a partner (Sherman & Simonton, 1999). People struggling to adapt to an empty nest following the departure of their children may be relieved to be back in the familiar role of caretaking, or they may feel particularly resentful. Although older couples appear to adapt more easily to the diagnosis of an illness, plans for retirement may need to be set aside (Power, Hershenson, & Schlossberg, 1991).

Finally, time since diagnosis has been thought to play a role in a person's or couple's adjustment to illness. Again, the evidence is equivocal. Wenzel, Berkowitz, Robinson, Bernstein, and Goldstein (1992) sought to examine various psychosocial stressors following the diagnosis and treatment of gestational trophoblastic disease, a cancerous growth of cells diagnosed during pregnancy. The authors found that there were no significant differences in reported mood disturbance, marital satisfaction, or sexual functioning from diagnosis to less than 1 year, 1–2 years, or 3–5 years postdiagnosis. However, despite the fact that time with a disease may not play a role in adjustment, a recurrence of a disease can have considerable effects. A recurrence of a disease may cause greater distress than an initial diagnosis. For example, Silberfarb, Maurer, and Crouthamel (1978) found that women in the recurrent phase of breast cancer illness reported significantly more psychological distress than women in either their primary treatment or in their final or palliative treatment. Interestingly, disturbance in the partner role was the most common problem reported in the recurrent phase of treatment, and this was most stressful during the first recurrence. In addition, women in the recurrent group had more problems with social isolation, role disruption, and sexual difficulties than women in the primary treatment group. Similarly, patients in the final or palliative stages of treatment reported less depression and anxiety, as well as a lower incidence of social isolation and impairment in daily routine than either the primary or recurrent treatment groups.

For all these differences among couples, we advocate an individual differences approach to both assessment and treatment. That is, instead of planning services to fit a particular group (e.g., women patients, or older patients), we advocate assessing, for each couple and each individual, what personality attributes will interact with the treatment, what needs are most pressing, what resources the couple have available to them, what beliefs each person has surrounding illness or care, and what factors might inhibit the couple from benefiting from the services that are offered. Although we rarely use formal or structured assessment techniques for these purposes, our interviews and interventions are geared toward obtaining this information. We then tailor the intervention to address the needs of each individual and each couple as they are presented.

ROLE CHANGES AND ILLNESS

Adjustment to a chronic illness, and sometimes even to an acute illness, requires a reevaluation of established roles and expectations (Baider &

Kaplan De-Nour, 1998). A serious illness in one partner elicits dramatically altered roles for the other. Old patterns of complementarity (e.g., one arranges social events, the other does the finances; one is the comedian, the other is serious and sensitive) may undergo shifts. For example, in terms of adapting to a chronic illness, concerns about being able to carry out their previously defined roles within and outside the home have been cited as dominant among cancer patients. Among cancer patients especially, patients report worry over their burden on the family and friends, and their abilities to continue in their roles at home, work, and in the community (Mahon, Cella, & Donovan, 1990). Additionally, cancer patients report a loss of pride and self-esteem as their ability to work becomes progressively limited. Physical decline that prevents patients from fulfilling their former duties in the home also leads to frustration and anxiety. Patients of both sexes also lament the loss of domestic roles (Vess, Moreland, Schwebel, & Kraut, 1988).

In response to these changes, the therapist can help the couple negotiate new roles or renegotiate old ones. Again, techniques such as emotional expressiveness training to express and hear feelings regarding partners' roles, and problem solving to help with the behaviors associated with each role, are typically helpful.

Sexual Changes

In addition to social role changes, couples also often experience changes in sexual behavior during and after an illness. These changes include a change in sexual behaviors consistent with a new disability, a decrease in sexual frequency due to fatigue or discomfort, and a distancing in the relationship overall that is also evident in a couple's sexual behavior due to fear, withdrawal, or anxiety. Anxiety surrounding sexual contact has a number of roots (Schover, 1989). In the cancer literature, there is evidence that a couple's sexual relationship is often adversely affected by the cancer experience, especially for breast and testicular cancers (Lavery & Clark, 1999). For example, patients or partners sometimes worry that cancer can be sexually transmitted. After a heart attack or stroke, a common fear is that sex could provoke another cardiovascular episode.

Research and clinical experience suggest that often there are gender differences in how an illness affects the sexual functioning of a couple. For example, many men are socialized to believe that their self-worth is measured by their ability to provide for their families financially and their ability to please their partners sexually. Disease can impact both of these abilities and therefore severely impact the man's feelings of masculinity, worth, or importance in their relationship. Men also are more likely to withdraw emotionally and sexually if they feel ashamed at being dependent on a wife because of their illness. Women, on the other hand, tend to focus more on changes in physical appearance than on sexual performance (Andersen & Jochimsen, 1985; Derogatis & King, 1981, as cited in Schover, 1989; Liss-Levinson, 1982; Schover, Evans, & Von Eschenbach, 1987). Therefore, disfiguring cancers might be more likely to change sexual desire for women, whereas diseases or medications affecting sexual performance (e.g., testicular cancer, heart disease) might be more difficult for men.

In terms of intervention, couples can be encouraged to work out changes in their sexual relationships due to a medical illness. Sex therapy can be offered to patients who feel they are unhappy with the sexual intimacy in their relationship. Therapists can help couples to learn to work around the illness in order to accommodate sexual relationships. Often an attitude change about sex can help a couple to work out their problems. Some couples feel that lovemaking should only be spontaneous. If so, they have no way to cope with pain, fatigue, or medication effects except to wait for a better time. For couples to remain sexually active during an illness, more planning may be necessary than they are accustomed to. For example, a woman on hemodialysis may only have normal energy level on one day out of three, a man with a colostomy may prefer sex at a time of day when his bowels are less active, or a terminally ill cancer patient may have a small "window" of time when pain medications are effective but drowsiness has not set it (Schover, 1989).

Couples can be taught to communicate around sexual needs and wants and can be given the tools to engage in such discussions. One client with multiple sclerosis poignantly noted the following to her husband in a conjoint session:

> "I have to decide every day whether to wash the dishes or make love to you. On some days, the dishes may be more important. On others, you are, but nobody can make that decision for me."

For this couple, the wife's willingness to communicate such feelings was the first step toward problem solving around sexual issues. The next step involved helping the couple figure out how to get both of their needs met without resentment or hurt feelings.

Caregiver Burden

In addressing roles and role changes in the face of a chronic illness, it is important to consider the burden imposed on the partner in their new role as caregiver. Whetten-Goldstein, Sloan, Kulas, Cutson, and

Schenkman (1997) examined the burden of Parkinson's disease. They estimated that of the patients who received informal care, the caregiver, usually the partner, provided an average of 22 hours of care per week. In addition to direct caregiving duties, partners of patients who were previously stay-at-home parents often have to return to work and become primary wage earners in the face of an illness; alternatively, other wage-earner caregivers may need to reduce their work hours in order to accommodate caretaking demands.

This care comes at both a physical and emotional cost for the caregiver. Chekryn (1984) reported that partners were concerned when they became caregivers about the changes in family roles and relationships, as well as the restrictions they experienced in leisure time activities. These changes are often accompanied by depression, anxiety, feelings of helplessness, guilt for the patient, and anger or hostility in both partners as well as marital strain (Beery et al., 1997; Lewis, Woods, Hough, & Bensley, 1989; Sommers & Shields, 1987). As Beery and colleagues report, according to a 1984 Senate report by the Select Committee on Aging, caregivers were three times more likely to be depressed, two to three times more likely to take psychotropic drugs (e.g., tranquilizers), and 12% more likely to use alcohol as a way to cope with stress than the general population. Additionally, caregiving often results in loneliness or isolation because it takes precedence over other social activities (Hannappel, Calsyn, & Allen, 1993).

In addition to caregiving responsibilities and changes in wage-earning responsibilities, caregivers also find themselves serving as "buffers" by which they filter and reduce stresses of day-to-day living to protect their loved one in the wake of an illness (Wilson & Morse, 1991). The partner of a patient with a serious illness may try to hide that their child received a bad grade on a test or that the roof has a leak, in order to spare the patient from worrying about the daily stresses. Partners may also begin to hide their emotions in order to spare the patient from excessive stresses. Although the intention of these efforts is to shield the patient from additional stress, the effect of this buffering can also lead to the patient feeling excluded from family business and day-to-day activities and the partner to feel emotionally overwhelmed. Vess et al. (1988) found in their study of oncology patients that some families seemed to close ranks during the patient's absence, reallocating roles to the point where the patient no longer felt needed. This is seen more commonly in families with older children and may lead to increased anxiety in the patient.

Time may play a role in how a partner adapts to a caregiving role. Most partners are highly supportive in the wake of cancer, but some can undermine treatment, minimize the illness, criticize the patient, or withdraw from the relationship (Vinokur & Vinokur-Kaplan, 1990). Given and Given (1992) found that caregivers of patients with recurrent disease were especially vulnerable to the impact of the illness. Caregivers of patients with recurrent disease reported more depression than caregivers of patients with newly diagnosed breast cancer. In addition, caregivers of patients with recurrent disease experienced a greater impact of the illness on their daily schedules and on their health.

Ethical and Legal Issues

Working within a couple-based approach to illness requires addressing additional ethical and legal questions. For example, clinicians often can provide support and guidance for couples addressing issues such as advanced directives (e.g., "do not resuscitate" orders), durable power of attorney for medical decisions, and issues related to wills and finances during the illness or after death. Our experience with these issues is that the clinician is best served to facilitate the process of communication about these issues. A referral to the legal or medical communities is often recommended for help with the content of such discussions.

An interesting question in working with patients with a medical illness and their partner is who is the identified patient. Although a couple may seek out treatment as a unit, often the individual with the illness seeks help, and throughout treatment their partner is brought in only as necessary. If an individual seeks treatment, they are the patient and questions about confidentiality become increasingly important. Can a psychologist or physician discuss the medical history of a patient with their partner, or is that a violation of the patient's confidentiality? Does that same clinician have a responsibility to discuss the care of the patient with their partner if the patient is not present at the session? In our work, we have taken the approach of "following the patient's lead." If the patient presents for treatment with his or her partner, the two of them are considered the unit of treatment, with all associated rights and privileges. In other cases, a patient may ask if their partner can accompany him or her to some of the sessions to learn more about their illness, its treatment, or related implications. In that case, the patient remains the client and only what the patient wants known or discussed is the focus of couple sessions; outside telephone or in-person contact is then discouraged with the partner. Finally, as in all cases, if no previous arrangements have been made and the partner seeks out the therapist for information, the therapist is obligated not to reveal anything without prior permission from the patient.

Another ethical question regarding treatment with couples concerns the extent of followthrough for which a therapist is responsible. If recommendations to begin exercise and dietary change to prevent developing a heart condition are not followed by the patient, can a clinician contact the patient's partner to express concern? If the clinician chooses not to contact the patient's partner, could the therapist be held accountable if a medical crisis arises? These issues are complex in that they are not easily decided by traditional ethical principals.

Another example involves patients who are fearful about following up on a symptom that may indicate a recurrence or worsening of their disease. Certainly, this is a therapeutic issue that should be addressed in treatment. However, restricting intervention to discussion in therapy and not following up with the appropriate medical personnel in a timely fashion could lead to more serious consequences of the symptom. For example, consider a breast cancer patient who has been in remission for the last year. She mentions that she has noticed a lump in her other breast but explains that she is not going to bring this to the attention of her doctor because she is "sure it is nothing." In this situation, we recommend that the therapist discuss the importance of symptom follow-up and the costs of not proceeding in this manner. However, it is important to remember that the woman is the one who must make the choice, no matter how much the therapist might disagree with a decision to wait. To deny her this right would be a message that she does not have control over her own care. Additionally, she could argue that it is a breech of confidentiality if the issue were discussed with other members of her medical team without her permission.

CONCLUSIONS

There are many issues related to taking a couple-based approach to illness. Our goal is not to intimidate therapists about doing such work. Instead, by highlighting these issues and offering some recommendations for intervention, we encourage health psychologists to incorporate a couple perspective. Similarly, we hope that those accustomed to working with couples will incorporate a behavioral medicine perspective as the need arises. Our experience is that a couple-based approach to illness is extremely rewarding. The clinician has direct access to the environment that can encourage or hinder efforts to feel better. He or she can facilitate health-promoting attitudes and behaviors and develop plans to extinguish other attitudes or behaviors found to be detrimental for both the patient and their partner.

When possible, we advocate a multidisciplinary approach to caring for couples struggling with illness. Teams comprised of nurses, doctors, psychiatrists, psychologists, social workers, physical therapists, occupational therapists, hospice staff, and chaplains can be brought together to allow the couple to receive all of the information, support, and care that they need. Research is necessary regarding the integration of these disciplines and the effects such teamwork has on patients and their partners. Each discipline brings specific knowledge about distinct areas of patient care. Working together, professionals from diverse backgrounds may be better able to serve patients and family members.

Like the disease process itself, therapy with medical patients and their partners is a dynamic process. Partners' ability to handle the illness themselves and with each other is often variable both within and among couples. Therefore, a couple approach to illness must take into account the uncertainty of the illness process, the changing needs of patients and their partners, and the fact that no one solution fits all couples.

Nick and Anita Revisited

How was a couple-based approach implemented with Nick and Anita, the couple described at the outset of this chapter? The immediate issues facing them—medical, financial, psychological, and familial—were overlapping and overwhelming for both of them. First, therapy took a problem-solving approach to help the two of them with medical concerns such as how they should go about finding a surgeon and the right hospital for the transplant. Problem solving also helped them delineate and solve financial and logistical problems such as dealing with insurance, disability issues, and childcare costs given the amount of time that Anita wanted to be at the hospital. Finally, they used problem solving to decide if and when Anita should return to work. What was decided was that Anita would postpone her return to work. Instead, she would focus on obtaining information about hospitals, doctors, and transplants because she wanted all the information she could obtain and because Nick took a more passive approach to his care. They also decided to have Nick's parents move in with them. In this way, Anita and they could trade off childcare responsibilities and visits to Nick as well as keeping Nick's parents closer to their son and his care.

Psychologically, both Nick and Anita were overwhelmed. Their therapist met with them together and taught them emotional expressiveness to help them express the issues confronting them emotionally. Nick was frightened by mortality issues, leaving the children with one parent, and the burden of his illness on their relationship. He also feared that Anita would leave the relationship because he could no longer serve as a provider. Anita was anxious about the possibility that Nick might die and angry that such a serious illness could strike them at a relatively young age. She also expressed resentment at the burden of being well and trying to balance Nick's needs with those of their children, the house, the bills, and the medical details. Additionally, both expressed increasing frustration with the uncertainty of Nick's illness, the probability of obtaining a heart, and what life would be like following such a surgery. Problem solving was integrated into the sessions again to help them find respite from each other when bitterness built up and to develop a plan for how and when to talk about these types of issues.

As Nick's condition worsened and his hopes for obtaining a heart decreased, therapy moved to grief counseling. Their therapist met with them together and individually to help them express their fears, concerns for each other, and wishes following Nick's anticipated death.

Throughout therapy, progress was not always smooth. There were times when each felt resentful of the therapy and its inability to provide answers or guarantees. At other times, a medical focus took precedence over a psychological focus. Overall, however, the couple approach with Nick and Anita allowed them to identify and face the numerous difficult issues that were confronting them, many of which otherwise might have remained covert and unresolved.

REFERENCES

Badger, T. A. (1992). Coping, life-style changes, health perceptions, and marital adjustment in middle-aged women and men with cardiovascular disease and their spouses. *Health Care for Women International, 13,* 43–45.

Baider, L., Kaplan De-Nour (1988). Adjustment to cancer: Who is the patient—the husband or the wife? *Israel Journal of Medical Science, 24,* 631–636.

Beach, D. L. (1995). Caregiver discourse: Perceptions of illness-related dialogue. *The Hospice Journal, 10,* 13–25.

Beery, L. C., Prigerson, H. G., Bierhals, A. J., Santucci, L. M., Newson, J. T., Maciejewski, P. K., Rapp, S. R., Fasiczka, A., & Reynolds, C. F. (1997). Traumatic grief, depression and caregiving in elderly spouses of the terminally ill. *Omega, 35,* 261–279.

Bramwell, L. (1986). Wives' experiences in the support role after husbands' first myocardial infarction. *Heart and Lung, 15,* 578–584.

Brotzman, G. L., & Butler, D. J. (1991). Cross-cultural issues in the disclosure of a terminal diagnosis: A case report. *Journal of Family Practice, 32,* 426–427.

Chekryn, J. (1984). Cancer recurrence: Personal meaning, communication, and marital adjustment. *Cancer Nursing, 7,* 491–498.

Counselman, E. F. (1997). Self-disclosure, tears, and the dying patient. *Psychotherapy, 34,* 233–237.

Coyne, J. C., & Smith, D. A. (1991). Couples coping with a myocardial infarction: A contextual perspective on wifes' distress. *Journal of Personality and Social Psychology, 61,* 404–412.

Epstein, N., & Baucom, D. H. (2002). *Treating couples in context: Innovations in cognitive-behavioral therapy.* Washington, DC: American Psychological Association.

Fiske, V., Coyne, J. C., & Smith, D. A. (1991). Couples coping with myocardial infarction: an empirical reconsideration of the role of overprotectiveness. *Journal of Family Psychology, 5,* 4–20.

Given, B., & Given C.W. (1992). Patient and family caregiver reaction to new and recurrent breast cancer. *Journal of the American Women's Medical Association, 47,* 201–205.

Hannappel, M., Calsyn, R. J., & Allen, G. (1993). Does social support alleviate the depression of caregivers of dementia patients? *Journal of Gerontological Social Work, 20,* 35–51.

Hart, L., Reese, J., & Fearing, M. (1981). *Concepts common to acute illness.* St. Louis, MO: Mosby.

Kiecolt-Glaser, J. K., & Newton, T. L. (2001). Marriage and health: His and hers. *Psychological Bulletin, 127,* 472–503.

Lavery, J. F., & Clarke, V. A. (1999). Prostate cancer: Patients' and spouses' coping and marital adjustment. *Psychology, Health, and Medicine, 4,* 289–302

Lewis, F. M., Woods, N. F., Hough, E. E., & Bensley, L. S. (1989). The family's functioning with chronic illness in the mother: The spouse's perspective. *Social Science and Medicine, 29,* 1261–1269.

Liss-Levinson, W. S. (1982). Reality perspectives for psychological services in a hospice program. *American Psychologist, 37*(11), 1266–1270.

Mahon, S. M., Cella, D. F., & Donovan, M. I. (1990). Psychosocial adjustment to recurrent cancer. *Oncology Nursing Forum, 17*(3, Suppl.), 47–54.

Miller, S. M. (1987). Monitoring and blunting: Validation of a questionnaire to assess styles of information seeking under threat. *Journal of Personality and Social Psychology, 52,* 345–353.

Morse, S. R., & Fife, B. (1998). Coping with a partner's cancer: Adjustment at four stages of the illness trajectory. *Oncology Nursing Forum, 25,* 751–760.

Northouse, L. L., Mood, D., Templin, T., Mellon, S., & George, T. (2000). Couples' patterns of adjustment to colon cancer. *Social Science and Medicine, 50,* 271–284.

Payne, S. A. (1992). A study of quality of life in cancer patients receiving palliative chemotherapy. *Social Science and Medicine, 35,* 1505–1509.

Power, P. W., Hershenson, D. B. & Schlossberg, N. K. (1991). Midlife transition and disability. In R. P. Marinelli & A. E. Dell Onto (Eds.). *The psychological and social impact of disability* (3rd ed., pp. 100–111). New York: Springer.

Ptacek, J. T., Pierce, G. R., Ptacek, J. J., & Nogel, C. (1999). Stress and coping process in men with prostate cancer: The divergent views of husbands and wives. *Journal of Social and Clinical Psychology, 18,* 299–324.

Revenson, T. (1990). All other things are not equal: An ecological approach to personality and disease. In H. S. Friedman (Ed.), *Personality and disease* (pp. 65–94). New York: Wiley.

Richman, J. (1995). From despair to integrity: An Eriksonian approach to psychotherapy for the terminally ill patient. *Psychotherapy, 32,* 317–322.

Rolland, J. (1994). In sickness and in health: The impact of illness on couples' relationships. *Journal of Marital and Family Therapy, 20,* 327–347.

Rose, M., Scholler, G., Jorres, A., Danzer, G., & Klapp, B. F. (2000). Patients' expressions of complaints as a predictor of the course of acute hepatitis A. *Journal of Psychosomatic Research, 48,* 107–113.

Schmaling, K. B., & Sher, T. G. (1997). Physical health and relationships. In W. K. Halford & H. J. Markman (Eds.), *Clinical handbook of marriage and couples interventions* (pp. 323–345). New York: Wiley.

Schoevers, R., Beekman, A., Deeg, D., Geerlings, C., Jonker, C., VanTilburg, W. (2000). Risk factors for depression in later life: Results of a prospective community based study (AMSTEL). *Journal of Affective Disorders, 59,* 127–137.

Schover, L. R. (1989). Sexual problems in chronic illness. In S. R. Leiblum & R. C. Rosen (Eds.), *Principles and practice of sex therapy: Update for the 1990s* (pp. 319–351). New York: Guilford Press.

Schover, L. R., Evans, R. B., & Von Eschenbach, A. C. (1987). Sexual rehabilitation in a cancer center: Diagnosis and outcome in 384 consultations. *Archives of Sexual Behavior, 16*(6), 455–461.

Sherman, A. C., & Simonton, S. (1999). Family therapy for cancer patients: Clinical issues and interventions. *Family Journal, 7*(1), 39–50.

Silberfarb, P. M., Maurer, H., & Crouthamel, C. S. (1978). Psychosocial aspects of neoplastic disease: I. Functional status of breast cancer patients during different treatment regimens. *American Journal of Psychiatry, 137,* 450–455.

Sommers, T. & Shields, L. (1987). *Women take care: The consequences of caregiving in today's society.* Gainesville, FL: Triad.

Spencer, S., Lehman, J., Wynings, C., Arena, P., Carver, C., Antoni, M., Derhagopian, R., Ironson, G., and Love, N. (1999). Concerns about breast cancer and relations to psychosocial well-being in a multiethnic sample of early-stage patients. *Health Psychology, 18,* 159–168.

Stedeford, A. (1981a). Couples facing death: Psychosocial aspects. *British Medical Journal, 283,* 1033–1036.

Stedeford, A. (1981b). Couples facing death: Unsatisfactory communication. *British Medical Journal, 283,* 1098–1101.

Talamantes, M. A., Lawler, W. R., & Espino, D. V. (1995). Hispanic American elders: Caregiving norms surrounding dying and the use of hospice services. *The Hospice Journal, 10,* 35–49.

Tong, K. L. & Spicer, B. J. (1994). The Chinese palliative patient family in North America: A cultural perspective. *Journal of Palliative Care, 10,* 26–28.

Van Zuuren, F., & Hanewald, G. (1993). Cognitive toenadering en vermijding in medisch bedreigende situaties [Cognitive confrontation and avoidance in threatening medical situations: The development of an inventory]. *Gedragstherapie, 25*(1), 33–48.

Vess, J. D. Jr., Moreland, J. R., Schwebel, A. I., & Kraut, E. (1988). Psychosocial needs of cancer patients: Learning from patients and their spouses. *Journal of Psychosocial Oncology, 6*(1/2), 31–51.

Vinokur, A. D., & Vinokur-Kaplan, D. (1990). "In sickness and in health": Patterns of social support and undermining in older married couples. *Journal of Aging and Health, 2,* 215–241.

Wenzel, L., Berkowitz, R., Robinson, S., Bernstein, M., & Goldstein, D. (1992). The psychological, social, and sexual consequences of gestational trophoblastic disease. *Gynecologic Oncology, 46,* 74–81.

Whetten-Goldstein, K., Sloan, F., Kulas, E., Cutson, T., & Schenkman, M. (1997). The burden of Parkinson's disease on society, family, and the individual. *Journal of the American Geriatrics Society, 45,* 844–849.

Willert, M. G., Beckwith, B. E., Holm, J. E., & Beckwith, S. K. (1995). A preliminary study of the impact of terminal illness on spouses: Social support and coping strategies. *The Hospice Journal, 10,* 35–48.

Wilson, S., & Morse, J. M. (1991). Living with a wife undergoing chemotherapy. *Image, 23,* 78–84.

CHAPTER 16

Aging and Cognitive Impairment

SARA HONN QUALLS

Of all of the aspects of aging that are viewed negatively, cognitive impairment inspires the most terror. One commonly hears, "I would rather die than be unable to know what I am doing so I am a burden on others." The fear of burdening a partner is especially poignant. What happens when one partner develops dementia? How can mental health professionals assist these couples to adjust to the dramatic losses and retain a meaningful relationship? This chapter begins by distinguishing among the different types of cognitive impairment and their primary effects on individuals and families. Ways in which cognitive impairments challenge intimate relationships are then described, along with suggestions on how to focus couple assessment and how to structure useful interventions. Finally, a case study illustrates interventions with a couple confronting dementia.

COGNITIVE IMPAIRMENT

Cognitive impairment (CI) encompasses a range of diseases and disorders, many common in later life, that cause a deterioration in cognitive functioning sufficient to impair the ability to accomplish day-to-day activities. In later life, several diseases, disorders, and conditions can produce impairments that vary widely in their impact on the functioning of the patient and family. The focus of this chapter is on chronic, nontreatable conditions such as dementia and poststroke CI. Reversible conditions such as delirium and pseudodementia caused by depression will be noted below because they are important to consider when working with any cognitively impaired older adult.

Global Cognitive Impairment: Dementia

Dementia, the most common chronic cognitive impairment, is defined as a progressive, deteriorating process produced by diseases that permanently impair multiple functions within the brain. Found in 5–6% of persons over age 65, dementia increases in prevalence dramatically with advancing age, approximately doubling in prevalence with every 5 years of advancing age (Jorm, Korten, & Henderson, 1987). Although estimates vary, in community-dwelling older adults, persons over age 85 show prevalence of dementia in the 25–50% range (Gallo & Lebowitz, 1999). Within acute or long-term care settings, the rates are even higher, reaching 75% in many nursing homes (Rovner et al., 1990). The most common dementias are Alzheimer's disease and vascular dementia, with less common dementias including Pick's, Creutzfeldt-Jakob, and Huntington's.

Dementia typically becomes evident to families when the person shows impaired ability to perform complex functions such as job tasks, balancing the checkbook, maintaining the car, or preparing a multicourse meal. However, one of the most confusing aspects of dementia is the ambiguity that is often present early in the process of deterioration. Some individuals appear to family members as if they have simply become more cantankerous, perhaps even a mere exaggeration of previous personality characteristics. Others present with memory problems, personality changes, depression, or interpersonal conflict. Family members are often somewhat confused as to whether they are witnessing normal changes with age, maladaptation to difficult losses that accompany aging, adverse effects of medication or illness, or a truly new disease process such as Alzheimer's.

Focal Cognitive Impairment: Strokes and Tumors

The other major category of chronic CI includes strokes and tumors. These conditions produce focal damage that impairs specific cognitive functions. Depending on the location of the stroke, or the area of brain tissue damaged by tumor, CI may include speech, attention, memory, executive functions (e.g., planning and sequencing of events), initiation or motivation of action, pattern recognition, or a host of other specific cognitive functions. Often, recovery of cognitive function occurs for months after a stroke or brain surgery to remove a tumor, leveling off after 6 months to a year at a stable level of functioning that can be assessed with some accuracy. Further deterioration is not expected unless the tumor returns or other disease processes are operating, as is often common, for example, with a poststroke patient who also experiences ongoing mild transient ischemic attacks that continue to erode cognitive function over time.

Reversible Cognitive Impairment

The two major categories of reversible sources of cognitive impairment are delirium and depression-induced cognitive impairment, often referred to as pseudodementia. One of the most common differential diagnosis questions faced by clinicians working with older adults is discriminating among the "3 D's"—dementia, delirium, and depression. They present very similarly, and are often confused by clients and their families. Couple therapists might not perform the differential diagnosis but need to be aware of the importance of a thorough assessment.

Delirium

Delirium is "characterized by a disturbance of consciousness and a change in cognition that develops over a short period of time" (American Psychiatric Association, 1994). Common causes of delirium in later life include medications (e.g., toxicity, interactions, adverse reactions, or withdrawal), medical illness, substance intoxication or withdrawal, malnutrition, or some combination of factors. Thus, delirium can, and commonly does, occur in persons with chronic CI as well. For example, a person with dementia may develop a delirium when infected with urinary tract infection.

Depression

Clinical depression appears among community-dwelling older adults at a slightly lower prevalence rate than among midlife and young adults. Rates of clinically significant symptom levels are higher in later life, however, even though the criteria for diagnoses may not be met. Furthermore, rates of depression increase significantly in medical and long-term care settings (Blazer, 1994). Depression is quite common among persons with dementia and among those caring for persons with CI (Frazer, Leicht, & Baker, 1996).

Common presenting symptoms of depression in older adults include lack of interest in normally pleasurable activities, difficulty concentrating, and memory complaints. These obviously mimic effects of CI in ways that are quite confusing and lead to misdiagnosis. Indeed, the term "pseudodementia" was coined to reflect the similarity in presentation between dementia and depression. However, Depression is highly treatable in older adults by both nonpharmacological and pharmacological means (Gerson, Belin, Kaufman, Mintz, & Jarvik, 1999), and thus should not be considered a long-term cause of CI.

CHALLENGES TO THE COUPLE'S RELATIONSHIP

CI alters almost every function of a couple's relationship. Several of these domains are discussed below, along with ways to assess and treat the changes.

Giving It a Name

The pervasive negative effects of dementia on all aspects of cognitive function mean that over time the individual experiences "loss of self" (Cohen & Eisdorfer, 1986). An inevitable consequence is that both partners ultimately lose their relationship as well. Although the legal and moral bond may remain in tact, the historical, emotional, and social relationship is essentially lost. The loss process is slow, often insidious, and fraught with ambiguity.

The onset of dementia is characterized by symptoms a layperson may not recognize as CI. Families often describe their loved one as "not himself," "depressed," "just different," "difficult to get along with," or "lazy." Obviously, the person with CI and family members will make an attribution for what they experience, and the attributions will affect directly the strategies for handling the changes. For example, personality attributions often do not lead to aggressive medical evaluations whereas presuming that the unusual behavior represents a medical condition can lead to multiple physician visits to pursue the source of vague complaints, a chase that may produce no definitive answer.

Frequently, a key turning point in family members' adjustment is the point at which someone gives "it" a name. Far too often, dementia is not given a name, even if one or two medications are prescribed to see if they will help. Given a name, the family can begin the process of adjusting to the chronicity or inevitable deterioration that is part of dementia, and plan for the legal and financial changes ahead. Spousal caregivers recall the point at which a dementia diagnosis is first given as the loneliest moment in their journey. At that moment, they often experience their future as doomed although they are often not sure exactly how the specifics of the picture will unfold. The patient him- or herself may also be highly distressed by the application of a label, although the patient may also deny the problem vehemently. CI with a focal cause, such as stroke or tumor, may be given a name, which offers the family a reason for the problem, but may offer little in terms of help making sense of the observed changes in the loved one.

Understanding the Impact on Daily Function

The first step in understanding the impact of the CI on daily function is to discriminate among the specific types of cognitive dysfunction. Neuropsychological assessment details the nature of the deficits. From this information, a therapist can anticipate some of the problems that will be reported and demonstrated. Despite general commonalities, however, the pattern of deficits experienced by persons with the same disease or the same focal damage can be amazingly variable.

A therapist should ask very specifically about how the person is functioning in daily life. Activities of daily living include the abilities to provide self-care by feeding, bathing, toileting, dressing, grooming, transferring (e.g., bed to chair to standing), and walking short distances. More complex skills known as instrumental activities of daily living are also needed to live independently, including skills for handling medications, housework, meals, money, the telephone, and transportation (Lawton, 1988). Therapists working with a couple experiencing CI need to obtain a clear picture of both persons' abilities to accomplish these skills, whether independently or with assistance.

Persons with CI often display behavior problems that present significant intrusions into everyday life. Because many types of CI produce difficulty initiating tasks, family members struggle to figure out when a person is being "lazy" and when he or she really cannot initiate tasks for one of these other reasons. Sleep patterns are important to examine because poor sleep can lead quickly to caregiver burnout. Eating patterns can also be disrupted by CI in a variety of ways including poor appetite, confusion about how or when to eat, forgetfulness about how much was eaten, inability to eat a full meal at one sitting, or inability to sit to eat.

Changes in daily function affect the caregiver as well as the care recipient. Caregivers can become burdened and frustrated over seemingly small tasks of daily living. When small tasks add up to a full-time job of managing the home and person, or when the incapacity experienced by the person with CI places serious burden on their partner for physically or psychologically taxing tasks, relief is needed. Changes in daily routine also have a significant impact on the psychosocial well-being of the person with CI. When the entire morning is devoted to basic self-care routines, little time remains for pleasurable aspects of life. Loss of capability to contribute to household functioning can be particularly discouraging to persons with CI because it robs them of roles, interpersonal power, a sense of contribution, and an opportunity to do things for their partner.

Reorganizing Couple Dynamics

Marriage to a person with CI is a state often referred to as "married but not married," or what could be described to couples as "marital purgatory" or "marital limbo." Boss (1999) and her colleagues have discussed this phenomenon in terms of *boundary ambiguity* that leaves the family unclear whether the person with the CI is an insider or an outsider to core family functions.

Perhaps the most obvious dynamic change is in how power is redistributed. Regardless of the balance of power that existed in the previous life structure, the balance will inevitably tilt away from the partner with CI. The redistribution is an emotionally laden process that easily leads to depression for either partner. The caregiver may feel burdened by work, guilty about taking away another's rights, privileges, and roles, as well as grief at the loss of a more mutual relationship. The person with CI may also experience a wide variety of feelings including guilt, sadness, frustration, and helplessness.

Each CI couple renegotiates power in specific domains that are salient in their relationship and its history. The domains include money, driving, sex, social communication, meal choice and preparation, travel, and a seemingly endless series of small day-to-day components of daily life that underscore the changes. In an effort to minimize how much power is redistributed, a caregiver may let his or her partner with CI retain control over a domain long after it is convenient or even safe. On the other hand, a caregiver may step in very early in the process in the name of safety and demand the right to take nearly full control over all aspects of shared existence.

Intimacy is also renegotiated. Many types of CI impair a person's ability to plan, execute, and follow up with actions in ways that are sensitive to context and social nuance. Caregivers often report that their partner with CI no longer initiates small signs of affection such as hugs, kisses, or smiles. The loss of mutuality in initiating affection or intimacy is a true loss.

Sexual intimacy can be fraught with challenges such as underarousal or overarousal that frightens either or both members of the couple if it launches aggressive behavior (very rarely), grief for familiar and satisfying patterns that are no longer possible, and guilt over enjoying sex with a partner who does not fully participate (Davies, Zeiss, & Tinklenberg, 1992). Many of the age-related changes in physiological functioning caused by diseases and medications are also experienced by persons with CI. Couple therapists are encouraged to be particularly forthright about investigating what has changed in the sexual aspects of the relationship because caregivers often do not initiate the conversation about this topic and persons with CI often cannot (Zeiss, Zeiss, & Davies, 2000).

Phases of Adjustment

The couple's relationship is reorganized over time in what could be characterized as a series of phases. Just as caregiving has been conceptualized as a career that proceeds through predictable phases over time (Aneshensel, Pearlin, Mullan, Zarit, & Whitlatch, 1995), so, also, the couple's relationship must make predictable transitions.

Phase 1: Figuring It Out

Initially, when the disease or disorder is becoming manifest, the couple is unclear about what functions have changed and often flounder in efforts to adapt. In addition to struggles with other domains of daily life, partners often report frustration, anger, or hurt about aspects of their relationship that have changed. What further confuses matters is that the CI-partner's "problem behavior" may be his or her own effort to compensate for the CI, albeit in ineffective or hurtful ways. Thus, there obviously is a willful component to it, adding validity to the non-CI partner's attribution. The behavior may be consistent with long-term behaviors that were never satisfactorily negotiated within the relationship. Furthermore, the person with CI often denies the problem, requiring their partner to be very creative in engaging the person with CI in appropriate behaviors regardless of the desire to cooperate (e.g., going to the doctor or changing clothes). During this phase the person with CI is still viewed as an autonomous agent who is expected to contribute to the relationship and daily life, but the non-CI partner is increasingly a caregiver who must at least monitor personal and relationship care.

Phase 2: Restructuring Roles

In the second phase during which the CI is labeled and at least to some extent understood, the caregiving partner often experiences role overload as he or she picks up roles previously filled by the person with CI. Initially, the caregiver may struggle with competence in the new roles, and he or she may benefit from education and support (Aneshensel et al., 1995). New skills that relate specifically to the needs of the person with CI must be acquired (e.g., assisting with toileting and bathing, managing problem behavior). Furthermore, the progressiveness of dementia means that about the time the caregiver has learned to provide care competently and comfortably, the CI person's functioning deteriorates and new skills are needed.

For the caregiver, perhaps the most discomforting aspect of adding these roles is the sense that one is taking over, or stealing, his or her partner's dignity. Many caregivers express their agony about how to make the necessary changes while retaining as much of the old role structure for their partner as possible. This period brings confusion to both partners about how to view their respective roles in their relationship.

Phase 3: Caregiving

During the third phase, the couple's relationship is often defined by caregiving interactions. For the partner with CI, this is a period when defining a role, giving nurturance, communicating desires, and participating in decisions are cognitively taxing. For the caregiving partner, the most salient characteristic of the relationship is commitment, with intimacy and passion often unavailable or unsatisfying. Both persons' well-being is at risk if the caregiver suffers from excessive burden from care demands and the sense of being trapped. The caregiver's feeling of being stuck in a role that lacks sufficient satisfaction also increases the likelihood of placing their CI partner in a nursing home. The commitment that defines the couple's relationship can also become the trap that constrains well-being.

It is especially challenging to maintain meaning within the relationship once one's partner is so low functioning that institutionalization is needed (Kaplan, 2001). By this stage, there is often no reciprocity in communication, nurturance, or responsibility for the relationship. Although the community-dwelling partner maintains many of the caregiving roles, he or she is likely to be both relieved by the reduction in responsibility for moment-to-moment care while being surprised at how much responsibility is retained. The institutionalized partner's behavior problems continue to bring distress (Stephens, Ogrocki, & Kinney, 1991). The caregiving partner is likely to feel fully responsible for the other person (although not in full control of day-to-day events and care). Guilt is a common experience of caregivers (Aneshensel et al., 1995).

Many caregivers fear that others will question their commitment to their partner with CI because they have initiated or at least cooperated with institutionalization. The fear of "being put away" is quite primitive and dramatic. Caregivers often feel compelled to make their commitment to their institutionalized partner very explicit to their social network and the facility where their ill partner lives. However, the caregiver also needs to begin exploring a new life structure as a person who will function alone socially and personally, at least for a while. Often, caregivers struggle with who they are as individuals, as is evident in their struggles over how often to visit, what to do with the institutionalized person's clothing and personal effects that remain at home, or how to structure a social life as "a married single person." Caregivers need affirmation; they need to know that others understand and can validate their need to be seen both as a devoted partner and as a new kind of creature (e.g., "semiwidow") that is as yet undefined.

Caregiving decisions are fraught with basic ethical dilemmas related to their relationship during this period. To what extent "should" the caregiver make decisions about the couple's home as "he would have if he were able" versus "as I want to now that I have to focus on caring for myself" or "as he would want me to decide, given his situation"? How should the caregiver handle the dreaded question from their institutionalized partner, "When can I go home?" Should the person with CI attend large family gatherings on holidays? How should a caregiver handle knowing that the partner with CI has developed a "special relationship" with another resident of the facility of the opposite sex? How should a caregiver handle his or her own desires for a confidant, dancing partner, sexual partner, or companion?

Phase 4: Affirming and Moving On

The final phase of the couple's changing relationship is widow(er)hood when the surviving partner must work through grief and figure out what kind of final narrative he or she will write about their relationship. Released from the responsibilities of caregiving, the individual can feel lost when it comes to defining the meaning of their previous relationship. In the preceding months or years, most of the focus was on commitment. Now, however, the surviving partner often needs to revisit their relationship's entire history for the purpose of writing a final couple narrative that integrates disappointments, sources of joy and pride, ways in which one was known and not known, intimacies, losses, opportunities taken and not, and the impact of the CI on the final phases that led to separation through death.

ASSESSMENT

Causes and Consequences of the CI

Cognitive impairment produces multiple problems for the couple, requiring the assessment to be multidisciplinary. The first steps in assessment are to gather data that provide as clear a picture as possible of the neurology, cognitive deficits and strengths, and rehabilitative efforts. Key points to clarify include diagnostic issues, comorbidity, stability of CI, and cognitive strengths and weaknesses. The family's report is insufficient to clarify these points; contact with other health providers is imperative.

What Does the Family Believe and Know?

Regardless of what is in the medical chart, the family will use a belief structure to make sense of what is happening. The name of the illness is only a small piece of the cognitive framework that will shape action and attitude. Most of the families I have seen clinically have had very little or no idea about how Alzheimer's disease or stroke really works to influence everyday cognition. In the absence of clear information, family members generate a variety of explanations, many of which lead them to handle problem behaviors in ineffective, inefficient, or hurtful ways. Beliefs and attributions can be elicited directly by asking about both partners' understanding about the illness, the prognosis, and the effects of the brain impairment on thought processes and everyday functioning. A therapist also can assess frameworks indirectly by observing the attributions made in the course of normal conversation.

Current Challenges

The problem that the couple brings to a therapist needs to be examined in the context of the normative challenges discussed above, the neurological information, and the couple's unique relationship. In many cases, the therapist may have to poke around a bit into various practical aspects of the couple's life in order to find the full range of problems. Various tools exist to guide a therapist to ask about the full range of possible behavior problems and their impact on the caregiver. One self-report measure that is quite useful is the Memory and Behavior Checklist (Teri, Truax, Logsdon, Uomoto, Zarit, & Vitaliano, 1992; Zarit, Orr, & Zarit, 1985). The caregiver provides two ratings for 24 problem behaviors that are commonly part of dementia: a frequency rating and the degree to which the behavior bothers or upsets the caregiver. In very few minutes, a clinician can have a picture of the daily behavior problems as well as their impact on the caregiver.

Relationship History

In order to understand the effects of an illness on any particular couple, it is most useful to learn something about the couple's story. A developmental review of the couple's relationship helps elucidate how this family is going to interpret and write this episode into a lifelong storyline. One should inquire about how partners' relative power was balanced prior to the illness, and how much intimacy was available. These aspects of history influence the caregiver's commitment to the relationship (e.g., how much sacrifice he or she is willing to make; how new role burdens are experienced), the caregiver's grief process (i.e., how much and what is lost), and the caregiver's rebuilding process (e.g., what parts of the self were never cared for in the couple's relationship).

Financial and Social Resources

Pragmatic information about the couple's resources is also very important to obtain. Financial and social resources dictate options for supplementing or replacing a partner's care with formal providers. Therapists working with these couples need to understand the funding streams that support various service delivery networks (e.g., Medicaid, Medicare, aging services, and disability programs). Social resources are also critically important. Who exists in the real network? What ties do they have (e.g., obligations, affection)? What limitations in availability are relevant (e.g., geographic distance, financial resources to support travel, work and family constraints)? How supported does the caregiving partner *feel* when the children or siblings visit? What influences those feelings of support? How capable is the caregiver of asking for assistance?

Health History

The patient's health history provides information about comorbidity complications to the current source of CI. The health history of the caregiving partner is equally important to assess. Caregiver sustainability will be directly influenced by his or her health. The caregiving partner should be reminded that self-care is of primary importance because two people's well-being depends on it!

Caregiver Burden

The two components of a caregiver's burden are (1) the problems being handled, and (2) the stress experienced. Although a heavier load of work certainly adds to a sense of burden, the specific tasks that produce a feeling of burden are subjectively determined. Research indicates that behavior problems that break meaningful social rules or threaten safety are especially likely to weigh heavily on the caregiving partner (Aneshensel et al., 1995). Constant questioning, although annoying, is less likely to burden than explosive outbursts in public or inappropriate toileting behavior. However, burden is ultimately a subjectively determined variable that requires individual assessment.

The Process of Assessment

The assessment is primarily conducted in an interview format, although occasionally inventories can be used to measure caregiver burden, as described above. It is usually preferable to see both members of the couple together, although there are exceptions to this (e.g., when CI is significant or when one person denies their CI). The therapist should consult with other providers such as physicians or, preferably, hands-on providers such as home health aides, nursing home staff, or an adult child who serves as secondary caregiver. A few sessions are spent with both members of the couple, gradually transitioning into work with the caregiving partner. This way of working also symbolizes the reality that the responsibility for care will fall more and more to the caregiving person.

Interviewing a couple together is tricky if they view the CI differently, as is often the case because CI often reduces insight into one's own deficits and capacities. One should begin by inquiring into the impaired person's perceptions of problems. Attention should be paid to the ways the CI deficits appear in normal conversation, the ways in which the person with CI responds to information shared from other health providers (e.g., diagnosis, nature of deficits as evident in other evaluations), and how his or her partner responds to any distortions that are presented. In some ways, this is like dealing with any relationship in which two people have two different views of a problem. In this case, however, the CI can be expected to produce distortions that may endanger the individuals or couple. Thus, the therapist has a different role maintaining some kind of objective truth and providing guidance about how to deal with the very real challenges of living daily life without full cognitive capacity. Therapists' expertise also allows them to label problems that the couple has not yet recognized.

INTERVENTION

Information, Information, Information

A key piece of advice for mental health professionals who work with chronic CI is to have information readily available and to share it generously. Many myths, fears, and misattributions can be addressed quickly with brochures that are readily available to lay readers from national organizations such as the Alzheimer's Association (*www.alz.org*) or the National Stroke Association (*www.stroke.org*). One should attempt to convince the family to go to the local organization's office to become familiar with the local resources and to make themselves known to the staff of a local association who are likely to engage them in a wide variety of helpful services including support groups, educational seminars, and disease-focused counseling that can be invaluable to them.

Provide Labels and Clarify Attributions

An extension of the therapist's role as informational advocate for these couples is the role as interpreter. It is helpful to educate the person with the CI as well as the caregiver about the causes and implications of their condition or illness. Causal attributions, such as laziness, provide reasons for problem behavior that can provoke significant conflict between the couple. The caregiving partner, already burdened by the pragmatic and subjectively troubling aspects of care, can become chronically angry with his or her partner with CI whom the caregiver believes is simply being lazy or uncaring. For example, when provided with an explanation about the effects of frontal lobe impairment on initiation of activities, the caregiver can shift to an illness-based attribution that reduces anger.

Common themes appear repeatedly in the attributions made for behavior of persons with CI. Within the category of attributions for *poor initiation* of activity are attributions for failure to initiate affection, social interactions with friends and relatives, and problem solving. Personality deficits, depression, or lack of personal caring are often invoked to explain the failure to initiate appropriate behavior in these situations. *Fluctuations in functioning* are often attributed to conscious choices and willful behavior rather than CI. This issue is tricky, of course, because willful use of CI behavior can indeed be intended to manipulate other family members into the desired caretaking behaviors. Therapists have to assess carefully the specifics of the fluctuating behavior in order to discriminate those that are truly neurological from those that may indeed be purposeful. *Problem behaviors* that are the cognitively impaired person's effort to cope with the limitations are commonly seen as primary rather than secondary to the CI. Viewing a problem as the person's best effort to solve another problem can direct a search for more effective alternative solutions to the primary problem. Both partners benefit from seeing that the person with CI is actually engaging in problem solving.

Fostering Positive Interactions

Living with CI can be so disorganizing to old patterns of affection and pleasurable activities that both partners succumb to an existence centered around illness and impairment. Not only are the individuals at risk for depression when this happens, but the couple loses the ability to generate positive interactions. A therapeutic goal is to ensure that each couple includes in their daily repertoire positive couple interactions as well as the necessary individually meaningful pleasant activities.

Behavioral strategies can be used to increase the frequency of specific affection behaviors (e.g., hugging, holding hands, sitting close on the couch). Behavioral cues (e.g., a note on the dresser mirror or bedside table) can help the person with CI initiate a desirable behavior. The caregiver can learn to initiate interactions that may lead to the person with CI participating actively enough that it feels to the caregiving partner as though he or she is the recipient of caring action. For example, sitting on the couch holding hands may be a cue to a sequence of cuddling and kissing that the person with CI can carry through once the initial step is launched. Interventions can be undertaken to improve the hygiene of the person with CI if he or she no longer attends to it, because poor hygiene makes physical closeness unpleasant for the caregiving partner.

With some couples it is helpful to identify long-term couple behavior patterns that affirmed the couple's identity as a couple. Although the CI may now interfere with some aspect of previous patterns, small adaptations may make it possible to enjoy a form of an activity that evokes in the couple an affirmation of their relationship. For example, it may not be easy to go to a large dance hall, but it may be possible to dance in the living room. Simpler games, a different restaurant (or picnic in a park) that has characteristics that make the CI less impairing (e.g., less noisy, more tolerant of odd behavior), or shared music with less expectation to talk about the story line of the opera may still be quite mutually enjoyable.

Sexuality is a domain of positive interaction that is often fraught with complex feelings and confusing behaviors. The issues are diverse and often left unspoken unless specifically investigated by a therapist. Interventions may be needed to address guilt, anger, disappointment, fear, or physical awkwardness. In addition, inappropriate sexual behaviors or behaviors with persons other than the spouse may need to be addressed with the CI partner or formal care providers (e.g., nursing home staff).

Build Positive Roles for the Partner with CI

One of the more devastating losses experienced by the person with CI is the alteration or loss of roles. Although the social roles are more obvious, the loss of familiar roles within a relationship can also be significant to both partners. The caregiver loses the sense that someone is there to share the load, and to do tasks for which one's own skills are inadequate. The caregiver's losses must be addressed through assistance with grief and skill development. The care recipient, however, also warrants focused intervention.

Filling waking hours with meaningful activity is often a problem for persons with CI. Partners of persons with CI can be so overwhelmed with lost sources of pleasure and meaning that they do not recognize new possibilities. Usually the person with CI cannot generate options, and their partner is often struggling to come up with creative ideas. There are several ways to identify new or adapted activities that can be meaningful. In some cases, a consultation with an occupational therapist can be quite helpful. Books and journals for activity therapists in institutional settings provide interesting ideas for home settings as well. Alzheimer's and stroke associations maintain listings of good resources. In addition, one can use the Older Persons Pleasant Events Schedule (Teri & Lewinsohn, 1982) or the Pleasant Events Schedule—AD (Alzheimer's disease) version (Teri & Logsdon, 1991) to help couples identify activities with low physical and cognitive demand that can be sources of pleasure (e.g., watching clouds). Often, the caregiver is as surprised as the person with CI to discover that many sources of pleasure remain available.

Another option that is often appropriate to introduce is a day program especially designed for persons with CI. The social interaction and activities appropriate for the cognitive abilities not only fill the day pleasantly and meaningfully, but offer the partners something to discuss over dinner at night. Although it may not be winning a golf tournament at the country club, singing with a karaoke machine with friends at a day center may generate a sense of satisfaction and pride. Most communities now offer day programs that operate at a fraction of the cost of residential care.

When stymied in the search for options, one might recall the wisdom of a woman who arranged for her mother-in-law to peel 10 pounds of potatoes per day because it generated such a sense of accomplishment, participation, and pride in the woman whose dementia rendered her incapable of producing the lovely big meals for which she was renowned. The potatoes were taken to the local soup kitchen, and the cost of potatoes was negligible compared to the benefits in self-esteem and kitchen camaraderie among members of the family. That principle can be adapted by couples as well. Laundry can be folded and refolded many times a day, if that addresses the need for purposeful activity.

Rewriting the Relationship Narrative

Throughout the process of adjusting to CI, and especially in the final fourth phase of grieving, the caregiving partner will tell and retell the story of their relationship to integrate the very altered structure of their current situation within the longer narrative. Many specific tasks can foster as well as symbolize this process: writing the obituary; preparing for family holidays and visits without the partner's presence; establishing new daily life structures for eating, sleeping, or scheduling activities; organizing pictures and scrapbooks for the next generations; sorting clothes and artifacts that belonged to their partner who is now dead; and possibly opening one's self to new relationships.

Many persons are initially reluctant to speak of disappointments or weaknesses related to their deceased partner. Once given permission, however, the ambivalent feelings surface, leading to some degree of struggle over what kind of narrative to write. Their ambivalence is important because the question of identity during widow(er)hood almost inevitably leads to recognizing parts of the self that were not nurtured within the relationship and are now ready for exploration. Furthermore, the final pieces of guilt seem to resolve once the individual examines directly the limitations of their partner, their previous relationship, and his or her own inability to make it perfect.

Impact of the Larger Family System

Couples are usually embedded within a larger family system that warrants a therapist's attention. Children or siblings bring potential resources as well as potential conflicts to the process of adjusting to CI. It can be useful simply to be curious about how the larger family system interacts with the couple, and to remain open to renegotiating therapy to include significant family members as needed (Qualls, 1999a, 1999b).

Here and Now, Then and There

A final focus for intervention in cases of deteriorating CI is planning for the future as a widow(er). Long before death, the caregiving partner is aware of semisingleness and future widowhood. Their looming future status is part of the current reality of caregiving partners, even those most entrenched in responsibilities for massive daily caregiving tasks. A therapist can begin by labeling the inevitable future. Often, a caregiving partner will shudder, verbally balk, or in another way show their dislike of the topic. It can be useful to look for other points to introduce this reality in a gentle but firm way. For example, a rationale for talking about this stark future reality is to remind caregivers that they must balance the needs of their partner with CI with their own needs in order to prepare for a future that will extend beyond the life of their partner. Once they move beyond any initial resistance, most individuals acknowledge that they have thought about this, and have some kind of concern. The range of concerns is quite broad and includes financial fears, resentment for loss of time to caregiving tasks, worry about loneliness, and anticipation of freedom to focus life around pleasure again. What is consistent is the caregiver's sense that he or she "should" not talk about the future, as if it somehow discounts the present.

Thus, one treatment goal is to help a caregiver, and if possible their partner with CI, to talk about the "then and there" as well as the "here and now." The goal is to introduce hope, understanding that it will be tempered with grief and a range of other emotions (e.g., guilt, regret, relief, loneliness). One can use the future image to help identify parts of that lifestyle that perhaps could be initiated now such as hobbies, exercise, eating preferences, and social contacts. To the extent that balancing needs between the partners is important to maintain the well-being of one or both, the future image can serve as a beacon to guide the search for ways to care for the caregiver.

CASE ILLUSTRATION

Madge asked for psychotherapy for her 75-year-old husband, Dale, who she believed was experiencing depression as well as "senility." She chose to participate in the therapy as well because she was concerned that any interventions would need to be managed by her. The key problems they identified were his intensive anger outbursts and lack of investment in shared activities. They acknowledged that in their 15-year marriage (a second marriage for both) she had overshadowed him with her more extraverted style of interacting in a broad range of community activities. Now, he was insisting on slowing down to the point of almost no activity, and she was worried that he was depressed.

After the first session I obtained medical records to determine that Dale was diagnosed with probable Alzheimer's disease. His interaction style, description of home activity patterns, and response to a brief mental status examination suggested he was probably just moving into the middle stage of the disease. In my view, until Madge began to accept his illness as terminal and progressive, she would continue to engage in their partnership in ways that she had valued throughout the marriage, to meet her needs for a confidant, and intellectual and social partner.

He was clearly overwhelmed by her verbiage and felt increasingly inadequate as a person because he could not process the content of her monologues. He was disturbed by her distress but could not respond. My initial treatment plan included (1) educating the couple about the cognitive changes common in Alzheimer's disease and the behavior patterns that accompany it; (2) helping Madge form appropriate attributions for Dale's behavior; (3) helping Madge accept increasing separateness as part of the path ahead because Dale was both unable and uninterested in participating in the same shared activities; (4) ensuring a marital role for Dale by helping Madge structure appropriate activities for Dale to address the growing depression and by finding ways for him to support Madge; and (5) teaching Madge and Dale strategies for helping him deal with frustration and anger.

In the second visit, we again discussed his perception that she was moving too fast for him, leaving him frustrated with his cognitive deficits. The angry interchanges that followed from this frustration were given different attributions by the two: Madge experienced him as not caring about her needs while Dale experienced her verbal exchanges as disrespectful in tone. We slowly reviewed the interchange to note each step for the purpose of identifying alternative responses that they could each try. Based on that work, homework assignments were given to each. Dale's assignments were written down with the instruction for him to rehearse them regularly through the week. He was to (1) signal Madge when he thought she was going too fast *before* he got angry, and (2) on two occasions tell her what he likes about her. Madge was to (1) notice Dale's signals (both the purposeful ones and the subtler signs of increasing frustration), and (2) write in a journal rather than telling him all of her thoughts and inner analyses about their interactions.

The next two sessions were focused on the major role transitions they were experiencing but not acknowledging. I saw Madge and Dale together for one session and separately for the other. Madge clearly did not perceive Dale's incapacities accurately. She continued to set expectations for him that were beyond his current capacities, and experienced frustration and personal rejection when he did not rise to meet them. We spoke frankly about how she was becoming an unequal partner, a caregiver. In order to sustain her mental health in that role, she needed to begin thinking of her own interests and desires separately from her caregiving role in the marriage. Madge resisted accepting the changing roles for fear that she would prematurely increase his dependency. She was overgeneralizing the hard lessons she had learned about fostering independence when raising her developmentally disabled daughter. She also simply did not want to begin the grief process. Dale continued to focus on signaling his frustrations and engaging in the useful role of complimenting Madge's strengths.

At this point, I worked with Madge alone so I could work more directly on her transition to caregiver. Madge acknowledged that she was depressed due to the changing lifestyle that had fewer stimulating conversations and inadequate social contact. She affirmed her commitment to care for Dale at home as long as possible, however, and resisted efforts to use formal providers to relieve her to spend more time with friends and in community activities. In an effort to identify factors that influenced her mood fluctuations, I assigned her a daily mood rating sheet (rate mood on a 1–9 scale daily and give two reasons for that rating), and an Older Adult Pleasant Events Schedule as homework. When she brought them back she thanked me for my help and asked to end our work for now. She felt that she had come to grips better with Dale's illness and her changing roles. She acknowledged that she was struggling with her mood but was unwilling to alter the caregiving role she had structured for herself, preferring instead to appreciate what she could of Dale's companionship for as long as possible. Although abrupt, I believed her decision was sound because she needed time to work with the new perspectives we had forged.

One year later, Madge requested a session to get advice about how to handle Dale's recent rapid deterioration. She continued to struggle with his anger outbursts. Behaviorally, she was handling them better, although she continued to attribute to him more willful control over them than was realistic. We reviewed the nature of the illness and its impact on self-regulation of anger in an effort to focus her attributions on the illness rather than his lack of caring for her. She used the "booster" session well, and left feeling encouraged and not in need of further work at that time.

Three months later, when Dale died, Madge sought assistance with her grief process. She was entrenched in guilt, believing she should have provided more and better care. In the two sessions we had at that time, we did an abbreviated marital life review to assist the grief resolution, dwelling longest on the period of Dale's illness. We focused on the ambiguity of the illness onset and the variable course of the behavior deterioration in order to help her respect her own struggles with how to help him. She now feared that she had not provided enough support (the opposite side of her ambivalence about dealing with his dependency from what she expressed in the earlier sessions). I began to query her about the aspects of her life that had been on hold, and which ones she thought she might want to reinitiate in the succeeding months. My goal was not to rush her through the grief, but to remind her that she had made progress on establishing a separate lifestyle long before his death.

That earlier work on separateness was now the groundwork for this transition. Madge wrote me a note several months later describing the progress she had made in establishing a life again. She was quick to recognize the ongoing impact of her grief, yet noted that she had indeed established a meaningful life structure.

This case illustrates a common therapy process for couples dealing with cognitive impairment. Common themes that did not appear in this particular case include complicated interactions with other family members (e.g., children), management of other medical illnesses, historical difficulties in the marriage (e.g., abuse), and institutionalization. However, the sequence, timing, themes, and mixture of individual and couple sessions are prototypical.

Therapy with a couple experiencing cognitive impairment involves an intensive process of renegotiating every major aspect of their relationship. Roles, family rules, and familiar patterns of intimacy and conflict resolution almost always change dramatically. Depending on the nature of the CI, the change may be abrupt (e.g., due to stroke) or chronic and deteriorating (e.g., as happens with dementias like Alzheimer's disease). In either case, the couple is vulnerable to depression, anger, and increased conflict if they lack the ability to adapt. A careful assessment of the CI, its impact on the individuals and their relationship, and the context of this stage in their relationship is necessary. Therapists can offer meaningful assistance by providing education, labeling problems and clarifying the attributions for them, fostering positive interactions, building positive roles for both partners, and helping the well partner rewrite the relationship narrative to incorporate this very challenging final stage. Although primarily focused on the present challenges, the therapist must help the couple to anticipate an unattractive future and to find the strengths within themselves and their relationship to face it. Work with later life couples often challenges therapists to confront life challenges that are "off time" to their own life; such challenges are outside what anyone hopes will be part of his or her own life experience. Thus, work with these couples can be both highly satisfying and deeply poignant, as the therapist faces individuals' worst fears of later life.

REFERENCES

American Psychiatric Association. (1994). *Diagnostic and statistical manual of mental disorders* (4th ed.). Washington, DC: Author.

Aneshensel, C. S., Pearlin, L. I., Mullan, J. T., Zarit, S. H., & Whitlatch, C. J. (1995). *Profiles in caregiving: The unexpected career*. San Diego, CA: Academic Press.

Blazer, D. G. (1994). Epidemiology of late life depression. In L. S. Schneider, C. F. Reynolds III, B. D. Lebowitz, & A. J. Friedhoff (Eds.), *Diagnosis and treatment of depression in late life* (pp. 9–19). Washington, DC: American Psychiatric Press.

Boss, P. (1999). *Ambiguous loss: Living with unresolved grief.* Cambridge, MA: Harvard University Press.

Cohen, D., & Eisdorfer, C. (1986). *The loss of self.* New York: Norton.

Davies, H., Zeiss, A., & Tinklenberg, J. (1992). 'Til death do us part: Intimacy and sexuality in the marriages of Alzheimer's patients. *Journal of Psychosocial Nursing, 30,* 5–10.

Frazer, D. W., Leicht, M. L., & Baker, M. D. (1996). Psychological manifestations of physical disease in the elderly. In L. L. Carstensen, B. A. Edelstein, & L. Dornbrand (Eds.), *The practical handbook of clinical gerontology* (pp. 217–235). Thousand Oaks, CA: Sage.

Gallo, J. J., & Lebowitz, B. D. (1999). The epidemiology of common late-life mental disorders in the community: New themes for the new century. *Psychiatric Services, 50,* 1158–1166.

Gerson, S., Belin, T. R., Kaufman, A., Mintz, J., & Jarvik, L. (1999). Pharmacological and psychological treatments for depressed older patients: A meta-analysis and overview of recent findings. *Harvard Review of Psychiatry, 7,* 1–28.

Jorm, A. F., Korten, A. E., Henderson, A. S. (1987). The prevalence of dementia: A quantitative integration of the literature. *Acta Psychiatrica Scandinavica, 76,* 465–479.

Kaplan, L. (2001). A couplehood typology for spouses of institutionalized persons with Alzheimer's disease: Perceptions of "We"–"I." *Family Relations, 50,* 87–98.

Lawton, M. P. (1988). Scales to measure competence in everyday activities. *Psychopharmacology Bulletin, 24,* 609–614.

Qualls, S. Honn (1999a). Family therapy with older adult clients. In *Session: Psychotherapy in Practice, 55*(8), 1–14.

Qualls, S. Honn (1999b). Realizing power in intergenerational family hierarchies: Family reorganization when older adults decline. In M. Duffy (Ed.), *Handbook of counseling and psychotherapy with older adults* (pp. 228–241). New York: Wiley.

Rovner, B. W., German, P. S., Broadhead, J., Morriss, R. K., Brant, L. J., Blaustein, J., & Folstein, M. F. (1990). The prevalence and management of dementia and other psychiatric disorders in nursing homes. *International Psychogeriatrics, 2,* 13–24.

Stephens, M. A., Ogrocki, P. K., & Kinney, J. M. (1991). Sources of stress for family caregivers of institutionalized dementia patients. *Journal of Applied Gerontology, 10,* 328–342.

Teri, L., & Lewinsohn, P. M. (1982). Modification of the pleasant and unpleasant events schedules for use with the elderly. *Journal of Consulting and Clinical Psychology, 50,* 444–445.

Teri, L., & Logsdon, R. (1991). Identifying pleasant activities for individuals with Alzheimer's disease: The pleasant events schedule-AD. *The Gerontologist, 31,* 124–127.

Teri, L., Truax, P., Logsdon, R., Uomoto, J., Zarit, S., & Vitaliano, P. P. (1992). Assessment of behavioral problems in dementia: The Revised Memory and Behavior Problems Checklist. *Psychology and Aging, 7,* 622–631.

Zarit, S. H., Orr, N. K., & Zarit, J. M. (1985). *The hidden victims of Alzheimer's disease: families under stress.* New York: NYU Press.

Zeiss, A., Zeiss, R. A. & Davies, H. (2000). In P. Lichtenberg (Ed.), *Handbook of geriatric assessment* (pp. 270–296). New York: Wiley.

CHAPTER 17

Bereavement and Complicated Grief

ROBERT M. WILLS

For years, grief, bereavement, and mourning have been considered the domain of individual therapy. Therapists adept in couple therapy may very well believe that the proper way to handle cases of acute bereavement is to see the mourner individually or to refer to a bereavement specialist using an individual format, thereby ignoring important interpersonal and systemic issues. Part of the reason for this has been the dearth of articles discussing bereaved couples and their treatment. More recently, a few interpersonal and family systems therapists have begun to conceptualize grief from a family systems or family developmental perspective (Shapiro, 1994; Walsh & McGoldrick, 1995). Still neglected in this discussion are the conceptualization of couple bereavement and the adaptation of couple therapy to relationships impacted by profound loss.

In this chapter, I propose that couple therapists frequently observe the effects of bereavement on couples and that knowledge of bereavement from three perspectives—individual, family systems, and the couple system—is needed to address the therapeutic needs of bereaved couples. For the sake of simplicity, this chapter is written as if death is the source of bereavement. However, bereavement may follow many life events and circumstances other than death such as termination from a job, financial setback, injury or illness, the "launching" of children, or infertility; not all losses involve something once possessed, but instead may involve the loss of hopes or dreams. Moreover, grief is a profoundly unique experience, so that bereavement in a specific individual may follow an event that others would not recognize as traumatic or morbid (Rando, 1988). This chapter considers bereavement from both individual and family systems perspectives and suggests concrete steps couple therapists can take to address both acute and protracted grief responses in couples.

GRIEF FROM AN INDIVIDUAL PERSPECTIVE

The traditional conceptualization of bereavement, focusing on the individual, suggests that mourning proceeds in three phases or stages (Nolan-Hoeksema & Larson, 1999; Rando, 1988). The first phase is that of initial shock. It may last anywhere from moments to weeks, and is particularly pronounced when death is unexpected or traumatic. The bereaved person is likely to experience intensely painful emotions including sadness, anger, anxiety and fear; cognitive problems such as confusion, disorganized thinking, or feelings of unreality; behavioral reactions such as crying, angry outbursts, and hyperactivity; and somatic experiences such as gastrointestinal distress, dizziness, and numbness. The second phase is one of acute mourning in which depression, sleep and appetite disturbance, and intense yearning for the lost loved one may occur. During this phase, a person may feel helpless and unable to make decisions, may withdraw from others, and is often preoccupied with his or her loss. The person may become very dependent, seeking help from others, or withdrawn. The final phase is ushered in when the bereaved achieves an understanding of the loss and finds some way to accept it. This is frequently referred to as a restorative phase in which the bereaved person returns to a feeling of well-being and resumes ordinary tasks of living. Nevertheless, feelings of grief may reappear for years or throughout life (Nolen-Hoeksema & Larson, 1999).

Complicated grief occurs when the bereaved individual is overwhelmed by painful feelings, unable to function adequately, develops serious physical or psychological symptoms, or remains in a chronic state of grief. In other words, complicated, pathological, or unresolved grief exists on a continuum with normal grief—the difference residing in the intensity and the duration of the reaction, with the mechanism presumed to be a failure of the individual to progress through the prescribed tasks of grief work (Worden, 1991). A person whose grief response is pathological may refuse to face the fact that the loved one is gone, experience intense grief for years, refuse to adapt to the absence of the loved one and form new relationships, and underfunction or become dysfunctional and dependent on others. Many factors may be implicated in a person's failure to resolve grief (Rando, 1986, 1988). The pathological griever may have had a highly ambivalent relationship with the deceased, or the deceased may have represented a necessary part of the griever's self. Pathological grievers often have distorted or conflict-ual relationships with the deceased, or such grievers may have been overly dependent on the deceased and unable to function independently. The more traumatic, unexpected, or ambiguous the circumstances of death, the more difficulty people have with completing the grief process (Rando, 1988; Raphael, 1983). Persons with profound or multiple losses in the past may be at risk for complications in the grieving process. Finally, the less healthy the personality of the griever, the less capable of making the adaptations and changes necessary to accomplish the task of grieving (Worden, 1991).

Pathological bereavement as formulated in the fourth edition of the *Diagnostic and Statistical Manual of Mental Disorders* (American Psychiatric Association, 1994) is focused on abnormal or excessive reactions to death in the individual. According to DSM-IV, depressive symptoms are normal in bereavement as long as they resolve within a 2-month period. However, the following seven conditions denote abnormal or complicated grief:

1. Guilt about things other than actions taken or not taken by the survivor at the time of the death.
2. Thoughts of death other than the survivor feeling that he or she would be better off dead or should have died with the deceased person.
3. Morbid preoccupation with worthlessness.
4. Marked psychomotor retardation.
5. Prolonged and marked functional impairment.
6. Hallucinatory experiences other than thinking that he or she hears the voice of, or transiently sees the image of, the deceased person.
7. The presence of characteristic symptoms of a major depressive episode persisting more than 2 months after the loss.

Nolen-Hoeksema and Larson (1999) point out that the traditional models of bereavement rest on three clinically derived assumptions that (1) bereaved people go through predictable stages of grief; (2) some form of pathology typically results from a failure to grieve; and (3) recovery from grief is predicated on a process of working through grief that involves an examination of one's relationship to the deceased, experiencing anger toward the deceased, accepting the loss as permanent, and incorporating a place for the deceased in an expanded view of self.

Examining the empirical literature and drawing on their own research, Nolen-Hoeksema and Larson (1999) conclude that there is little empirical evidence to support any of the three assumptions. Regarding the assumption of predictable stages of grief, research by Osterweis, Soloman, and Green (1984) and Silver and Wortman (1980) depicts tremendous variability in the order, manner, and duration that bereaved individuals experience grief. This finding is of major importance because the common assumption held by many therapists and even the bereaved themselves is that one must experience grief in a particular manner to be healthy. If the stage model becomes the yardstick of healthy grief management, then those who fail to progress along its markers are deemed abnormal and at risk for breakdown at some later time.

Regarding the assumption that failure to grieve will result in pathology, although various studies of widows find a high prevalence of depression during the grief process (from 70 to 88%; Glick, Weiss, & Parkes, 1974; Vachon, Rogers, Lyall, Lancee, Sheldon, & Freeman, 1982); studies also indicate that widows who do not develop depression or high degrees of distress are less likely to develop distress later on than those who suffer greatly in the aftermath of loss (Clayton, Kalikas, Maurice, & Robins, 1973; Vachon et al., 1982). Reviewing the empirical literature, Nolen-Hoekseman and Larson failed to find evidence that low distress survivors of loss become highly distressed at a later time.

The third assumption, that working through the loss is essential to recovery, is hard to operationalize empirically. However, Nolen-Hoekseman and Larson (1999) cite earlier studies, supported by their own research, which suggest that people who quickly come to terms with their loss are the least likely to show pathology later on, whereas those who enter into prolonged yearning or ruminating about the loss show higher levels of distress several months later. The "working-through" hypothesis is also challenged by empirical literature suggesting that for 20–40% of survivors of significant loss, grief is experienced for many years, or it may never entirely cease to be a part of their lives (Vachon et al., 1982; Parks & Weiss, 1983; Zisook & Shuchter, 1986).

Therapists may do great disservice to clients by suggesting that recovery from grief is merely a matter of going through "grief work" in the proper manner—an underlying premise of traditional models of mourning. Nevertheless, Nolen-Hoekseman and Larson (1999) credit the traditional grief models with identifying several "poor risk" factors for those dealing with grief, including an ambivalent relationship with the deceased, excessive dependency, assuming inordinate responsibility for the loss, and denying emotions or engaging in avoidant behavior. Furthermore, traditional models of grief correctly posited that not all losses are equal; for example, people have much more difficulty recovering from the loss of a child or from traumatic or ambiguous losses (Nolen-Hoeksema & Larson, 1999; Rando, 1986).

GRIEF FROM A FAMILY SYSTEMS PERSPECTIVE

Family systems theorists assert that loss is a transactional process impacting the entire family. It expresses itself not merely in personal and subjective symptoms, but by becoming part of the interpersonal fabric of couples' relationships and the dynamics of family life. Various authors over the past 25 years have noted the interplay of family processes and family bereavement (Bowen, 1976; Herz, 1980, 1988; Kuhn, 1981; Paul & Paul, 1982, 1989; Pinkus, 1974); however, only recently has grief been conceptualized from an interpersonal/systemic perspective in a rigorous manner (Herz, 1988; Shapiro, 1994; Walsh & McGoldrick, 1995).

Although the impact of profound loss involves all family members and is often prolonged, it is frequently not associated by the family with the loss. Thus families may struggle with symptoms, difficulties, or conflict directly or indirectly related to death or other major losses without being aware that at the core, their experience is a grief reaction. Herz (1988) postulated that the mechanism whereby grief creates family disturbance is through disruption of the family life cycle. Thus, untimely death is more disrupting to the family than death in old age because a person who dies out of the natural order is a person whose loss deprives the family of essential interactional or symbolic functions. Herz suggests that there is a 20-year span in the life of the nuclear family when untimely death to any member creates the greatest amount of disorganization. The most emotionally unsettling death in any family is the death of a child because children represent the most critical aspect of the parent's dreams and hopes and purpose in life, so that "the loss of the child is an existential wound of the worst kind" (Herz, 1988, p. 466). The death of a parent in a young nuclear family is also extremely disruptive because the surviving parent must deal with his or her own grief, the grief of remaining children, often a loss of income, and the assumption of the deceased parent's roles and functions. The death of one's own parent is less disruptive because it has the least effect on the family life cycle. However, a long debilitating illness preceding the death of a parent may disrupt the family life cycle significantly, especially if one of the parents must divide time between the usual tasks of parenting and family life, and the additional tasks of caring for one's own, or one's spouse's, parent in the terminal stages of life.

From a family systems perspective, a family is both an interactional and a transgenerational entity. Loss can be experienced as either a present happening or a legacy from the past. Bowen (1976) described profound loss as an emotional shock wave that reverberates throughout the family system for generations. Loss in the family causes far more than grief; it may precipitate a realignment of relationships, a reorganization of functions, or a change in the family's definition of itself or its belief system.

According to Walsh and McGoldrick (1995), the ability to accept loss and make the requisite adaptations in family processes is at the heart of healthy family functioning. By contrast, family dysfunction results from denying loss, becoming locked in time, rigidifying relationships, and escaping reality by use of alcohol, drugs, or fantasy. Risk factors include traumatic deaths (accidents, homicide, suicide), deaths that severely disrupt the family life cycle, premorbid family disorganization (rigidity, disengagement, or enmeshment), dysfunctional belief systems (pervasive paranoia or pessimism), conflicted or estranged relationships at the time of death, previously unresolved grief (including grief from past generations) and, above all, closed or faulty communication patterns (McGoldrick, 1999; Walsh & McGoldrick, 1999).

Shapiro (1994) combined family systems theory with developmental theory, discerning in grief a family developmental crisis affecting both attachment and identity, and disrupting family stability in the short run while having the potential to radically redirect the future course of family development in the long run. For Shapiro, grief can either constrain growth by disrupting family stability, or enhance growth by gradually promoting a new sense of family organization and creative opportunities. Death and profound loss tend to transform family relationships, not only among the living, but including relationships to the deceased whose image is integrated into both psychic and interactional structures that support ongoing family development. Thus, family bereavement is not merely something to survive or from which to recover. Family bereavement can be a positive force for directing the flow of development. Healthy grief enhances family stability, strengthens family coping skills so as to better master future losses, redefines personal identities, and enhances collaborative skills in the complex dynamics of family life. Thus, increased development and health can be the ultimate outcome of the family bereavement process.

Shapiro asserted that following a traumatic family loss, it may take many years to achieve the reconstruction of both personal and family processes in order to achieve stability and reintegration. Internal change and transformation of family processes occur simultaneously, recursively supporting and fostering one another. Grief is not a time-limited process followed by the mourner's return to life as it was before the loss. Rather, the loss is permanent and becomes a lasting reality that the bereaved must integrate into new structures and new realities. Recovery from grief is a misnomer. Persons don't recover; instead, they reestablish themselves with their identities altered and relationships inevitably changed (Shapiro, 1994).

GRIEF FROM A COUPLE RELATIONSHIP PERSPECTIVE

Very little can be found in the literature that conceptualizes bereavement in couples, except in the case of parents who lose a child (Rando, 1986) or among gay male couples where one is dying from AIDS (Nolen-Hoeksema & Larson, 1999; Sowell, Bramlett, Gueldner, Gritzmacher, & Martin, 1991). It is reasonable to surmise that grief comes to the couple subsystem incorporating features described from the individual perspective as well as features from the family systems perspective. Yet couple bereavement has its own distinctive character. Profound grief disturbs not only one's internal sense of coherence, but also the boundaries and cohesiveness of the dyad as well. Schnarch (1991, 1997) asserts that the core task of marriage is the ability to balance two separate and competing forces—the need for space and individuality on the one hand, and the need for closeness or togetherness on the other. Partners distressed by bereavement typically move in one direction or the other, seeking more space or demanding more closeness. What may be a fairly wide latitude in the couple's style of relating under normal circumstances narrows to an intensified demand for being alone or being together as a way of coping with bereavement. But both partners are unlikely to want the same thing, at the same time, in the same manner. Imbalance in the couple's style of relating leads to emotional distance, disappointment, or conflict.

Grief may launch a pursuer–distancer cycle with the pursuing spouse, frequently the wife, seeking solace and comfort from the partner who handles his own grief by withdrawing and comforting himself. The walls erected during prolonged pursuing and distancing typically result in increased criticism, defensiveness, and contempt (Guerin, Fay, Burden, & Kautto, 1987; Heyman, 2001).

Couples may experience grief very differently (Rosenblatt, 2000). The partners may encounter a different intensity in their feelings, one being overwhelmed with emotions while the other remains impassive. Partners may have different ways of handling pain. One may want to be encircled by their family while the other prefers to be sequestered. One may need to remember sad or difficult times whereas the other needs to forget them. Typically, a strong emotional process such as grief in one's partner creates equally strong anxiety in one's self. Poorly differentiated couples tend to handle anxiety interpersonally, that is, intruding on the partner's feelings or behavior in the attempt to calm the partner or to punish the partner for making one uncomfortable. Better differentiated partners calm themselves, thus making themselves emotionally available as a resource to the other (Schnarch, 1991).

Individuals may pace themselves differently as they experience grief. One partner may have a prolonged grief reaction while the other is bereaved for only a short time. One person may experience continuous grief while the other transitions in and out of mourning. A husband may deal with grief through activity while his wife finds herself barely able to garner the energy to face the next day. The meaning of the loss may also be very different for each partner. A stillbirth may represent the loss of descendants to one partner while the other experiences the event as failure and is consumed with guilt. The couple's sexual relationship may suffer during bereavement, not only during the initial shock when feelings are numbed, but also during the long period of depression when the suppression of sexual desire is common. Some people feel it is inappropriate to experience sexual pleasure while mourning.

Faith may play a different role in grief for each partner, one relying on prayer and drawing closer to God while the other blames God and drops away from religious practices. One person may find worship a comfort during bereavement while the other finds it a painful reminder of the funeral. In bereavement one partner may sense the presence of the deceased while the other has no disposition for such experiences.

If the two members of the couple come from different cultural or ethnic backgrounds, they are likely to find crucial differences in the manner and extent to which they and their families of origin are involved in bereavement. Under the stress of bereavement, the couple's boundaries may shift so that parents and siblings, or even the entire extended family, may intrude on boundaries the couple had previously established. Of course, violations of relationship boundaries during bereavement are not confined to couples of dissimilar cultural origins. If the couple has had previous trouble establishing boundaries with extended family, such boundaries will likely be tested again as the family system reorganizes during the bereavement process.

Rosenblatt (2000) notes that most couples carry not only marital roles but parental responsibilities as well. Grief also impacts the children, causing unanticipated emotional or behavioral reactions. Grief challenges one's resources for parenting. It saps energy, it makes parents less patient and more irritable, conflict with children may increase, things may be said to children or by children that have never been said before, and any difficulties previously experienced in child rearing may only be magnified by bereavement.

Of course, disaffection, disharmony, and conflict are not inevitable consequences of a couple's bereavement. Many couples deal with bereavement smoothly, supporting one another and making the adaptations and adjustments necessary to keep their relationship strong. Some couples are drawn closer through their joint grief and find the bereavement process one in which they connect with and support one another in a way that binds them, emotionally and spiritually, closer than ever. Nolen-Hoeksema and Larson (1999) report that a majority of bereaved parents emerged from their loss with something positive, including prioritizing life goals, becoming more loving, sensitive, or tolerant, resolving old conflicts, renewing commitment to current relationships, learning to face death more calmly, and discovering strengths they did not realize they had.

Factors associated with the ability of couples to manage the pain associated with grief and to grow through this experience are explicitly related to the process of differentiation, that is, balancing separateness and togetherness (Schnarch, 1991). Couples who negotiate bereavement successfully have a strong sense of cohesion and value the support they mutually provide one another. At the same time, they have a deep respect for differences and neither expect nor demand that their partner will experience grief exactly as they do. They have the ability to remain open to each other's experience, even when feelings are painful and difficult. They can tolerate changes in one another and the temporary loss of important interpersonal exchanges, believing that in the long run the relationship will stabilize and good feelings will return. They adjust their activities and routines flexibly, making allowance for what is neglected and accommodating their partner's needs for greater support and understanding (Walsh & McGoldrick, 1995).

Some of the factors that benefit the bereaved couple are external to their relationship. The support of extended family and friends can be crucial. Adequate finances and stability in the supporting environment—work-related and social—can be very important. It is easier to handle one trauma than to have upheaval in many areas of life.

In addition, couples who cope successfully with bereavement tend to have a healthier belief system and outlook than those who are adversely affected. They understand that in case of profound grief, they may never "get over it"; rather, grief is given new meaning and a new place in life. Part of reconstructing life after grief is learning to live with pain and being able to share it with one's partner. In its most favorable outcome, grief works to transform the couple's intimacy in the direction of more openness, connection, and a deeper understanding of one's place in the cycle of life and death (Shapiro, 1994).

CLINICAL IMPLICATIONS FOR COUPLE THERAPY

Assessment

Assessment is the study of factors related to the presenting problem for the purpose of thoroughly understanding how the problem came about and what maintains it. Do couples seek help from a couple therapist for problems of bereavement? Yes, but generally not in the same way that bereaved individuals seeks help. In many cases, couples present with interpersonal difficulties related to a multitude of personal, relational, and family systems factors intertwined with grief from past loss or losses. This fact leads McGoldrick (1991) to suggest that therapists routinely screen for traumatic loss using a three-generational genogram and chronology or timeline of major stress events as part of every evaluation.

In the following assessment format, seven questions, liberally modified from those suggested in Raphael (1983) and Rando (1986), have been formulated to elicit crucial information about the loss as well as to facilitate the emotional expression and reappraisal necessary in grief work. For the sake of simplicity, these questions are written as though the couple is experiencing an acute grief reaction triggered by death. However, as noted earlier, many grief reactions are more chronic in nature and triggered by nondeath events. Examples of such nondeath loss have been included in the discussion below to underline the importance of this point. The reader should modify the proposed assessment framework to fit these principles to the vast array of special circumstances that grief experiences can encompass.

1. *Can you tell me about the death? What happened?* Bereavement can be complicated by the nature of the loss—for instance, when the loss occurs suddenly and unexpectedly, is "untimely," violent, the result of suicide or homicide, or when the body is not recovered (the ambiguous loss). Loss of a child or a hoped-for child is especially difficult for couples, including abortion and relinquishing a child for adoption. During the discussion it will become apparent how comfortably the partners can talk about the loss, and whether or not there are special issues for one or the other spouse.

2. *Can you tell me about the deceased and about your relationship with the deceased from the beginning?* In general, the risk of complications to loss

increases when the person lost played a significant role in the daily functioning of the survivor, was crucial to the survivor's identity or sense of adequacy, or had a strongly ambivalent or conflictual relationship with the survivor.

3. *How has this death affected you, your relationship, or your family? How have things changed for the two of you?* Not only are the couple's personal and subjective reactions to loss important, but also how the loss has affected their relationship and the functioning of the family. One couple continually referred to a significant change in their relationship beginning 8 years earlier, but could not identify any significant events that would account for this until by happenstance the wife mentioned that it was at about this time that her husband developed Peyronie's disease, a curvature of the erect penis that makes intercourse impossible. Once the Peyronie's disease was identified and the couple discussed how it affected their lives, it was obvious that both had suffered an important loss that they were previously unable to discuss. The inability to communicate feelings and concerns to one another impedes crucial adjustments a couple must make to accommodate new realities that affect their relationship.

4. *What about the timing of this death? What else was going on in your lives at this time? Were there other problems occurring simultaneously?* These questions make it clear that loss takes place in a context that may complicate the grief that ensues. The therapist wants to pay special attention to life cycle transitions that may have been interrupted by loss.

5. *What do you know about other significant deaths in your family, including past generations? Did any of them carry special significance or meaning for the family?* This inquiry underlines the presumption that the context in which death occurs is multigenerational. Death can lay down a legacy for the family that shapes and informs subsequent relationships and experiences with death.

6. *How have you struggled to cope with this loss thus far?* Coping involves the ability to adjust to new situations and manage emotion effectively. Emotional regulation is a key ingredient to coping well, because people who fail to deal effectively with their feelings are more likely to act impulsively, destructively, or fail to act altogether. Nolen-Hoeksema and Larson (1999) found that people who seek emotional support, express their emotions openly, and try to see something positive in their experience fare much better with grief than those who ruminate, worry, or avoid their feelings or anesthetize them with drugs and alcohol. Evidence further suggests that people who are more dependent on others for their self-esteem, those who are emotionally unstable, insecure, or neurotic, and those who are dispositionally pessimistic use less effective coping strategies than people who are better adjusted.

7. *Is there anything you would want to change about your manner of coping with this loss—either individually or as a couple?* This open-ended question invites the partners to look deeply into themselves and their relationship. Schnarch (1991) discusses the relationship among loss, self-awareness, and intimacy. The loss of someone or something important may create an acute awareness of loneliness within a person, as well as foster important changes in one's view of self and relationships. Furthermore, loss may result in new awareness of either the need for, or fear of, an intimate partnership with another person. Loss may provide the opportunity for a couple to examine their isolation from one another, and open them to the possibility of bonding with one another at a deeper level.

On the other hand, coping poorly with loss—withdrawing, ignoring, discounting, invalidating, overreacting, or negating the partner's grief—may drive a couple further apart. Refusing to make adjustments or accommodations to life changes and difficulties that accompany loss make couple and family transitions more difficult. When both partners are grieving, too much may be expected of one another; grieving partners may have too little energy, compassion, and patience to give the desired level of support to one another.

Couples who experience increased conflict and stress as a result of loss are at risk for triangulation. The more stressed partner may cope with the loss by looking outside the relationship for comfort and support while rejecting his or her mate as nonsupportive or annoying. When triangles become rigid and fixed over years, as when the relationship becomes emotionally depleted or chronically hostile and antagonistic, partners are less likely to resolve their differences and make the adjustments necessary between them.

In addition to the seven specific questions above, the couple therapist also needs to determine:

1. *The presence of complicated grief.* Major depression and serious distortions in the normal grief process require separate attention including medical intervention.
2. *The premorbid state of the relationship.* If the bereaved couple returns to their former level of functioning, will that be a satisfactory outcome or do preexisting interpersonal problems need to be addressed? Is helping the couple through the mourning process sufficient, or can bereavement function as a bridge to deeper issues of transformation and growth?
3. *The couple's current satisfaction with the relationship.* Couples who feel good about their relationship are more likely to support

each other's grieving, whereas grieving in dissatisfied relationships only breeds greater misunderstanding and distancing.

4. *The nature of the couple's commitment to the relationship.* Traumatic loss threatens the stability of a relationship because the relationship no longer feels as if it has the same purpose or fulfills the same needs. Does the couple have a sense of commitment to the relationship that transcends cycles of adversity and distress, or is one partner likely to "cash in the chips" when discouraged and hassled?

Treatment

Three different circumstances can bring bereaved couples to therapy: (1) both partners are grieving the same loss; (2) the loss causes one person to grieve and the other individual is having difficulty relating to or supporting the grief of this partner; or (3) both partners are grieving separate losses. The loss of a child is the typical example of the first situation, but miscarriages, stillbirths, abortions, and giving up a child for adoption can also represent situations in which both persons grieve the same loss. The loss of a parent, sibling, or best friend is a common example where only one partner grieves the loss. Both persons may experience acute grief involving separate losses, for instance when a parent of each partner dies in close temporal proximity.

The immediate decision facing the couple therapist is whether to see both partners conjointly, to see each partner separately, or to see one person and refer the other to a colleague. Individual sessions may provide greater support for the surging painful emotions present in acute grief and offer undivided attention, reassurance, and empathic regard to the grieving partner without attending to the more difficult and conflictual interpersonal processes. Individual sessions may also be the treatment of choice when one partner is too fragile or too reactive to tolerate the presence of the other in the therapy session. Finally, individual sessions may be offered to someone who is having a much more difficult grief experience, even when both partners are grieving.

Conjoint sessions offer the therapist a better opportunity to address separate styles of bereavement, grief-induced conflict, and old relationship conflicts stirred up by heightened dependency needs and changes in the family structure as a result of death or other loss. Conjoint sessions would be the treatment of choice when the emphasis is more on interpersonal issues than on internal processes. Many couple therapists combine conjoint and individual sessions, varying the proportion to meet changes in emphasis as acute grief abates and interpersonal issues emerge. The experience and competence of the therapist will also affect the decision regarding individual versus conjoint treatment; the more able the therapist is to manage conflict and control the tenor of the therapy session, the more feasible conjoint sessions become. Referring one partner to a colleague should be considered when the relationship is dissolving and issues of trust and confidentiality are foremost.

The second major decision facing the therapist is whether to mold the therapy around issues of acute mourning or issues emerging in the restoration phase of grief. This decision is governed by the presence of signs of acute mourning such as depression, helplessness, confusion, guilt, and preoccupation with the loss. During acute grief, problem-solving activities are generally suspended while attention is concentrated on emotion-focused coping. Worden (1991) described four tasks of acute grief: (1) to accept the reality of the loss; (2) to experience the pain and grief; (3) to adjust to an environment in which the deceased is missing; and (4) to withdraw emotional energy and reinvest it in another relationship. The following may also be of value during the phase of acute mourning:

Providing a Safe Environment for Handling Painful Feelings

Sometimes the painful feelings of loss are difficult to express to an intimate partner. Sometimes painful feelings frighten partners, creating either high reactivity or withdrawal. The therapy session can be a place where painful feelings are shared in a supportive environment and then set aside until the next session, rather than constantly erupting outside of therapy. Furthermore, the therapist can model and teach empathic listening skills, helping impassive partners to provide care and support to the griever. Finally, the therapist can support those who have great difficulty tolerating painful feelings in their partner.

Supporting Separate Coping Styles

Two partners seldom grieve alike. Each will grieve in his or her own, distinctive manner. Shapiro (1994) pointed out that shared coping is an enormously complex process requiring mutual awareness and responsiveness. Helping individuals to respect and tolerate the feelings of their grieving partner, or differences in how each partner grieves, is the first step in shared mourning.

Normalizing

Much help is offered the couple when the therapist is able to label the intense and unexpected internal processes of mourning as normal. De-

nial is very common in grieving, as is irritability. The partner of a bereaved person, as well as the griever, may struggle to comprehend what
is happening, and may receive great comfort in simply knowing that the
griever is not going crazy. Some people worry that grief has changed
them or their partner, turning them into someone they neither recognize nor like. It is helpful for grievers and their partners to recognize
that grief is a temporary state of being, not a change in personality or
character.

Addressing Irrational Thoughts

Survivors can be unrealistically harsh on themselves. In traumatic loss, a
survivor may develop notions that the loss could have been prevented if
he or she had done something differently. Frequently one partner will
attempt to argue the other out of an unrealistic belief, coming across as
dismissing the griever's feeling or experience. Often the therapist can
provide insight that helps resolve distorted thoughts. For instance, one
woman promised her mother that she would never allow the doctor to
put her on a respirator. But the day before her mother died, the doctor
suggested respiration as a temporary means to assist with breathing, believing that the patient would yet recover. When the patient didn't recover, the woman felt that she had betrayed her mother's request. The
therapist was able to help the woman understand the difference between using the respirator as temporary assistance for a patient expected to survive, and merely prolonging life in a terminally ill patient.

Developing New Coping Strategies

Nolen-Hoeksema and Larson (1999) discuss several categories in describing mechanisms that promote healthy coping with loss. *Emotional
expression,* such as crying or screaming, is the core coping mechanism
for grief. Both grieving persons and their partners are frequently confused by the intensity and range of the feelings that emerge in grief, or
they believe that such feelings are improper—for example, anger directed at the deceased. Some persons may not want to burden their
partner with their feelings, creating emotional distance instead. *Reappraisal,* such as remembering good times with the deceased and finding
a positive way to look at the loss, is also healthy. Appreciating one's remaining personal relationships and positive life experiences or opportunities may be an important ingredient in reappraisal. *Distraction,* defined as engaging in activities that get one's mind off the loss, is also
seen as positive when used as part of the overall coping strategy. *Seeking
support* from others can also be helpful, but only when the person from

whom support is sought is able to give it and doesn't discount the loss. Seeking support from a grief support group may be very helpful. Good coping strategies lead to lower levels of depression and bring about a healthy resolution of the loss. Ultimately, *taking action* to address the problems and choices made necessary by the loss helps to alleviate the helplessness and powerlessness often experienced in conjunction with the loss.

Projection and Displacement

The loss of a loved one, especially one who performed important care-giving and supportive functions, leaves a person bereft of the benefits provided through the relationship with the deceased. It can leave the person feeling incompetent and rejected. These feelings can easily be projected onto a partner who is blamed for making one feel like a fail-ure. The anger felt toward the deceased may be displaced onto the part-ner, who may then react to the projected and displaced feelings in a re-jecting way that confirms the griever's sense of being discarded and unwanted—thereby creating a mutual downward spiral.

Understanding What It Means to "Heal" from Grief

Grievers and their partners need to understand that profound loss can result in pain that is felt for years, even for a lifetime. Rando (1986) re-ported that contrary to common sense, grief does not steadily decline, but instead sometimes grows more intense several months or a year after the loss, when the social supports drop off and one is increasingly reminded of how life has changed forever without the deceased. Rather than "healing" from profound loss, the griever comes to readjust and reshape his or her life, incorporating new behaviors, new relationships, and new meanings that make room for a positive remembrance of the deceased.

Renewing Spiritual Ties

Not infrequently, the grieving process is a time of heightened spiritual awareness or spiritual crisis; therefore the therapist may encourage the griever and his or her partner to strengthen or renew ties to faith com-munities during acute mourning. Simply listening and encouraging people in their struggle with questions concerning God, good and evil, and what happens after death can be helpful. Nolen-Hoeksema and Larson (1999) report that people who participate regularly in religious practices are more likely to find social support, increase active problem solving, and engage in positive reappraisal of their situation. Religious beliefs frequently become a source of hope and an important context for bringing new meaning to the loss.

Couple Therapy of Chronic Grief: A Personal Perspective

Although couple therapists are called on to help couples during periods of acute grief, couple therapists may even more frequently be sought to resolve relationship problems and conflicts long after the relationship has been disrupted by profound loss. Many of these couples may have no idea that their relationship difficulties are grief related, stemming from losses that are sometimes quite remote. One clue that such difficulties are part of a bereavement process is that the subject of past losses is avoided; alternatively, when the therapist directs attention to the loss, there is a change in affect that sweeps over the partners and the tone and content of the discussion shift markedly. It is less constructive to think of couples stuck in chronic grief as somehow involved in a process that is "incomplete" than to regard them as couples whose mourning has uncovered preexisting personal and interpersonal problems. Other opinions to the contrary, the task of treating chronic grief seems not merely to be to "empower and strengthen the [couple] to mourn their loss and move on" (McGoldrick, 1995, p. 54). Instead, the critical issue is that mourning forces a couple to face themselves and reality in a new way, stripping them of superficial adaptations that no longer work and uncovering flaws in their way of being a couple. It is not simply "moving on" that is required, but a deeper coming to terms with who they are and what their relationship requires of them. It is seldom sufficient to merely recover what was; rather, it is necessary to grow and restructure their relationship as something new. More often than not, chronically bereaved couples have reestablished their previous equilibrium and found it wanting.

During acute grief, the couple has been forced to live in closer proximity with painful feelings than ever before. Bereaved partners cry more, show sadness, become melancholic, and get irritable. When acute grief subsides, partners may have difficulty becoming intimate again. Most couples believe that intimacy is composed exclusively of good feelings. However, being with a partner whose feelings have made one uncomfortable is very much a part of being intimate. It is in learning to tolerate the unpleasant affects in one's partner, and to manage one's own reactivity, that one becomes truly intimate. Bereavement is never easy for a couple to share, but partners who pass through it together and maintain a strong connection with one another grow more intimate.

Whether in the midst of one's own grief, or living with a grief-stricken partner, one's ability to remain loving and caring has been tested. Undoubtedly, each person has said and done things that have injured the other. Part of the restoration of the couple's relationship after acute grief is the acknowledgment of responsibility for hurts rendered and support not given. It takes maturity to ask forgiveness from one's partner for one's failings and wrongdoing. Immature partners believe that a relationship is constantly loving, and any failure to feel *in love* is a failure in the marriage. Mature partners understand that loving feelings come and go, that love is easy or difficult depending on the circumstances, and that it is one's commitment to the relationship and to being a loving person that ultimately makes a long-term relationship work.

Many couples fail to distinguish misbehavior from behavior that is merely annoying or disappointing. A partner's failure to provide sufficient comfort, attention, and closeness during acute grief is not necessarily a character flaw. Over the course of a relationship, individuals have to come to terms with the fact that their partner is not the "prince" or "princess" they initially thought. The real issue is whether or not they can love the partner they have chosen. Mature persons learn to love the partner they have, weaknesses and all. Crises in relationships force people to look at whether or not their ability to love is sufficient, not merely whether or not their partner is lovable. Gaining a new level of maturity in their relationship is part of the task of restoration following bereavement.

Unfortunately, some persons exhibit hurtful or destructive behavior during the phase of acute grief. Affairs, alcohol and drug abuse, and abusive behavior are examples of wrongdoing that jeopardize a partner's well-being. Although individuals may be expected to manage their own feelings and adjust to their partner's irritating behavior, a partner's hurtful or destructive behavior represents a serious character issue that must be addressed. However, individuals cannot rehabilitate their partners. A person has to address his or her own character flaws. People with significant character issues often have to be confronted with the possible loss of their relationship in order to take their own deficits seriously. I have found it a powerful intervention to address the distinction between behavior that is merely annoying and behavior that represents character fault. For example, a man who had numerous affairs and blamed it on his grieving wife's depression, saying that his unhappiness in marriage caused him to be unfaithful, was simply confronted with the statement, "That is what character is for. It keeps you doing the right thing during difficult times. If your character failed you when doing the right thing was tough, then the problem is in your character, not in the situation." In order to straighten up one's character, a person needs to revisit in therapy incidents of wrongdoing and then make amends to all who have been hurt by misbehavior. Strengthening character also means that the person learns to articulate the values and principles that govern their relationship, and commit themselves to living by those principles. Failure to live by those principles means the likely loss of their relationship.

CASE ILLUSTRATION

Katherine and John were a couple in their mid-30s who had been married 8 years. They had an adopted son, Russell, who was 2 years old. John was a roofer whose work was steady except during the three coldest months of the year. Katherine was the office manager for an independent insurance agency. Their combined incomes just barely provided them with a middle-class lifestyle. The couple came to me following Katherine's discovery of John's affair. Katherine was cleaning out the pockets of John's jeans when she found a note with a phone number. Already suspicious, Katherine dialed the number and discovered it belonged to Alice, a high school friend of John's. Alice admitted to an affair of 6 months with John. When confronted, John said he didn't want a divorce and agreed to end the affair with Alice and attend therapy.

Katherine described a growing distance between herself and John ever since Russell was adopted. She said that the couple's sexual relationship, poor since the first year of marriage due to John's transient problems with impotence, had become a source of great difficulty over the past 2 years. She said that if she did not initiate sexual relations, there were none. She complained that John showed little sexual interest in her and did what he could to avoid sexual intimacy. They seldom fought because John avoided conflict.

From John's perspective, he did not intend to have an affair, it just happened. He had bumped into Alice, an old high school acquaintance, at a restaurant one day when he stopped for lunch. Alice was recently divorced and had begun working out at a local gym. John worked out regularly and was soon arranging to meet Alice at her gym. Although the relationship was sexual from the beginning, John said that he really enjoyed talking with Alice more than anything. Alice and John shared a lot of disappointments and troubles with one another that they could not talk about with others. John said that he always felt guilty about the sex with Alice, but continued to see her because he enjoyed talking to her.

The background information about the marriage revealed that shortly after the couple began dating, Katherine became pregnant.

Since neither was ready to raise a child, emotionally or financially, the couple decided to abort the pregnancy. They continued to date for the next 4 years and then got married. Katherine wanted babies immediately and John, although ambivalent, acquiesced. But the babies did not come, and Katherine was found to have fertility problems. Fertility treatment followed and Katherine conceived immediately. However, the couple's baby girl, also named Katherine, was stillborn. John declined to view the baby, something he continued to regret. The couple's next pregnancy ended in miscarriage. The third pregnancy after marriage resulted in twins, a boy and a girl, born very prematurely. The boy lived 3 days, and the girl lived 5 days, dying in John's arms. The couple's fourth pregnancy ended in a late-term miscarriage. The couple decided to stop further fertility treatment and adopted Russell. In total, the couple had experienced one abortion, two miscarriages, a stillbirth and two infant deaths. Before they were 35 years old, the couple owned three gravesites that John visited frequently, usually alone.

Background information revealed Katherine and John to come from intact but very different homes. Katherine was close to her father, a businessman, who was very loving but passive. Katherine's mother was an abrasive and intrusive woman who dominated the home. Katherine kept her mother at a distance after marrying John until Russell was adopted. Then Katherine's mother became Russell's back-up childcare service and increasingly intruded into Katherine's life again. John was so resentful toward his mother-in-law that he refused to talk to her.

To the degree that Katherine's mother was intrusive, John's parents were uninvolved in his life. Both of John's parents worked long hours and were seldom home. He described his father as mean and his mother as "having virtually no maternal feelings." John was left to his own devices growing up, and as a youngster frequently visited his aunt and uncle who lived six blocks away for nurturing and for meals. When John was 12 his uncle was killed when he took John's bicycle for a ride.

From the beginning of therapy, Katherine wanted to address John's affair, but John was very defensive and unwilling to reveal much. To John, the affair was over and further discussion only felt like badgering. Furthermore, it caused Katherine pain, and John didn't want to cause Katherine more suffering.

Initially, John had a similar approach to his feelings about the multiple losses in his life, from the tragic death of his uncle through the abortion, miscarriages, stillbirth, and infant deaths. All of these were extremely painful for John and he did not see any sense in discussing them. However, in the fourth session, John began to express deep sadness about the death of his babies. He blamed himself for the death of the twins because he did not insist that Katherine stop working during her pregnancy. He blamed Katherine for the miscarriages and the still-born child because she was a smoker. He felt he had let his wife down when he refused to see the stillborn baby. And he had deep guilt over the abortion of the couple's pregnancy prior to marriage. The feelings associated with these losses were still painfully alive in John, much to the surprise of Katherine. He admitted to years of feeling depressed and dejected. He looked tired and defeated. At one point in the session John said, "What we do best is make and kill babies." At another point, he referred to the irony of putting roofs over the heads of babies for a living, but not being able to keep his own babies alive. John revealed how often he visited the cemetery, much more frequently than Katherine knew. His mood swung between morose and angry. He talked about being afraid of getting close to Russell, and fearing that Russell would also suddenly die. He worried that, like his mother, he lacked the instinct to be a good parent and to be involved in his child's life. John was asked to consider medication for his depression but because he had abused drugs as a teenager, he did not want anything to do with drugs now, even if prescription drugs.

Over the next few sessions, Katherine became less angry with John for the affair and more aware of John's distress. She began to understand that after adopting Russell, she too had become overly concerned about keeping Russell alive and had become absorbed in her baby, overlooking her marriage. The couple found that for the first time they could talk about their shared losses, and began to support rather than blame each other. John let go of irrational beliefs—that he was responsible for his uncle's death, that he was only good at "making and killing babies," and that Russell might die if John allowed himself to get close to him. John also became aware of a deep paternal instinct through his frequent visits to the cemetery. As John and Katherine drew closer to each other emotionally and learned that they could talk about painful things, they began to address their sexual relationship. They found that they could also discuss other issues without avoidance or anger, eventually reestablishing the boundary between their family and Katherine's intrusive mother. Finally, John was also able to address the affair and take greater responsibility for his wrongdoing and the suffering he had caused Katherine. The couple reaffirmed their commitment to their marriage and to a monogamous relationship. The remembrance of their tragic losses was still painful, but they learned to face suffering together and that together, they could bear much more than alone.

Opening the issues around unfinished bereavement with John and Katherine appeared to help them grieve more successfully and move on with their lives. Yet much more happened to Katherine and John than merely resuming their lives. The restoration phase of John and Katherine's bereavement involved significant internal and interpersonal changes. John was able to establish a more positive identity; he was not merely someone who "killed babies" but instead, he was a husband and father. He learned to deal constructively with his pain. He affirmed values that supported becoming a good husband and a role model for his son. He experienced the sharing of powerful emotions with his partner within the boundaries of an intimate relationship, not outside of it. Katherine and John paid better attention to their connection with each other and to nurturing their togetherness. They learned to better define and safeguard their marital boundary, protecting it from an intrusive grandmother. They structured their lives around their shared roles as parents, and compartmentalized their grief so that it did not dominate their family life. Their ability to deal constructively with their mutual grief opened the path for John and Katherine to address many issues, internal and interpersonal, which had previously constrained a healthy marital relationship.

CONCLUSION

Death and profound loss affect not only the internal state of an individual, but also the interpersonal fabric of couples' relationships and the dynamics of family life. Grief may precipitate a realignment of relationships, a reorganization of individual and family functioning, and a change in the family's definition of itself and its belief system. Thus, although an individual may appear to "recover" from the symptoms of grief, systemic and interpersonal changes resulting from bereavement frequently continue to affect a person, couple, or family for the rest of their lives or even across successive generations.

Grief is a uniquely individual reaction to death and traumatic loss; recovery varies according to the coping mechanisms used by the individual as well as the subjective meaning of the loss and its surrounding circumstances. Hence, intimate partners do not experience losses in the same way, nor do they follow the same path to recovery.

Clinicians need to be attuned to the long term effects that bereavement has on the couple's relationship and the manner in which core relationship processes—balancing autonomy and togetherness, establishing intimacy, managing intense emotions, and sharing without losing oneself—are challenged during bereavement, leading to protracted relationship problems. Locating the source of bereavement-driven problems in the context of grief and its aftereffects often frees up blocked emotional processes and destructive beliefs that have prevented individuals from completing the bereavement process. As a result, couples' struggles that emerge during bereavement may be the "crucible" (Schnarch, 1991) in which each partner is challenged to grow and to address those core relationship processes that lead to health and wholeness. Thus, couple therapy is an appropriate and frequently necessary intervention for handling both acute and chronic bereavement.

REFERENCES

American Psychiatric Association. (1994). *Diagnostic and statistical manual of mental disorders* (4th ed.). Washington, DC: Author.

Bowen, M. (1976). Family reaction to death. In P. Guerin (Ed.), *Family therapy* (pp. 335–348). New York: Gardner.

Clayton, P. J., Kalikas, J. A., Maurice, W. L., & Robins, E. (1973). Anticipatory grief and widowhood. *British Journal of Psychiatry, 122,* 47–51.

Glick, I. O., Weiss, R. S., & Parkes, C. M. (1974). *The first year of bereavement.* New York: Wiley.

Guerin, Jr., P. J., Fay, L. F., Burden, S. L., Kautto, J. G. (1987). *The evaluation and treatment of marital conflict: A four-stage approach.* New York: Basic Books.

Herz, F. (1980). The impact of death and serious illness on the family life cycle. In E. A. Carter & M. McGoldrick (Eds.), *The family life cycle: A framework for family therapy* (pp. 223–240). New York: Gardner.

Herz, F. (1988). The impact of death and serious illness on the family life cycle. In B. Carter & M. McGoldrick (Eds.), *The changing family life cycle: A framework for family therapy* (2nd ed., pp. 457–482). New York: Gardner.

Heyman, R. E. (2001). Observation of couple conflicts: Clinical assessment applications, stubborn truths, and shaky foundations. *Psychological Assessment, 13,* 5–35.

Kuhn, J. (1981). Realignment of emotional forces following loss. *The Family, 5,* 19–24.

McGoldrick, M. (1995). Echoes from the past: Helping families mourn their losses. In F. Walsh & M. McGoldrick (Eds.), *Living beyond loss: Death in the family* (pp. 50–78). New York: Norton.

Nolen-Hoeksema, S., & Larson, J. (1999). *Coping with loss.* Mahwah, NJ: Erlbaum.

Osterweis, M., Soloman, F., & Green, M. (1984). Death at a distance: A study of family survivors. *Omega: Journal of Death and Dying, 13,* 191–225.

Parks, C. M., & Weiss, R. (1983). *Recovery from bereavement.* New York: Basic Books.

Paul, N., & Paul, B. (1982). Death and changes in sexual behavior. In F. Walsh (Ed.), *Normal family processes* (pp. 229–250). New York: Guilford Press.

Paul, N., & Paul, B. (1989). *A marital puzzle.* Boston: Allyn & Bacon.

Pinkus, L. (1974). *Death and the family: The importance of mourning.* New York: Pantheon.

Rando, T. A. (1983). An investigation of grief and adaptation in parents whose children have died from cancer. *Journal of Pediatric Psychology, 8,* 3–20.

Rando, T. A. (1986). Individual and couples treatment following the death of a child. In T. A. Rando (Ed.), *Parental loss of a child* (pp. 341–413). Champaign, IL: Research Press.

Rando, T.A. (1988). *Grieving: How to go on living when someone you love dies.* Lexington, MA: Lexington Books.

Raphael, B. (1983). *The anatomy of bereavement.* New York: Basic Books.

Rosenblatt, P. C. (2000). *Help your marriage survive the death of a child.* Philadelphia: Temple University Press.

Schnarch, D. M. (1991). *Constructing the sexual crucible: An integration of sexual and marital therapy.* New York: Norton.

Schnarch, D. M. (1997). *Passionate marriage.* New York: Norton.

Shapiro, E. R. (1994). *Grief as a family process: A developmental approach to clinical practice.* New York: Guilford Press.

Silver, R. L., & Wortman, C. B. (1980). Coping with undesirable life events. In J. Garber & M. E. P. Seligman (Eds.), *Human helplessness: Theory and applications* (pp. 279–375). New York: Academic Press.

Sowell, R. L., Bramlett, M. H., Gueldner, S. H., Gritzmacher, D., & Martin, G. (1991). The lived experience of survival and bereavement following the death of a lover from AIDS. *Image, 23,* 89–94.

Vachon, M. L. S., Rogers, J., Lyall, W. A. L., Lancee, W. J., Sheldon, A. R., & Freeman, S. J. J. (1982). Predictors and correlates of adaptation to conjugal bereavement. *American Journal of Pyshciatry, 139,* 998–1002.

Walsh, F., & McGoldrick, M. (1995). Loss and the family: A systemic perspective. In F. Walsh & M. McGoldrick (Eds.), *Living beyond loss: Death in the family* (pp. 1–29). New York: Norton.

Worden, J. W. (1991). *Grief counseling and grief therapy: A handbook for the mental health practitioner* (2nd ed.). New York: Springer.

Zisook, S., & Shuchter, S. R. (1986). First four years of widowhood. *Psychiatric Annals, 16,* 288–294.

PART IV

Integration

In this final part, the editors discuss implications of previous chapters for clinical practice, training, and research. A consistent theme in this part emphasizes that effective treatment of both individuals and couples requires assessment and intervention strategies targeting both intrapersonal as well as interpersonal components of functioning. Therapists should be competent in recognizing the recursive influences of individual and couple difficulties. They also need to exercise both technical and theoretical flexibility in drawing on specific interventions addressing the full spectrum of individual and relationship functioning and must possess an organizing conceptual framework for integrating these interventions effectively.

To achieve this objective, additional research needs to delineate the impact of relationship functioning on the treatment of mental and physical disorders, and the impact of individual functioning on the treatment of couple distress, including therapeutic processes, mechanisms of change, and both intermediate and long-term outcomes. Empirical findings from such research need to be incorporated throughout the broader healthcare system to ensure the utilization of couple-based interventions that have been demonstrated to be equally or more effective than traditional individual treatment modalities in treating or preventing clients' emotional and behavioral disorders.

Based on the previous chapters in this volume, the editors delineate 12 imperatives for clinical practice, training, and research. Pursuit of this "12-step" program promises to enhance the ability of both individual and couple therapists to recognize and intervene in their clients' emotional and behavioral difficulties across multiple levels of the family system.

CHAPTER 18

Understanding Psychopathology and Couple Dysfunction

Implications for Clinical Practice, Training, and Research

DOUGLAS K. SNYDER
MARK A. WHISMAN

Couple therapy has entered a new era. Both theoretical and empirical developments have made increasingly clear not only that couple therapy represents a viable intervention for a broad spectrum of individual emotional and behavioral disorders but that, in many cases, couple therapy comprises the preferred treatment. Individual and relationship distress interact in a recursive and mutually reinforcing manner. Rarely would one anticipate encountering someone with significant psychopathology or physical illness for whom there are not also significant implications for that person's intimate relationships. Hence, providers of mental or physical health services need to address the role of couple dysfunction both as a contributing factor and consequence of individual emotional, behavioral, and health problems.

Similarly, findings regarding the comorbidity of individual and relationship dysfunction emphasize that couple therapists should anticipate a strong likelihood that many of the partners they treat will also exhibit significant individual dysfunction historically neglected in many previous formulations of couple therapy (Whisman & Uebelacker, Chapter 1, this volume). At the very least, individual psychopathology and physical health problems render couple therapy more difficult. Individual difficulties in either partner may cause or exacerbate existing relationship problems, may interfere with or detract from couple therapies targeting interpersonal functioning, or may require specific interventions aimed at individual emotional or health problems before interventions emphasizing relationship issues can be effective. Consequently, it is essential that couple therapists become more skillful in recognizing and treating individual difficulties that accompany and interact with relationship distress.

Understanding the relation of psychopathology to couple therapy has distinct implications for clinical practice, training, and research. Although in the discussion below we separate implications for practice and training from those for research, clearly each relates to the other. Ultimately, neither clinical practice nor training in couple therapy can proceed from an empirically informed perspective without an adequate research base that delineates the covariation of individual and relationship difficulties and evaluates interventions targeting both.

IMPLICATIONS FOR CLINICAL PRACTICE AND TRAINING

• *Effective treatment of individuals and couples requires comprehensive assessment of intrapersonal and interpersonal functioning throughout affective, behavioral, and cognitive domains across multiple levels of the family and socioecological system.* Couples presenting with primary complaints of relationship difficulties often fail to recognize, understand, or acknowledge the role of individual problems in their interpersonal distress. Similarly, individuals seeking treatment for their own emotional or health problems may neglect or minimize the interaction of these concerns with interpersonal functioning in their intimate or broader social relationships. Practitioners are similarly vulnerable to viewing presenting complaints through the filtering lens of their own preferred theoretical or treatment modality—whether from an individual perspective or from an interpersonal and relational perspective.

Effective treatment of individuals and couples requires understanding of *what* to assess. Specifically, practitioners need to assess their clients' emotional, behavioral, and health functioning and the functioning of their intimate partners across a broad spectrum of individual and system domains (Snyder, Cozzi, & Mangrum, 2002). This includes the onset, course, and previous treatment of partners' individual difficulties and the manner in which these contribute to, result from, or interact with relationship problems. Separate from any individual concerns, clients' relationships need to be assessed in terms of their over-all dysfunction or well-being. This includes partners' relationship strengths and vulnerabilities, adaptation or deterioration, fears and aspirations, and frustration or fulfillment.

Approaches regarding *how* to assess both intrapersonal and interpersonal functioning vary as a function of theoretical assumptions. The clinical interview remains the primary mode of clinical assessment for most practitioners, but can only be as good as the clinician's knowledge regarding specific indicators of individual and relationship functioning (Snyder & Abbott, 2002). Structured interviews ensure systematic attention to domains and social system levels of functioning often neglected or overlooked in typical practice; so too do more formal observational and self-report assessment techniques. Clinical assessment will be facilitated by understanding the comorbidity of individual and relationship problems both within and between partners. For example, given empirical findings in both community and clinical samples, it seems almost unimaginable that a practitioner would treat individual depression without investigating the role of relationship distress, would conduct couple therapy without carefully assessing for potential substance abuse or physical aggression, or would intervene with severe emotional dysregulation in one or both partners without screening for early childhood abuse or neglect, and considering its effects in other areas of both individual and relationship functioning.

Additionally, assessment of individual and relationship functioning essential to effective treatment requires recognizing heterogeneity both in the patterns of characteristics defining individual and relationship problems and in their levels of intensity. For example, research has documented variation in the patterns of partners' physical aggression with respect to frequency and severity of aggression and related cognitive and affective components—with individual differences in this regard linked to alternative intervention strategies and differential outcome (Holtzworth-Munroe, Marshall, Meehan, & Rehman, Chapter 9, this volume). Similarly, subdromal expressions of individual or relationship disorders may warrant consideration of treatment approaches similar to those developed for their more intensive clinical counterparts.

For these implications to be realized, training programs in the allied health and related human service professions need to ensure that all practitioners achieve at least a minimum level of proficiency in assessing and recognizing recursive interactions between individual and relationship functioning. Physicians, clergy, and individual therapists need to be trained in basic principles of relationship assessment and intervention and they need to be familiar with the role of relationship quality in mental and physical health, compliance with medication and related treatment regimens, and vulnerability or resistance to relapse. Similarly, couple and family therapists need to be schooled in psychopathology and principles of individual assessment and treatment, including biological interventions for relationship difficulties rooted at least in part in physical or mental illness of one or both partners.

• *Therapy will be most effective when individuals and couples are matched to treatments for which they possess prerequisite attributes and are excluded from treatments for which they are particularly ill suited.* For assessment to influence treatment, individual differences in intrapersonal and interpersonal functioning need to be linked to alternative models and modalities of intervention. For example, couple-based interventions for individual emotional and behavioral problems may follow one of three approaches: (1) general couple therapy and reduction of relationship distress causing or contributing to individual difficulties; (2) disorder-specific interventions targeting specific aspects of relationship functioning resulting from, contributing to, or maintaining individual concerns; or (3) partner-assisted treatments in which one partner offers support, guidance, or response contingencies aimed at modifying the behavior or alleviating the distress of the other (Baucom, Shoham, Mueser, Daiuto, & Stickle, 1998). Although the development and evaluation of disorder-specific and partner-assisted couple treatments for individual problems comprise a relatively recent phenomenon, continued advances along these lines promise to alter substantially the practice of couple therapy. No longer will generic relationship-enhancement techniques suffice as more effective approaches to working with difficult couples are articulated.

It will continue to be the case that, for some disorders, the clinical challenge will not be which specific treatment to select for the disorder but, rather, how to adapt existing treatments to individual difficulties. For example, regardless of the practitioner's preferred theoretical approach to treating relationship distress, both the content and pacing of interventions will likely need to be modified when one or both partners exhibit significant levels of interpersonal hypervigilance, emotional dysregulation, or disruption of cognitive processes associated with aging or posttraumatic stress, physical health problems, or unresolved grief.

In addition to matching variation in individual and relationship characteristics to differences in treatment modality, so too should these be matched to differences in treatment *goals*. In some cases, adaptations of couple therapy may be undertaken to *contain* individual difficulties—as when working with partners exhibiting a narcissistic or paranoid disorder. In other cases, as when treating complicated grief, the goal may be to *restore* previously healthy levels of individual and relationship functioning disrupted by traumatic loss. In other cases, the goal may be to *enhance* the relationship. Enhancement is distinguished from restoration among couples whose well-being has persistently been compromised by individual difficulties and the goal is to help partners achieve a new and more satisfying level of intrapersonal and relationship functioning. For some couples, such as those confronting terminal illness, treatment objectives may emphasize minimizing or *preventing* comorbid individual emotional and relationship difficulties that may develop in response to the health problem.

To a large extent, both the clinical literature and clinical practice have emphasized inclusionary criteria to the neglect of exclusionary criteria for treatment selection. For example, individuals presenting with depression tend to be offered individual treatments, independent of comorbid relationship problems resulting from or contributing to the person's depression. Similarly, couples presenting with relationship distress typically receive couple-based interventions, regardless of whether specific characteristics of one or the other partner require interventions targeting individual difficulties prior to relationship therapy. Descriptions of specific approaches to couple therapy sometimes incorporate a promotional zeal emphasizing a broad spectrum of individuals or disorders for which that specific approach is advocated while overlooking individual or relationship characteristics contraindicating or reducing the treatment's likely effectiveness. Clinicians need to be as attentive to exclusionary characteristics influencing treatment selection as they are to inclusionary criteria. Moreover, they need to be sufficiently trained both in theory and research methods to be discerning consumers of the literature in evaluating diverse treatment modalities.

- *Empirical findings regarding the efficacy of couple- and family-based interventions for individual emotional, behavioral, and health problems should influence practice guidelines at the corporate level.* By "corporate" we mean practice beyond the individual practitioner. At the simplest corporate level, this implies collaboration among practitioners varying in discipline and level of expertise. Clinicians preferring to practice primarily through the modality of individual interventions need to develop collaborative alliances with colleagues having special expertise in dealing with aspects of relationship functioning that interact with individual difficulties. Similarly, couple therapists working with difficult couples experiencing physical health problems or major psychopathology need to form close working relationships with physicians for managing medical treatment or pharmacological interventions, and with therapists skilled in treating individual emotional or behavioral disorders that lie outside the scope of couple-based techniques.

Both individual and couple or family practitioners need to extend system-based formulations to the broader socioecological context to incorporate interventions from the legal, medical, educational, social, and religious communities. Collaborative, multidisciplinary treatment rarely proceeds on its own and requires initiation and sustained coordination of efforts. Practitioners need to be trained in handling complex issues of confidentiality when participating in collaborative treatment (Osterman, Sher, Hales, Canar, Singla, & Tilton, Chapter 15, this volume).

A higher order of corporate response involves institutional policies formalizing multidisciplinary interventions across individual and couple or family levels. For example, within medical settings this involves systematic attention to relationship phenomena on primary care units and inclusion of couple interventions to treat individual health problems or contain their secondary effects. Within psychiatric settings—including substance abuse treatment facilities—it implies placing couple and family interventions at the forefront of treatment rather than relegating them to elective collateral interventions. Within the legal community, corporate response implies discerning when couple interventions are either advantageous or essential to remediation for individual legal violations (as in substance abuse, sexual offenses, or domestic violence) and ensuring that sentencing guidelines—including mandatory involvement in couple- or family-based interventions—reflect empirical findings. It also implies recognizing when couple-based interventions are *not* appropriate—as in severe physical violence—and avoiding well intentioned but misguided referral to mandated couple therapy as a means to deter divorce.

Finally, corporate response among health maintenance organizations and third-party payers requires eliminating clinical service and reimbursement policies that discourage couple- and family-based treatments. In their effort to contain costs and avoid paying benefits for elective "relationship enhancement" interventions, insurers have discouraged couple-based interventions that have been demonstrated to be equally or more effective than traditional individual treatment modalities in treating or preventing clients' emotional and behavioral disorders. Couple therapy remains essential for reducing relationship distress that may function as a precursor or the cause of significant emotional, behavioral, or health problems. Moreover, couple-based interventions may serve as a critical component of a comprehensive treatment regimen for a variety of disorders requiring intervention at multiple levels of the individual's psychosocial system.

• *Differences in urgency of individual and relationship issues and their progression during therapy require an organizational conceptual framework for selecting, sequencing, and pacing interventions.* Although virtually all approaches to couple therapy possess an implicit progression of individual treatment components, difficult couples demand special attention to the selection, sequencing, and pacing of specific interventions. For some couples this consideration is mandated by individual or relationship issues that impede an initial working alliance between partners or with the therapist—as in severely antagonistic relationships or with narcissistic or paranoid clients. For other couples the modal sequencing of interventions must be modified to contend with such crises as suicidality, alcohol or drug dependence, major psychopathology, infidelity, violence, or other trauma including recent diagnosis of a terminal illness. Because such crises may emerge at any point during couple therapy, practitioners need an organizational framework for integrating concurrent individual and relationship interventions, and linking immediate responses to crisis to therapeutic strategies that both preceded and follow these events.

The intensity of affect exchanged between partners and other family members in couple and family therapy can present special challenges to the clinician in managing his or her own affect. Therapists need to be trained to incorporate their own emotional responses as an assessment technique in understanding the complex and sometimes subtle interplay of emotional dynamics in a couple or family system (Scharff & Bagnini, Chapter 12, this volume). Similarly, because the challenge of responding to affective components at both the individual and relationship level can be particularly daunting with difficult couples, ongoing consultation or supervision from peers or a multidisciplinary treatment team can be vital.

Beyond the level of individual crises, the nature of systems to resist change also influences the organization of treatment components when working with difficult couples. There is a long-standing perspective that once a system has accommodated to individual or relationship dysfunction, improvements in one or more members or relationships within a system result in changes across the whole system (Jackson, 1957). Hence, treatment of particularly difficult couples often requires alternating attention between partners and their relationship with each other or other family members in promoting growth in one individual or relationship and then working with other members to promote their adaptation to this change. The interaction between individual and relationship problems accentuates the importance of an organizational framework for attending to such system dynamics.

Practitioners' organization of interventions also needs to be tailored to the inherent progression of the specific challenges facing partners and their relationship. For example, with major mental illness such as schizophrenia or a bipolar disorder the modal function may be phasic and recurrent—where the goals of treatment may involve preparation for relapse, recognition of prodromal indicators, and containment of symptoms when they recur (Miklowitz & Morris, Chapter 5, and Mueser & Brunette, Chapter 6, this volume). In other cases, as in Alzheimer's disease or terminal illness, the expected course may involve progressive deterioration for one individual and the sequencing of interventions may evolve from initial treatment targeting the identified patient to interventions designed to help the couple adapt to changing roles, and ultimately transitioning to individual therapy provided to the surviving partner (Osterman et al., Chapter 15, and Qualls, Chapter 16, this volume).

• *Effective treatment of difficult couples often requires therapists to conceptualize and practice integratively across diverse theoretical orientations.* Difficult couples often require thinking outside the parameters of any one theoretical orientation—in part because theoretical approaches to both individual and couple therapy vary in their attention to cognitive, affective, and behavioral components of intrapersonal and interpersonal functioning. The more difficult the couple, the greater the need may be to draw on increasingly diverse intervention strategies to address multiple individual and relationship problems. Integrative practice may be pursued in two ways (Lebow, 1987). One path involves training in, and use of, theoretically integrative models described in the literature. An alternative to adopting an existing integrative approach is to practice pluralistically across multiple theoretical modalities, but to pursue technical integration by incorporating a conceptual organizational framework tailored to couple differences in individual and relationship functioning (Snyder, Schneider, & Castellani, Chapter 2, this volume). Technical integration within a theoretically pluralistic approach presents a greater challenge to the therapist because it demands familiarity with both specific intervention techniques and conceptual underpinnings across a broad spectrum of theoretical approaches, and then systematically selecting specific treatment components in a coherent and synthetic manner in tailoring these in unique fashion to each couple.

Training programs need to focus explicitly on instructing developing therapists in the principles and strategies of integrative practice—ensuring a technical understanding of specific therapeutic techniques, the theoretical context in which these evolved, and their demonstrated efficacy for particular problems in specific populations (Norcross & Beutler, 2000). Well-trained clinicians require explicit and internally consistent theories of integrative practice. At a minimum, such theories need to specify relevant domains of experience, parameters of functional and dysfunctional behavior, intermediate and long-term treatment objectives, and multiple processes of change at both the intrapersonal and interpersonal or systemic level.

IMPLICATIONS FOR RESEARCH

• *The co-occurrence of relationship and mental or physical health problems and their recursive interactions need to be explicated in both community and clinical populations.* The extant literature regarding co-occurrence of relationship dysfunction and health problems varies in its attention to Axis I versus II disorders as well as acute versus chronic physical health problems. Indeed, there are numerous mental and physical health problems for which their covariation with relationship functioning has rarely, if ever, been studied. Furthermore, research on the co-occurrence of relationship dysfunction and health problems is needed in both community and clinical samples because epidemiological findings indicate that clinical samples represent a minority of individuals with psychiatric disorders (Kessler et al., 1994), and there may be important differences between people who seek treatment from those who do not.

Much of the existing literature has focused on the association between a target disorder in one person and their own relationship functioning. However, because most persons having one psychiatric disorder also have other co-occurring disorders (Kessler et al., 1994), investigators need to consider the issue of comorbidity in evaluating whether relationship functioning is associated with the target disorder, a co-occurring disorder, or the comorbidity between disorders. Furthermore, because research has shown that partners of people with psychiatric disorders are more likely themselves to meet criteria for disorders (e.g., McLeod, 1995), additional research is needed on the relational impact of co-occurring disorders across partners, or more generally regarding the impact of dysfunction in one partner on the well-being of the other. Finally, in addition to evaluating the bidirectional association between relationship functioning and psychiatric disorders, there is an additional need for evaluating this association for subdromal expressions of clinical disorders or variations within such spectrum disorders as schizophrenia or paranoia.

In addition to redressing these limitations, research on the co-occurrence of relationship dysfunction and health problems needs to attend to such methodological considerations as evaluating a person's functioning within their intimate relationship in comparison with their social support and functioning in other kinds of relationships (Whisman, Sheldon, & Goering, 2000). Furthermore, there is a need for research evaluating this covariation that also takes into account the role of other disorders or other characteristics such as stage of individual or family development. For example, the comorbidity of cognitive impairment, depression, or sexual dysfunction with relationship quality may vary considerably as a function of age.

In addition to explicating the co-occurrence of relationship dysfunction and mental or physical health problems, researchers should aim to identify common mechanisms potentially underlying their covariation and stimulate theoretical models for these recursive relationships that would lend themselves to specific clinical interventions. Exemplars of the latter include interpersonal models of depression and research examining the role of families' expressed emotion in relapse in schizophrenia and bipolar disorders (Miklowitz & Morris, Chapter 5, this volume). Potential domains for exploring common mechanisms include the role of cognitive distortions in depression, emotional dysregulation in borderline personality disorder, hypervigilance in paranoid disorder, dominance and intimacy in sexual functioning, childhood sexual abuse in posttraumatic disorder, and the shared impact of each of these factors on couple distress.

• *Research needs to delineate the impact of relationship functioning on the treatment of mental and physical disorders, and the impact of individual functioning on the treatment of couple distress—including therapeutic processes, mechanisms of change, and both intermediate and long-term outcomes.* Inherent in this guideline is determining those recursive interactions of individual and relationship functioning that cause some couples to be particularly difficult to treat. In some domains the moderating effects of relationship dysfunction and mental or physical health problems on treatment outcome have been well substantiated. For example, untreated relationship problems predict poorer individual response to alcohol and drug abuse treatment, and poor response to substance abuse treatment predicts ongoing couple distress (Fals-Stewart, Birchler, & O'Farrell, Chapter 7, this volume). In other domains such research has been sparse or nonexistent. Little is known regarding the effects of comorbid disorders (e.g., borderline personality disorder and substance abuse, or sexual disorders and depression) on treatments developed for either disorder alone. Almost nothing is known about the interactive effects of comorbid disorders across partners on treatment processes or outcomes. Similarly, research has neglected individual differences in severity of intrapersonal dysfunction or couple distress; for example, there are few data regarding the effectiveness of couple therapy for depression when couples report only low levels of conflict (Beach & Gupta, Chapter 4, this volume).

Equally important as examining moderating effects of relationship dysfunction and health problems on treatment outcome is research explicating those features of intrapersonal and interpersonal functioning that buffer individuals from distress, facilitate treatment when difficulties arise, and reduce vulnerability to relapse. Individual and relationship strengths involve more than freedom from dysfunction. Do the factors that protect couples' relationships from generalized effects of individual emotional or health problems mirror those moderator variables identified for couple therapy in general? Do such protective factors reflect individual differences in relationship processes (e.g., trust, intimacy, or commitment), individual well-being and developmental history (e.g., exposure and adaptation to previous stressors), or psychological processes (e.g., attributional style or spirituality)?

Further research should also critically examine theoretical assumptions regarding the symptomatology and etiology of psychiatric disorders and their implications for processes of change. For example, assertions regarding disease processes underlying alcohol and other substance abuse potentially constrain the composition and application of couple-based prevention or treatment interventions (Fals-Stewart et al., Chapter 7, this volume); so too do assumptions regarding the role of repressed memories and the importance of confronting the perpetrator when intervening with couples for whom one partner continues to struggle with posttraumatic stress from childhood sexual abuse (McCarthy & Sypeck, Chapter 14, this volume). Even long-honored but unsubstantiated clinical lore regarding individual grief processes may misdirect interventions for couples struggling with complicated bereavement (Wills, Chapter 17, this volume). Hence, investigations of couple treatments for specific disorders need to be complemented by more basic research on the nature of these disorders themselves.

• *Greater attention needs to be focused on the generalizability of research findings across such potential moderators as age, family life stage, gender, culture and ethnicity (including interethnic couples), family structure (including composition of stepfamily and extended family systems), and nontraditional relationships (including cohabiting and same-gender couples).* There is ample evidence to indicate the importance of sociodemographic domains in moderating the linkage of individual and relationship functioning and their respective effects on treatment. For example, both young and old couples may become more socially isolated when confronting physical illnesses compared to their middle-aged counterparts—younger couples because there may be fewer other couples their age experiencing such illness, and older couples because of their decreased mobility and greater general isolation. Difficulties with infertility may have quite different impact on individuals and their relationship depending on their age, the presence of other children, and whether or not this is the partners' first marriage.

Similarly, increased consideration of gender and ethnicity in studies of mental and physical health has not translated into comparable attention to such moderator effects in research on relationship functioning and treatment. For example, there is relatively little research on couple-based interventions for depression where the husband is depressed (Beach & Gupta, Chapter 4, this volume). Cross-cultural comparisons of couple therapy—particularly couple-based treatments of individual emotional or health problems—are rare, despite documented differences in how couples of diverse cultural backgrounds contend with mental and physical illness (Osterman et al., Chapter 15, this volume). Also missing from the literature are treatment studies as well as more basic research on individual and relationship functioning in nontraditional couples including nonmarried cohabiting dyads in committed relationships and same-gender couples (Means-Christensen, Snyder, & Negy, 2003).

The importance of identifying moderators of linkages between individual and relationship functioning and their impact on treatment processes and outcome will require special consideration in designing clinical studies. To date, most clinical trials have involved samples insufficiently large to afford statistical power for detecting moderating effects. Couples reporting high rates of physical aggression or partners exhibiting such individual difficulties as personality disorders or substance abuse are frequently excluded from such trials, thereby precluding the ability to detect the moderating impact of such factors on treatment process or outcome. Measurement strategies often neglect important components of intrapersonal functioning, particularly as these relate to individual strengths. Treatment samples in research environments often fail to mirror the diversity of couple characteristics found in various practice settings. Addressing these limitations will likely require more extensive, collaborative, multisite studies supported through federal funding.

• *Research needs to examine the effectiveness of couple-based interventions for diverse disorders and for specific components within disorders.* This guideline has multiple implications. First, there needs to be further research on the effectiveness of existing couple treatments for specific disorders. In most cases, few controlled outcome studies have been conducted for any particular approach to a given disorder; comparisons among alternative couple-based treatments for a given emotional or behavioral disorder are rare (Christensen & Heavey, 1999). Most controlled studies for a specific disorder exclude individuals with comorbid conditions despite their prevalence in community or clinical samples, thereby limiting the generalizability of findings. Both comparisons among competing approaches and better articulation of exclusionary as well as inclusionary criteria should facilitate matching of couples to specific interventions and treatment modalities.

Second, the development and validation of couple-based interventions for emotional, behavioral, and health disorders not represented among existing treatments remains a priority. Across the spectrum of Axis I and particularly Axis II disorders, relatively few well-articulated couple treatments have been developed and empirically evaluated (Baucom et al., 1998). The application of couple-based interventions for physical health problems—including problems related to aging and cognitive decline—remains in its infancy. The absence of established couple treatment guidelines for emotional and physical disorders is striking given comorbidity studies and assorted findings regarding moderator effects in individual and couple therapy indicating the co-occurrence and recursive interactions of relationship and individual emotional and health concerns in diverse clinical populations and treatment settings.

Third, development of new treatments for specific disorders needs to complemented by studies examining the adaptation of existing approaches to couple distress when specific dysfunctions (e.g., narcissism, paranoia, or cognitive decline)—although not an explicit target of treatment—moderate both treatment process and outcome. Such adaptations should reflect the impact of specific disorders as well as specific components or subdromal expression of such disorders (e.g., emotional dysregulation or hypervigilance to specific trauma-related events).

There has been very little study of couple-based treatments for a given disorder across multiple settings such as structured laboratory research protocols versus flexible delivery by community practitioners. Virtually no research has examined critical issues of implementation across individual, concurrent, conjoint, or mixed-delivery modalities. For example, how effective are couple-based interventions for highly dysregulated couples with borderline personality functioning and concurrent suicidality or substance abuse as a stand-alone intervention versus delivery in combination with concurrent individual psychosocial and pharmacological interventions? When and how should combined treatments across multiple formats be conducted? Under what conditions might concurrent couple therapy enhance individual treatment?

When does individual therapy potentially enhance or detract from couple-based interventions? Research needs to examine not only the indicators and outcomes of combined intervention modalities with difficult couples but also the optimal sequencing, pacing, and coordination of interventions across these diverse approaches.

Investigations of couple-based interventions also need to expand the criteria by which treatments are evaluated. First, in terms of individual and relationship functioning, outcome measures need to move beyond reductions in individual and couple distress to examine promotion of such positive characteristics as hope, compassion, intimacy, playfulness, and creative pursuit of new opportunities for individual and relationship fulfillment. Second, research needs to consider outcomes for family members not specifically targeted by the treatment. For example, do couple treatments for partner violence generalize to reductions in parental verbal and physical aggression toward their children? Do couple-based interventions for Alzheimer's disease or other chronic or progressive physical illnesses promote positive outcomes for other caregivers within the extended family? Finally, couple treatment evaluations should address not only traditional markers of that treatment's effectiveness but also its costs relative to alternative interventions; research of this type may be the most compelling in influencing corporate policies toward third-party reimbursement for couple therapy.

• *Studies of treatment outcome need to be complemented by research on treatment processes, particularly as these relate to difficult couples.* Research on couple therapy process should begin with efforts to articulate both common factors in couple-based interventions and specific components that distinguish one approach from another (Wills, Faitler, & Snyder, 1987). To the extent that diverse treatment approaches share common attributes, this may facilitate shifting from one therapeutic modality to another to capture unique techniques specific to that approach when working with difficult couples. Because some techniques may require a set of interventions linked together in a specific constellation or sequence to be effective, research on articulating therapeutic components should identify the smallest unit of intervention that can be transported across approaches while retaining its efficacy.

Difficult couples disrupt the modal or prescriptive sequencing and pacing of interventions. For example, collaborative alliances may require a longer time to establish and may be more easily compromised or broken. Continuing or episodic crises may interrupt efforts to promote new relationship skills. Interventions promoting affective self-disclosure that might facilitate partners' emotional connectedness in healthier couples may instead trigger dysregulation and trauma in more disturbed couples. Consequently, process research needs to attend to variations in therapeutic processes within a theoretical model across couples varying in individual and relationship functioning, and delineate the specific intrapersonal and interpersonal attributes that drive these variations in process.

Research on variations in treatment process across individual and relationship factors should be integrated with studies of how specific intervention components and their variations are linked to within- and between-session responses of each of the participants. That is, process research interfaces with outcome research by emphasizing more immediate, proximal effects of therapist interventions on partners' behavior and partners' effects on the therapist and each other (Rice & Greenberg, 1984). For example, do cognitive reattributions or reframing interventions deescalate couples' negative interactions within session? Do interventions aimed at promoting insight into developmental components of individual and relationship distress promote partners' softened reactions to each other's behavior? Under what circumstances do therapeutic interventions promoting insight result in an increase in defensiveness or negative reactivity? When do vulnerable self-disclosures and partners' reciprocal soothing behaviors mutually reinforce each other, and for which couples or at which times do they not? What characteristics of partners' behavior or their interactions with each other lead to nontherapeutic responses by the couple therapist such as negative escalations or counterproductive struggles over control?

Research on such therapeutic event-related processes also needs to attend to changes in these linkages across the course of treatment. For example, the effects of interpreting developmental components of interpersonal distress may be very different if conducted early in therapy than later in treatment once collaborative alliances and constructive communication skills are more firmly established. Consequently, stages of couple therapy need to be defined not only by the composition or structure of clinical interventions, but also by their proximal effects on partners' responses and the therapeutic process. Although theoretical approaches to couple therapy often posit distinct treatment stages specific to that approach, it seems likely that any such stage progression in couple therapy is moderated by stages inherent in the progression of individual emotional or health problems that difficult couples sometimes present. For example, some disorders (e.g., bipolar affective disorder) have a long-term phasic course; others (e.g., posttraumatic stress disorder) exhibit episodic acute exacerbations; some (e.g., narcissistic, paranoid, or borderline personality disorders) involve enduring dispositions that may limit or delay the progression of couple interventions across modal stages; and still other disorders (e.g., dementia or physical illness) may involve progressive deterioration that substantially alters either the content, sequence, or pacing of couple therapy. Finally, studies of treatment process need to extend beyond termination to include couples' efforts or posttreatment interventions aimed at limiting or preventing relapse.

In addition to evaluating the impact of specific interventions on individual and relationship well-being, research is needed on the impact of interventions on treatment processes that can be viewed as outcomes in their own right. For example, one major challenge confronting therapists is that presenting clients often report that their partner will not attend therapy. How to get an unmotivated partner to come to therapy, therefore, is an important outcome in its own right, and research could be conducted at comparing different methods for engaging reluctant partners to attend therapy. For example, are reluctant partners more likely to attend therapy if the therapist speaks with them personally? Are there specific ways of introducing therapy that reduce partners' perception that they may be blamed for the problem? Attention to similar intermediate outcomes such as this would provide guidelines that are particularly useful to clinicians in working with difficult couples.

• *Research on treating difficult couples needs to move beyond existing therapies to examine integrative approaches—including indicators for selecting and sequencing specific treatment components, alternative integrative models, and moderators of therapeutic effectiveness.* Research on both the process and outcomes of traditional "pure-form" treatments should facilitate research on integrative approaches to couple therapy. Efforts to decompose couple-based interventions into their smallest transportable components should lead to research on the most effective ways of reassembling these in a manner uniquely tailored to couples' variation in individual and relationship functioning. For example, do narcissistic characteristics of individual functioning require interventions from a psychodynamic or object-relations approach? Do couples struggling with features of posttraumatic response in one or both partners require emotionally focused interventions promoting vulnerable self-disclosure and empathic understanding? Under what conditions does combining interventions from two alternative therapeutic approaches enhance or detract from the effectiveness of either approach administered by itself?

Each intervention incorporated into an integrative approach needs to be considered with respect to its necessity, sufficiency, and interactive effects. Issues of necessity involve delineating those individual and couple characteristics for which a given intervention or set of interventions is essential for reducing distress or promoting well-being. "More is better" may be the recommendation when some intervention is determined to be critical to producing a desired outcome, regardless of what other interventions may be included in the overall treatment strategy. By comparison, issues of sufficiency involve delineating those constellations of individual and relationship functioning for which a given intervention or set of interventions are enough to produce some desired therapeutic outcome, and "more yields the same." Determining sufficient conditions offers guidelines for when *not* to extend interventions in terms of number, length, or kind. Research on intervention interactions also needs to identify combinations of techniques that produce either positive or negative synergistic effects. For example, techniques of affective reconstruction may be beneficial only when combined with decision-making interventions outlining new interpersonal coping strategies; or vulnerable self-disclosures may promote intimacy only for couples already trained in empathic listening and responding skills. Because some treatment components may be interactively inconsistent, contradictory, neutralizing, or harmful, research also needs to identify when "more is worse." For example, interventions promoting vulnerable self-disclosure might be ineffective or harmful if combined with interventions aimed at reducing partners' enmeshment and promoting greater emotional individuation or autonomy. Research on integrative approaches to couple therapy needs to examine not only the combination of techniques but also their sequence and pacing.

In a related manner, research on necessary, sufficient, or deleterious interventions needs to articulate those aspects of partners' individual and relationship functioning as well as therapist characteristics that moderate couples' response to integrative approaches. For example, do level of integration and case complexity moderate the relationship between extent of eclecticism and treatment outcome (Snyder et al., Chapter 2, this volume)? Does level of therapist training or years of experience moderate the therapeutic effects of stepping outside structured pure-form approaches to pursue integrative practice? Which partner or couple characteristics demand integrative approaches? Do the same characteristics that require combining techniques from multiple theoretical modalities render their implementation in an effective integrative manner more difficult?

Research on integrative processes in couple therapy should examine the decision-making models of expert clinicians operating from a theoretically pluralistic perspective when working with difficult couples. Conversely, research should also seek to identify therapists' faulty case conceptualizations, theoretical misunderstandings, or logical thinking errors that impair integrative practice. Both integrative practice and training in integrative approaches are inherently more complex and difficult than for their respective pure-form therapeutic counterparts (Norcross et al., 1993). Hence, additional research should seek to identify those characteristics of both therapists and their trainers conducive to learning integrative couple therapy, as well as the content and processes of couple therapist training that maximize this potential.

• *Clinicians and researchers need to pursue more effective collaboration in identifying critical questions related to treating difficult couples, designing and conducting relevant research, and disseminating and incorporating findings germane to clinical practice.* Researchers need to be knowledgeable regarding both clinical and pragmatic issues of couple therapy in today's practice environment. This requires that they expose themselves to the challenges of working with individuals struggling with co-morbid individual and relationship dysfunction, couples for whom the costs of childcare or travel to the clinic cannot be offset by funds from a research grant, and treatment settings in which either the duration or modality of treatment is constrained by health care systems or other financial resources available to the couple. Researchers also bear responsibility for disseminating their findings in a format relevant to practitioners. This entails attending to multiple styles and media of communication including detailed treatment manuals, case-study publications, clinical workshops, and videotaped demonstrations. It also requires learning from practitioners what clinical and logistical issues present the greatest challenges in working with difficult couples.

Clinicians need to contribute to the scientific enterprise by collaborating with researchers in articulating issues critical to conducting couple therapy and by participating in the research process. The latter may involve willingness to administer structured treatments according to a research protocol in a community setting or assessing couples before and after "treatment-as-usual" in a treatment-comparison condition. Clinicians also bear responsibility for remaining abreast of both theoretical and empirical advances in couple treatment, reading both the clinical and research literature, availing themselves of clinical seminars and workshops by clinical researchers, and discerning new treatment approaches that are fashionable or cleverly marketed and those that are empirically supported.

Similar to couple interventions promoting the respective strengths of each partner, so too the field of couple therapy will advance when clinicians and researchers collaboratively encourage each other's respective professional pursuits in working with difficult couples in a more conceptually rich and clinically effective manner.

CONCLUSIONS

There have been many advances in understanding and treating co-occurring relational and mental or physical health difficulties. In this chapter, we have outlined some of the implications of these advances for practice, training, and research. We have also offered several suggestions that we believe would be fruitful for future advances in this area. Additional developments will serve to increase the understanding and effectiveness of interventions for couples who struggle with relationship difficulties and co-occurring emotional, behavior, and health problems.

REFERENCES

Baucom, D. H., Shoham, V., Mueser, K. T., Daiuto, A. D., & Stickle, T. R. (1998). Empirically supported couple and family interventions for marital distress and adult mental health problems. *Journal of Consulting and Clinical Psychology, 66,* 53–88.

Christensen, A., & Heavey, C. L. (1999). Interventions for couples. *Annual Review of Psychology, 50,* 165–190.

Jackson, D. D. (1957). The question of family homeostasis. *Psychiatric Quarterly, 31*(Suppl. 1), 79–90.

Kessler, R. C., McGonagle, K. A., Zhao, S., Nelson, C. B., Hughes, M., Eshleman, S., Wittchen, H.-U., & Kendler, K. S. (1994). Lifetime and 12-month prevalence of DSM-III-R psychiatric disorders in the United States: Results from the National Comorbidity Survey. *Archives of General Psychiatry, 51,* 8–19.

Lebow, J. L. (1987). Developing a personal integration in family therapy: Principles for model construction and practice. *Journal of Marital and Family Therapy, 13,* 1–14.

McLeod, J. D. (1995). Social and psychological bases of homogamy for common psychiatric disorders. *Journal of Marriage and the Family, 57,* 201–214.

Means-Christensen, A. J., Snyder, D. K., & Negy, C. (2003). Assessing nontraditional couples: Validity of the Marital Satisfaction Inventory-Revised (MSI-R) with gay, lesbian, and cohabiting heterosexual couples. *Journal of Marital and Family Therapy, 29,* 69–83.

Norcross, J. C., & Beutler, L. E. (2000). A prescriptive eclectic approach to psychotherapy training. *Journal of Psychotherapy Integration, 10,* 247–261.

Norcross, J. C., Glass, C. R., Arnkoff, D. B., Lambert, M. J., Shoham, V., Stiles, W. B., Shapiro, D. A., Barkham, M., & Strupp, H. H. (1993). Research directions for psychotherapy integration: A roundtable. *Journal of Psychotherapy Integration, 3,* 91–131.

Rice, L. N., & Greenberg, L. S. (1984). *Patterns of change: Intensive analysis of psychotherapy process.* New York: Guilford Press.

Snyder, D. K., & Abbott, B. V. (2002). Couple distress. In M. M. Antony & D. H.

Barlow (Eds.), *Handbook of assessment and treatment planning for psychological disorders* (pp. 341–374). New York: Guilford Press.

Snyder, D. K., Cozzi, J. J., & Mangrum, L. F. (2002). Conceptual issues in assessing couples and families. In H. A. Liddle, D. A. Santisteban, R. F. Levant, & J. H. Bray (Eds.), *Family psychology: Science-based interventions* (pp. 69–87). Washington, DC: American Psychological Association.

Whisman, M. A., Sheldon, C. T., & Goering, P. (2000). Psychiatric disorders and dissatisfaction with social relationships: Does type of relationship matter? *Journal of Abnormal Psychology, 109,* 803–808.

Wills, R. M., Faitler, S. M., & Snyder, D. K. (1987). Distinctiveness of behavioral versus insight-oriented marital therapy: An empirical analysis. *Journal of Consulting and Clinical Psychology, 55,* 685–690.

Index